MINDFULNESS

Also Available

Collaborative Case Conceptualization:
Working Effectively with Clients in Cognitive-Behavioral Therapy
Willem Kuyken, Christine A. Padesky, and Robert Dudley

MINDFULNESS

ANCIENT WISDOM MEETS MODERN PSYCHOLOGY

Christina Feldman
Willem Kuyken

Foreword by Zindel V. Segal

THE GUILFORD PRESS
New York   London

The authors have checked with sources believed to be reliable in their efforts to
provide information that is complete and generally in accord with the standards
of practice that are accepted at the time of publication. However, in view of the
possibility of human error or changes in behavioral, mental health, or medical
sciences, neither the authors, nor the editors and publisher, nor any other party who
has been involved in the preparation or publication of this work warrants that the
information contained herein is in every respect accurate or complete, and they are
not responsible for any errors or omissions or the results obtained from the use of such
information. Readers are encouraged to confirm the information contained in this
book with other sources.

Library of Congress Cataloging-in-Publication Data

Names: Feldman, Christina, author. | Kuyken, W. (Willem), 1968– author.
Title: Mindfulness : ancient wisdom meets modern psychology / Christina
   Feldman, Willem Kuyken ; foreword by Zindel V. Segal.
Description: New York, NY : The Guilford Press, 2019. | Includes
   bibliographical references and index.
Identifiers: LCCN 2019009790| ISBN 9781462540112 (hardback) | ISBN
   9781462540105 (paperback)
Subjects: LCSH: Self-actualization (Psychology) | Mindfulness (Psychology) |
   Self-acceptance. | BISAC: PSYCHOLOGY / Psychotherapy / General. | MEDICAL
   / Psychiatry / General. | SOCIAL SCIENCE / Social Work. | RELIGION /
   Counseling.
Classification: LCC BF637.S4 F4275 2019 | DDC 158.1/3—dc23
LC record available at https://lccn.loc.gov/2019009790

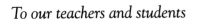

To our teachers and students

About the Authors

Christina Feldman is a leading senior teacher in the insight meditation community, offering retreats internationally. She is a contributing faculty member in several postgraduate mindfulness programs, including the University of Exeter in the United Kingdom and Radboud University in The Netherlands. She is a cofounder of Gaia House in the United Kingdom and a guiding teacher of the Insight Meditation Society in Barre, Massachusetts. The author of numerous books, Ms. Feldman is a core teacher at Bodhi College in the United Kingdom and is deeply engaged in the dialogue between Buddhist psychology and contemporary mindfulness.

Willem Kuyken, PhD, is Riblat Professor of Mindfulness and Psychological Science at the University of Oxford, United Kingdom, and Director of the Oxford Mindfulness Centre. His work focuses on depression and its prevention and treatment. In particular, his research examines how mindfulness and mindfulness-based programs can prevent depression and enhance human potential across the lifespan. Dr. Kuyken has published more than 100 journal articles, including key papers on the effectiveness, mechanisms, and implementation of mindfulness-based programs.

Foreword

In the poem "The Summer Day," Mary Oliver (2015) poignantly compares prayer to paying attention. After reading Christina Feldman and Willem Kuyken's wonderful book *Mindfulness: Ancient Wisdom Meets Modern Psychology*, I now see that these lines from Oliver's poem reflect the remarkable shift that has taken place in medicine, health care, and society over the past 25 years. What I am referring to, and what each of the authors has played a pivotal role in supporting, is the introduction of contemplative practices in mainstream health and social institutions as adjunctive means for addressing disease and suffering. Much as going to a yoga class is no longer considered esoteric, teaching people who are managing a mood disorder or cardiovascular condition how to practice mindfulness meditation is increasingly seen as integral to good quality care.

This book's particular value lies in providing a broader perspective on the two worlds—contemplative and secular—that undergird this movement. Where it succeeds most vividly is in synthesizing the varied research, clinical, and contemplative inputs into a framework that allows readers to fully appreciate how these domains are, in spite of their surface differences, implicitly linked. As well, this book could not have come at a better time. Most would agree that the mindfulness field is rapidly expanding; indeed, some would say it is becoming a global phenomenon. And yet with scale comes excess and the inevitable dilution of quality. Fortunately, *Mindfulness* invites us to pause and return to the sources that have informed this unique synthesis of modern science and ancient traditions, thereby allowing their shared intentionality to be revealed.

As guides through this material, I cannot think of two authors better suited to this task than Christina Feldman and Willem Kuyken. Christina is a world-renowned meditation teacher and cofounder of Gaia House in the United Kingdom, and Willem is a research psychologist who, as Director of the Oxford Mindfulness Centre, has published a number of our field's seminal papers. Their book provides the reader with a number of rare treasures, such as a contemplative teacher and scientist authorship team, or cognitive science and Buddhist psychology maps of "the mind."

At its most ambitious, *Mindfulness* is larger than the service of conceptual clarity and coherence it provides for our field. The book's core actually addresses a personal quest we each find ourselves on: how we can live with ease within the condition of our modern world. It is, true enough, a perennial question, and yet, here we find a novel set of answers that draw from the best that science and contemplative practice have to offer. For starters, it is vital to understand the roots of struggle and suffering that we all encounter. With this in hand, how can we use this knowledge to support greater moments of well-being and wholeness? Mindfulness has a central role to play here, both through its capacity to free the mind from the confines of habit and by creating an opening for the enactment of new choices and perceptions—in short, the possibility of real transformation. The living discussion among Buddhism, contemporary secular mindfulness, and psychological science that has been initiated across these pages helps draw us all closer to understanding how liberation is nearer to us than we might dare to imagine.

ZINDEL V. SEGAL, PhD

Preface

What does it mean to be happy and to live a good life?
How can we live a life that is free from suffering, in ways that support our
   well-being, the well-being of those around us, and the wider world?

These are questions that have been part of the human story for as long as we
have been able to reflect on the human condition. In one form or another,
they are questions we have all asked ourselves. They have been driving questions in the wisdom traditions, philosophy, and psychology for thousands of
years. Consider these words attributed to the Buddha:

> An undeveloped mind leads to great harm. . . . A developed mind leads to
> great benefit. . . . The mind when undeveloped and uncultivated entails
> great suffering. . . . The mind when developed and cultivated entails great
> happiness. (The Mind Is the Key; AN 1; in Bhikkhu Bodhi, 2005)

Translated into everyday language, the Buddha is suggesting that our
minds play a key role in creating both suffering and joy. And crucially, we can
actively cultivate our mind. These understandings have over time been rather
like water traveling down a mountain—they have had a powerful momentum,
taken the shape of whatever landscape they find themselves in, while largely
keeping their essence.

Now consider Zindel Segal, Mark Williams, and John Teasdale—three
contemporary applied psychologists—describing what is involved in the process of change and transformation during mindfulness training:

Both the research data and our clinical experience suggest to us that only when people learn to take a different stance in relation to the "battleground" of their thoughts and feelings will they be able in the future to recognize difficult situations early and deal with them skillfully. Taking this different stance involves sampling a different mode of mind from that which we normally inhabit. . . . (Segal, Williams, & Teasdale, 2013, p. 93)

The central thesis of our book is that Buddhist psychology and modern science together provide a helpful new perspective on these questions of how to live well in the contemporary world. We argue that they can help us chart the path from suffering to well-being and flourishing.

In the last 50 years there has been an important confluence of these ancient teachings with modern psychology, education, and medicine. Several notable examples in mainstream secular settings have been the work of Jon Kabat-Zinn, Marsha Linehan, and the triumvirate of Zindel Segal, Mark Williams, and John Teasdale.[1]

Jon Kabat–Zinn (1982, 1990) exhibited tremendous foresight and insight when he distilled the essence of the ancient pathway of transformation from several schools of Buddhism to create a program (mindfulness-based stress reduction) that was accessible to anyone—regardless of faith, background, class, or gender (Feldman, 2016).

Over approximately the same period of time, the psychologist Marsha Linehan was considering how to work with people who struggled with one of the most challenging psychological conditions: borderline personality disorder (a condition characterized by great and long-standing emotional and relationship instability). She had the same idea to distill ancient mindfulness practices into a form (dialectical behavior therapy) that people with borderline personality disorder could use (Linehan, 1993a, 1993b). Since then, an array of mindfulness-based programs has evolved intended to help people with a variety of issues and in a range of contexts.

Mindfulness-based cognitive therapy (MBCT) for recurrent depression is an example of such an adaptation. Depression is probably the most pressing mental health problem in the world; at some point in their lives, 1 billion of the world's population will likely suffer depression. Zindel Segal, Mark Williams, and John Teasdale (2013) have collectively produced some of the best psychological science that helps us understand what makes someone vulnerable to depression. They had the hypothesis that mindfulness training could be a vehicle for helping people who are vulnerable to depression learn how to work with the mind states that drive their vulnerability. It has now been evaluated in at least 10 randomized controlled trials and demonstrated its effectiveness in supporting recovery from recurrent depression. What all these mindfulness-based programs have in common is their commitment to using mindfulness training as a vehicle for healing suffering and supporting people to live a good life, realize their potential, and thrive.

Just as contemporary mindfulness teachers and trainings have benefited from the earliest teaching of mindfulness offered 2,500 years ago, many Buddhist teachers have found that their understanding and teaching has been enriched and deepened by what they learn from science, research, and psychology. In this book, we hope to demonstrate how this mutuality of learning and dialogue continues to serve the alleviation of distress, cool the fires of reactivity, and contribute to the deepening of understanding and compassion of individuals, communities, and societies.

The dialogue among Buddhism, contemporary mindfulness in secular settings, and psychology is not always easy. There is a critique that contemporary mindfulness is either too grounded in Buddhist psychology (Baer, 2015) or not grounded fully enough (Shonin, Van Gordon, & Griffiths, 2013; Van Gordon, Shonin, & Griffiths, 2016). Misgivings have been voiced by teachers and organizations—rooted in the Buddhist traditions—that mindfulness has been decontextualized and become a self-help tool rather than a path of awakening. Buddhist teachers have expressed concerns that contemporary mindfulness has stripped Buddhist teachings of their ethical base. On the other hand, there is a concern that many of the views, values, and more esoteric practices within Buddhism are hard to reconcile with science and contemporary mindfulness applications (Baer, 2015). Moreover, in mainstream professional settings, such as health care or educational systems, some have expressed concern that many mindfulness teachers do not have a professional qualification, and so are not supported by the ethics codes of medicine, education, and/or psychology. Perhaps mirroring the wider world, there is a fair amount of polarization in the mindfulness world and arrows are fired from camp to camp.

Throughout the book we consider and answer, as best we can, the following questions:

- "What is mindfulness? What are the attitudinal dimensions of mindfulness? Has it assumed such a myriad of meanings that its meaning has become muddied? Or is it like a diamond with several facets?"
- "There are already many effective psychological approaches for distress and suffering. What value does mindfulness training add?"
- "How does mindfulness provide us with ways of knowing, training, shaping, and liberating the mind?"

- "How does mindfulness support the path from suffering to flourishing? Is mindfulness a technique or a way of being in the world—or both? How does it enable transformation?"
- "What are the important questions around ethics and integrity for mindfulness practitioners, teachers, and the wider field? What supports this inquiry?"
- "For whom is mindfulness appropriate? For whom is it inappropriate?"
- "What is the purpose of a lifetime of mindfulness practice?"

We take you on a journey that explores not just the synergies and commonalities between Buddhist psychology and psychological science but also the tensions and the places where more than likely "never the twain shall meet."

The Story behind the Story

Christina and Willem: Our Shared Story

Like the confluence of ancient wisdom and modern psychological science, the paths of our lives converged in our friendship and collaboration. This book is the outcome of the decades we have spent in contemplative practice and psychological inquiry separately, and the years we have spent as friends and colleagues developing these ideas together. We both share the hope that mindfulness can be made more readily available in a world where many problems can be traced to the human heart and mind.

We became friends and colleagues at the turn of the century when we started collaborating in the establishment of one of the first academic master's-level mindfulness-based programs.[2] As the professor designing and leading the program, Willem approached Christina to explore the possibility of her contributing her understanding of the Buddhist psychological foundations of contemporary mindfulness to the course. Christina was somewhat surprised since she had never taught in a university context. She had the idea that "perhaps we could co-teach the psychological dimensions of the program." Willem raised his eyebrows and asked, "Do you really think we can do that?" Christina's answer was "Let's give it a go."

In the first run of the master's program, we taught within our roles, as a psychologist (Willem) and a Buddhist teacher (Christina). But with each iteration of the course, we started to more fully understand each other's perspectives, enabling us to see the landscape as a coherent whole. In retrospect, it was also an important step in bridging the divide between secular and nonsecular teachings of mindfulness. After three rounds of co-teaching the master's course, we decided it was time to commit the ideas to a book.

Christina and Willem: Our Individual Stories

Both of us began in our youth to undertake meditative training and contemplation. This training has been influential in both our work and our personal lives. We have come to understand the ways in which contemplative traditions and modern science can be powerful tools for training the mind and for positive change in the world.

Christina Feldman

I traveled to India as a teenager more than four decades ago. Arriving in Dharmashala, the home of the Dalai Lama and a community of Tibetan refugees, I was immediately struck by the poised, happy, and compassionate manner of these people who had endured untold suffering and lived in considerable deprivation. It was clear to me that they possessed inner resources unknown to me at that point in my life. I began studying with some of the most renowned teachers in that tradition—it was the beginning of a lifetime of contemplative study and meditative exploration.

Returning to the West in the mid-1970s, I began to be invited to teach mindfulness and insight meditation, and form centers where people could spend time in retreat. Although life can be difficult and challenging for many of us, the teaching stemmed from the principle that the key to our happiness, well-being, and freedom lay in our own minds and understanding. This teaching resonated with many, including the founders of mindfulness-based applications. As mainstream secular mindfulness began to develop, I felt increasingly drawn to understanding how these ancient and contemporary teachings converged. It has become clear to me that deeply understanding the roots of mindfulness in the classical teachings enriches the capacity to convey and embody mindfulness in contemporary teaching settings.

Willem Kuyken

As an academic clinical psychologist, my working life has pursued the question of how best to understand and prevent depression and enhance human potential across the lifespan. For as long as I can remember, these words from Einstein have been pinned to the board in my office: "Intellect has a keen eye for method and technique, but is blind to aim and value." In the way we have seen smallpox eradicated, my hope is that we can in time see a world without the devastating effects of depression. I have long been interested in how the broader perspectives of psychology, biology, philosophy, contemplative traditions, and social justice can help us to understand and find ways to prevent depression.

From an early age my inquiry was both academic and deeply personal. Like many people, my life has not been without struggle. My parents were exposed to unimaginable suffering in occupied Holland and Indonesia during World War II, and my uncle—who is my namesake—died in a Japanese concentration camp at the age of 4. As a young boy, I often felt a deep sense of empathy and compassion when I encountered pain and suffering. I was brought up in Nigeria and although my life was cocooned within the expatriate community, for a child it was impossible to not see the great suffering that was never far from view.

I first experienced depression myself as a young man and this experience has informed how I live and work. In my early 20s, I traveled extensively for my job at the World Health Organization. At a Bangkok airport, I picked up a book with the title *The Good Life: A Guide to Buddhism for the Westerner* (Roscoe, 1990). On the night flight back to Geneva, I read the book cover to cover. Toward the end of the flight I remember being in the cockpit of the plane looking out into the night sky (if you asked politely, you were allowed to sit up with the pilots in those days!) and having an extraordinary sense of identification with the teachings, a sense of common humanity, and a sort of awakening. The teachings resonated on two levels: my personal experience and my work as a young scientist. The ideas informed not only my understanding of my mind and life but also the research program I was developing. The end of the book included further resources, which I sought out with ardor and started on a path of mindfulness practice and learning. A few years later, at a conference entitled "East Meets West," I was exposed to some inspiring people and ideas who in different ways were working at the same interface. Jon Kabat-Zinn gave a masterful 3-hour opening keynote; Francisco Varela used philosophy, Buddhism, and cognition to work on embodiment; and Stephen Batchelor worked on making Buddhist psychology accessible and secular. Over a drink in the bar, John Teasdale, an academic clinical psychologist, encouraged me to bring my work on depression together with my personal interest in mindfulness. This was an extraordinary moment of convergence and set the direction for my career and life ever since.

Our deepest intention in writing this book has been our commitment to the transformative potential of bridging modern psychology and Buddhist psychology:

- This confluence of perspectives can suggest some new answers, or at least new perspectives on major challenges in the contemporary world.
- Buddhist psychology and modern science have much to learn from each other.
- Looking for bridges and synergies is more constructive than building fences and creating silos.

The ideas in this book are not original—we draw on rich ancient lineages as well as large bodies of modern science. We draw on many people's work and stand on the shoulders of both giants and the collaborators and teams with whom we have worked over the years. The Acknowledgments section lists many of these, but we know there are others we will have missed.

How to Get the Most Out of This Book

The book is organized sequentially, a bit like building blocks. Chapters build on one another, with earlier chapters informing the synthesis in later chapters. We start in Chapter 1 by unpacking mindfulness. We consider what we mean by mindfulness and offer a working definition that sets the stage for the rest of the book.

We then set out a map of how distress and suffering are created and maintained, using the frameworks of psychological science (Chapters 2 and 3) and Buddhist psychology (Chapter 4). Chapter 5 combines these Buddhist and psychological frameworks into a single map. This chapter is intended to be the sort of map that mindfulness teachers and students can use to better understand how distress and suffering are created and perpetuated.

We then use the earlier ideas-based chapters (Chapters 2–5) to provide practical route maps of how mindfulness training helps people move from distress and suffering to resilience and flourishing (Chapters 6–8). These chapters are more applied and grounded in mindfulness-based programs. In the penultimate chapter, we conclude by considering the ethics of mindfulness-based programs and how they support living with purpose, meaning, and integrity. Chapter 10 is a final word of summary and conclusion. Throughout the chapters we introduce you to four case studies (Mohammed, Ling, Sophia, and Sam). These are composites of people we have worked with and our intention is to bring the ideas to life.

It may be that you have greater or less familiarity with the topic of particular chapters, so some will be more novel and others more familiar. For example, if you're already a psychologist, the chapters on psychological science may well be familiar, or if you've studied Buddhism, the chapters on Buddhist psychology will be the most familiar. Finally, each chapter ends with a synopsis, so the headlines are easily accessible to you. The whole book also ends with a synopsis, with the headlines of our thesis summarized as a set of bullet points.

We have tried to use mainstream, consistent language throughout. Inevitably, when different ancient and contemporary approaches converge, there is a need to identify a common terminology and language. In Appendix 1, we set out some words and terms that we use consistently throughout the book with the particular meanings we intend. The cultural context and language in which the Buddhist ideas were developed were, of course, different from those of today, and in some cases, this means translation has nuances and complexities that cannot be readily conveyed. If a more precise Pali word (the language of the foundational teachings) or scientific word is needed, notes are used to explain and elaborate. Buddhist psychology often uses images, similes, allegories, and metaphors. We have adopted these when they connote richer meaning more effectively. For example, we sometimes use terms such as *shaping the mind* and *cultivating awareness* that build from the extensive references to artisans, farmers, and surgeons in the ancient Buddhist texts. This proposed lexicon and set of definitions provides a way of drawing together some of the etymology of language in Buddhist texts with the precision of psychological science. We refer throughout to mindfulness training and mindfulness-based programs. We define mindfulness training and set out the defining core and essential characteristics of mindfulness-based programs in Appendix 2. Our intention is to have a flow in our thesis that is uninterrupted by detailed considerations of etymology, definitions of key terms, or considerations of cultural context or history. We acknowledge how important these considerations are, but our primary focus is the bridging of ancient and contemporary teaching of mindfulness as a means of bringing distress to an end.

To support your reading we use a system of numbered notes to provide sources and elaborations. This is to ensure that the main text remains uncluttered. Interested readers can refer to the Notes section at the end of the book for elaborations of some of the ideas—the notes are organized by chapter. We use standard approaches to citing and referencing our sources and interested readers may wish to read some of the primary sources to find out more. To support learning, we suggest forming reading groups to discuss and explore the ideas and consider the applications of the ideas. The references provide ideas for further study.

Finally, our teachers and students have been in our minds and hearts throughout the writing of this book, first during the 7 years we taught together and then during the 3 years we have spent writing together. Their ideas and feedback, on what was helpful, what was formative, and what was more challenging but worth the effort—all of these have informed our work. We hope you, our readers, will find this book as rewarding and enjoyable to read as we found it to write. We hope the ideas will enrich your lives as much as they have enriched ours.

Acknowledgments

There are probably few important people in our lives who have not shaped this book in some way. It gestated over 10 years, was written over 3 years, and featured many moments of wonder, struggle, and joy. We'd like to thank and acknowledge a number of the people and apologize if we inadvertently neglected anyone we should have mentioned.

First and foremost, we'd like to thank Halley Cohen, who carefully edited the manuscript through several drafts. At The Guilford Press, we thank Jim Nageotte, who provided editorial support at every stage.

We don't claim to have written an original treatise—rather, we have brought together the work of many colleagues in the fields of psychological science, mindfulness-based interventions, and Buddhist psychology. In particular, we'd like to recognize and thank Jon Kabat-Zinn for decades of tireless work to formulate how mindfulness can best serve in the mainstream of the contemporary world. Equally, we acknowledge a huge debt of gratitude to some of the Buddhist teachers who have done so much to carry the tributary of the ancient wisdom of Buddhism into the contemporary world with unswerving commitment and clarity of intention: Joseph Goldstein, Jack Kornfeld, John Peacock, and Sharon Salzberg. We also owe a debt of gratitude for the work and friendship of the colleagues who developed mindfulness-based cognitive therapy: Zindel Segal, Mark Williams, and John Teasdale. Many conversations as well as their collective and individual programs of research work have shaped the psychological science tributary in this book.

Several friends and colleagues read drafts—the book is immeasurably better as a result of their feedback: Ruth Baer, Madeleine Bunting, Rebecca

Crane, Chris Cullen, Tim Dalgleish, Alison Evans, Liz Lord, Christina Surawy, John Teasdale, Alison Yiangou, and Peter Yiangou. The Guilford Press also sent out the manuscript to two anonymous reviewers whose feedback was constructive and incisive. Finally, Barbara Watkins at Guilford provided exemplary editorial feedback on a near final manuscript.

I (CF) would like to acknowledge the many teachers I have been privileged to learn from over decades for their generosity and encouragement. My friendship with John Teasdale has been rich and joyful. I am grateful to my family for their love and encouragement. Willem Kuyken brought me into the world of contemporary mindfulness teaching and I appreciate our friendship, the road we have traveled together in creating this book, and our years of teaching together. Last, I thank the many students who have brought to their own learning pathways sincerity, dedication, and compassion.

I (WK) would like to acknowledge colleagues Ruth Baer, Shadi Beshai, Sarah Byford, Catherine Crane, Rebecca Crane, Chris Cullen, Tim Dalgleish, Barney Dunn, Alison Evans, Tamsin Ford, Mark Greenberg, Felicia Huppert, Anke Karl, Elizabeth Nuthall, Jo Rycroft-Malone, Zindel Segal, Anne Speckens, Clara Strauss, Obi Ukoumunne, and Mark Williams; my mentors in this field: Trish Bartley and Catherine McGee; and the students I have been privileged to mentor: Modi Alsubaie, Jenny Gu, Anne Maj van der Velden, Anna Abel, Mark Allen, Chantal Baillie, Lisa Baxter, Andrew Bromley, Rachael Carrick, Colin Greaves, Emma Griffiths, JJ Hill, Emily Holden, Vivienne Hopkins, Hans Kirschner, Kat Legge, Jo Mann, Nicola Motton, Meyrem Musa, Selina Nath, Dimitrious Tsivrikos, and Alice Weaver. My research has been supported by the National Institute for Health Research, Wellcome Trust, Medical Research Council, Oxford Mindfulness Foundation, and the University of Oxford. I am privileged and humbled to have had the opportunity to learn from and teach and write with Christina—it has been a high point of my career. Last and first, my wife, Halley, and daughters, Zoe and Ava, mean everything to me—I feel grateful to love and be loved by them in ways that are beyond words.

Contents

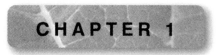

CHAPTER 1

Unpacking Mindfulness

If you didn't know ahead of time what your social status would be, what your race was, what your gender was or sexual orientation was, what country you were living in, and you asked what moment in history would you like to be born . . . you'd choose right now.
—BARACK OBAMA (in Gold, 2016)

The world is a better place today than in any time in history. This is according to various metrics, including greater life expectancy, lower infant mortality, better access to health care, a growing proportion of the world's population living outside of poverty, fewer deaths due to violence, improving access to education for children, and greater opportunity for young people (Rosling, Rosling, & Rosling-Ronnlund, 2018).[1] And still there is a chasm between improved metrics such as these and the suffering that is evident in the contemporary world.

Let's look at the good news of one metric: longer life expectancy. Better living conditions and health care improvements across much of the world means that more of us are living longer. But this has come with the cost of many of us living at least some of our years with chronic physical illness and pain, including arthritis, musculoskeletal conditions, dementia, diabetes, and coronary heart disease (GBD 2015 Disease and Injury Incidence and Prevalence Collaborators, 2016; Kings Fund, 2016). This means that we have to find ways to live with pain, discomfort, and limitations on our functioning, often for years, typically in the closing chapters of our lives. The scale of the problem across the world is huge. Fourteen percent of people over age 40 in developed countries have one or more chronic physical health conditions, and this rises to 50% in those over 65 (GBD 2015 Disease and Injury Incidence and Prevalence Collaborators, 2016; Kings Fund, 2016).

We introduce Mohammed, the first of our case studies.[2]

Mohammed broke his back playing sports at college. His life since has been marred by chronic, severe, and disabling pain. Doctors told him that they had done all they could medically. Like so many other people, Mohammed had to find a way to live his life productively while managing his pain as best he could.

Let's look at another metric: rates of mental health problems. One in four of us will experience significant mental health problems, such as depression and anxiety, at some point in our lives. Mental ill health is a *1 billion person problem*—that is, one in five of the world's population will suffer a mental health problem at some point in his or her life. The World Health Organization names depression as a leading cause of disability. It often develops in late adolescence or early adulthood and runs a recurrent course that can profoundly affect the ability to live a full life (Bockting, Hollon, Jarrett, Kuyken, & Dobson, 2015; GBD 2015 Disease and Injury Incidence and Prevalence Collaborators, 2016; World Health Organization, 2011).

We next introduce Ling, the second of our case studies.

Ling had suffered numerous bouts of depression in her life, which started in her early teens. While the first episode had been caused by many challenges at home and at school, more recently they would not have a clear trigger. Ling described her most recent episode of depression this way: "I had a plummeting feeling, I just went straight down, took to my bed, just slept, I couldn't do anything. I couldn't function." Like so many other people, Ling had to find a way to manage her recurring depression alongside working and being a single parent.

There are mental health challenges beyond depression, including anxiety disorders, addiction, and psychosis. For example, rates of eating disorders and self-harm in the developed world, particularly among the young, are alarming. Some 6.9% of young people in some countries are thought to self-harm as a way of managing their feelings (Hawton, Rodham, Evans, & Weatherall, 2002) and 13% have thought about dying or suicide (Klonsky, Oltmanns, & Turkheimer, 2003). Both physical and mental health problems affect those from more deprived backgrounds at higher rates (Barnett et al., 2012). There is a growing acknowledgment in the developed and developing world of the suffering and functional impairment caused by chronic physical and mental ill health.

It is human to want good physical and mental health, to be free from suffering, and to enjoy meaning, security, and ease of being, both for ourselves and for those we love. We can feel bewildered by the disconnection, unhappiness, or pathos we experience. We tend to blame the conditions in our lives for the despair and unhappiness we feel, and there is a relentless effort to change those conditions into an imagined, ideal reality that will deliver the happiness and meaning for which we long. It can feel discouraging when our happiness and success seem all too brief, altered by the inevitable tides of change. Bewilderment and disappointment follow, forming over time into familiar psychological states of distress, maintained by our understandable, but misguided attempts to change the unchangeable.

We introduce Sophia, the third of our case studies.

Sophia had suffered anxiety since childhood, which at times could be crippling. In her 20s she was out sick from work for several months, during which time she undertook psychotherapy. She came to see that her anxiety and much of the disconnection and exhaustion she experienced in her life was driven by a powerful inner critic that judged almost everything she did and found it wanting. At the suggestion of her therapist, she developed a regular mindfulness practice. Over several decades she worked on dismantling this inner critic— she even gave it a name: "Ms. Not Good Enough." She developed new ways of thinking about herself, her family, and her life. Later in life, Sophia developed Parkinson's disease, something she met with extraordinary courage and equanimity that she had learned through her life experience, alongside decades of mindfulness practice.

We all handle the challenges in our lives in different ways. When asked what he would like mentioned in his eulogy, Martin Luther King Jr. asked that they not mention his Nobel Prize, but instead that he lived a committed life of service to others, that his purpose was one of love. It is easy, of course, to reflect on heroic figures like Martin Luther King Jr., Mother Teresa, Desmond Tutu, Eleanor Roosevelt, and Nelson Mandela. However, in many ways, this heroism plays out for all of us, caring for our children before they are able to care for themselves, working long hours to provide food, shelter, and security for old age, and encountering the inevitable suffering of illness and old age in our parents and ourselves.

Mindfulness and Mindfulness-Based Programs

Some 40 years ago, Jon Kabat-Zinn—himself both a scientist and a dedicated contemplative—realized the transformative potential of mindfulness in Western medicine (Kabat-Zinn, 1982, 2011). With remarkable prescience and skill, he translated the ancient practices of cultivating mindfulness into a language and methodology appropriate for our contemporary concerns and Western medical contexts (Kabat-Zinn, 1990). Of course, distress, suffering, and confusion are human experiences, yet they are supported and compounded by the

preconditions of reactivity, forgetfulness, and lack of confidence and understanding. Kabat-Zinn began his work at the front lines of suffering, working in
a busy mainstream urban hospital with people with chronic pain and illness.
Many of his patients had exhausted all available strategies and treatments
and experienced mental health problems alongside their chronic pain and illness. He had no shortage of referrals because he offered his program to people
whose doctors had run out of options within mainstream medicine.

Participants in these mindfulness programs consciously developed mindfulness and compassion in the midst of pain, fear, and despair and began to
see changes (Kabat-Zinn, 1982). The program, called mindfulness-based stress
reduction (MBSR), was not a magical cure. What MBSR offered, importantly,
was the possibility of seeing that familiar pathways of fear and avoidance compound pain, and that pain could be responded to in radically new ways. MBSR
was first developed as a vehicle for people with chronic physical health problems
across eight weekly 2-hour sessions with a skilled teacher (Kabat-Zinn, 1990).

A large and growing body of research evidence suggests that MBSR is
effective in helping people learn to manage chronic physical health conditions (Gotink et al., 2015; Grossman, Niemann, Schmidt, & Walach, 2004).
People report living with these conditions with better mental health and
functioning. Mindfulness programs offer an integrated approach to the mind
and body and as such should help with both physical and mental health symptoms. There is promising evidence of positive outcomes in groups of people
with such coexisting conditions (Bohlmeijer, Prenger, Taal, & Cuijpers, 2010;
Khoury, Sharma, Rush, & Fournier, 2015; Lakhan & Schofield, 2013).

MBSR has been adapted to meet the needs of specific populations in different settings and Kabat-Zinn (2005, 2006) has broadened his description of
MBSR as a vehicle for understanding and transformation. In his foreword to
the 2015 *Mindful Nation Report*, Kabat-Zinn wrote:

> Interest in mindfulness within the mainstream of society and its institu-
> tions is rapidly becoming a global phenomenon, supported by increasingly
> rigorous scientific research, and driven by a longing for new models and
> practices that might help us individually and collectively to apprehend and
> solve the challenges facing our health as societies and as a species, optimiz-
> ing the preconditions for happiness and well-being, and minimizing the
> causes and preconditions for unhappiness and suffering. (Mindfulness All-
> Party Parliamentary Group, 2015)

There is a growing body of evidence that mindfulness and mindfulness-
based programs have transformative potential with other groups and in other
contexts. The following is just a small selection of the mindfulness-based programs tailored to specific populations and settings.

- *Depression and addiction.* Mindfulness-based cognitive therapy (MBCT) provides people suffering recurrent depression with an array of tools to stay well (Gu, Strauss, Bond, & Cavanagh, 2015; Kuyken et al., 2016). In another adaptation, mindfulness-based relapse prevention (MBRP) helps people struggling with substance abuse and dependence learn to relate differently to the triggers and cravings that feed addiction (Brewer, Elwafi, & Davis, 2013).

- *Children and adolescents.* Mindfulness-based programs have also been adapted and used with children and adolescents to support their social and emotional learning and ability to both manage challenges and to flourish. There are examples of this work in primary and secondary schools, clinical settings, and families (Greenberg & Harris, 2012; Kallapiran, Koo, Kirubakaran, & Hancock, 2015; Zenner, Herrnleben-Kurz, & Walach, 2014).

- *The criminal justice system.* Mindfulness is being used to teach skills of presence, compassion, equanimity, and patience—both to those held within the system and to those working in the system (Mindfulness All-Party Parliamentary Group, 2015).

- *The workplace.* A healthy workplace supported by mindfulness serves both the workers and the economy (Good et al., 2016). Yet in many countries there is a rising toll of work-related mental health problems, with high levels of absenteeism and presenteeism, where people turn up to work but are not productive. There is growing evidence that mindfulness is associated with staff well-being, skilled leadership, and the effectiveness of organizations (Good et al., 2016; Wolever et al., 2012).

The key insight is that mindfulness provides a way to understand the human mind and heart. Mindfulness training with a range of populations, across a range of contexts, provides a way of responding, at least in part, to some of the world's most pressing challenges.

Bridging Ancient Wisdom, Modern Science, and the Contemporary World

That which we frequently think about and
dwell upon, to this does the mind incline.[3]
—NANAMOLI AND BODHI (1995)

This ancient Buddhist teaching has been borne out by modern psychological science. Our minds shape and are shaped by our world. Our minds are the foundation upon which our world of experience is constructed. Our minds show *plasticity*[4] as we learn and adapt to the world, from birth into adulthood and into old age. We have an incredible capacity to shape and train our minds throughout our lives in ways that can help us better navigate our lives (Kok & Singer, 2017; Lutz et al., 2009; Slagter, Davidson, & Lutz, 2011).

Ancient Wisdom

Mindfulness and mindfulness training are embedded in most contemplative traditions. From 900 to 200 B.C.E., four distinct contemplative traditions evolved: Hinduism, Buddhism, and Jainism in the Indian subcontinent; Confucianism and Daoism in China; monotheism in the Middle East; and philosophical rationalism in Greece (Armstrong, 2011). During this intellectually and spiritually fertile period, the Buddha, Socrates, and Confucius developed their ideas. It was the ground on which Christ and Muhammed would a few hundred years later build their teachings. Although it is possible to outline how contemporary mindfulness draws upon the rich lineage of each of these early traditions, in this book, we draw primarily on Buddhism and, specifically, Buddhist psychology.

Buddhist teachings originated over 2,000 years ago in India with a young man, Siddhartha Gautama, whom we now refer to as the Buddha. He examined the world around him and his own psychological experience to develop a model of the mind and a methodology for training the mind (see Box 1.1). He was in many ways one of the first psychologists.

In the classic story of the Buddha's life, a young man leaves the fortress of his unrealistic views to seek the understanding that would provide a more reliable refuge. His experience opened his eyes to the understanding that distress, as much as joy, is integral to the human condition. He equally realized the limitations of hiding from reality and the inadequacy of the defenses we build to protect ourselves from uncertainty, discomfort, and change. Rather than pursuing what were in that time the traditional pathways (of transcendence, avoidance, and suppression) to overcome and escape affliction, he realized that suffering could be met fearlessly and that the origins of distress could be understood. Through that understanding much human distress could come to an end. It became apparent to him how much compounded human distress was borne of the incapacity or refusal to meet the inevitable moments of adversity in life with courage and understanding. The Buddha devised a comprehensive, practical pathway of turning toward life with all its joys and sorrows with curiosity, investigation, and care. He and a set of his monks communicated the teachings orally about 2,600 years ago. As the teachings spread to different cultures and languages (India, Sri Lanka, Burma, China, and later the West) the teachings evolved and changed. They were written down in several languages, originally Pali and Sanskrit. In the original teachings, they

---

BOX 1.1. Siddhartha Gautama: The Story of the Buddha

In the ancient teaching story familiar to many, the young man Siddhartha Gautama was cocooned by an overprotective father who sought to shield his precious son from the harsh realities of life. In his 20s, Siddhartha became restless and determined to venture out beyond the walls of his perfectly arranged environment. He was struck by the sight of a person diseased and ill, and then taken aback again by the sight of an old man, stooped and frail. The third sight that made him pause was to see a corpse lying on the side of the road. Each time he turned to his companion to ask, "Will this too also happen to me?" Each time he was given the same answer: "Yes, this too will be part of your life." The young man realized that all of his status, comfort, and possessions would not hold back the inevitable rhythms of life. He learned that all the love of his family would not protect him from aging, sickness, and death. Soon after, Siddhartha left his home and set out to find the abiding peace and freedom he longed for. The final sight Siddhartha encountered was a man in the crowd who embodied stillness, calm, and peace. This was the inspiration for Siddhartha to begin a path of inner exploration to understand distress, the origins of distress, and how to end distress and live a good life. It was this systematic quest that turned Siddhartha into one of the first scientists and psychologists.

---

were presented as a large number of discourses or *suttas* (>15,000).[5] This body of work has provided the foundation of contemporary mindfulness.[6]

Modern Psychological Science

Compared to the contemplative traditions, science is a relatively recent development. The current University of Oxford Museum of the History of Science started out as an *experimental philosophy* department in the 17th century, with chemistry laboratories in the basement and undergraduate teaching on the ground floor. Modern psychology is only a little over 100 years old, and neuroscience much younger still. Yet in that time, we have accumulated a wealth of knowledge about:

- How we see and experience the world (e.g., attention and perception);
- How we make sense of the world (e.g., learning and memory, language and thought, social perception);
- What supports mental health and human flourishing;
- What creates and maintains mental ill health (e.g., personality, psychopathology[7]); and
- How we can learn to use this understanding to lead our lives well.

There is, as yet, no unifying model of the mind, and arguably we are some distance from having one. In many ways, modern psychological science took a backward step when it accepted Descartes' conclusion that the mind and body were distinct, that consciousness was located in the mind, and, more recently, that consciousness could be reduced to the brain (Damasio, 1994). It seems increasingly clear that complex mind–body systems shape our experience, health, and well-being (Davidson et al., 2003; Kahneman, 2011; Sapolsky, 2017). It is likely that as we inch toward a unifying model of the mind we will need to integrate many disciplines besides psychology, including the understanding and perspectives from contemplative traditions such as Buddhist psychology.

The Confluence of Ancient Traditions and Modern Science

The architecture and functioning of the human mind and body has not evolved a great deal in the last few thousand years. Moreover, many of the fundamental challenges of life—negotiating childhood and adolescence, health and illness, old age and death—are the same challenges that people have faced throughout the history of the human species. The understanding and comprehensive pathways of transformation, mapped out by the Buddha, are as meaningful today as they were centuries ago. Rather like the confluence of two rivers, there has been a remarkable confluence of ancient Buddhist psychology with modern psychological science and neuroscience (e.g., Dalai Lama, 2002, 2011b; Kabat-Zinn, 2011). This confluence provides perspectives on and methods for working with some of the challenges of the contemporary world.

The key proposal we make is that ancient Buddhist psychology and modern psychology can be drawn together in ways that help us better understand the mind. Mindfulness training provides ways to train and shape the mind so we can better respond to challenges in our lives and help others respond to the challenges in their lives.

The last case study we introduce is Sam. His journey was from a life of addiction that nearly destroyed him, and those around him, to being an active, useful person.

Sam was a recovering addict. Through years of recovery in 12-step programs and then an MBRP program, he learned first to understand his addiction. He began to "tame his demons," and over time made some major life changes. Like many others, Sam was able to use what we know from psychology and 12-step programs to work with the cravings and self-destructive behavior that nearly killed him. After a few years in recovery and through sponsoring people in his 12-step fellowship, he decided to become an addiction counselor.

What Is Mindfulness?

Mindfulness is the unfailing master key for knowing the mind, and is thus the starting point; the perfect tool for shaping the mind, and is thus the focal point; and the lofty manifestation of the achieved freedom of the mind.
—NYANAPONIKA THERA (1962)

Mohammed experiences a searing stabbing sensation in his lower back for the hundredth time that day. He meets the pain with care and equanimity, choosing to do some small gentle stretches. Ling recognizes the negative thought "I don't think I can face the day, it's going to be too much," and says to herself, "This is a thought, not a fact." Sam has a powerful urge to drink when he sees a bottle of whiskey in the supermarket aisle; he surfs the waves of the urges until they pass. Sophia is sitting in the doctor's surgery waiting room worrying what her latest medical test results will say. She notices a spider spinning its web and intentionally allows herself to be immersed in the wonder of the spider at work. Mohammed's, Sam's, Ling's, and Sophia's experiences in these moments all illustrate mindfulness. When our phone's notifications demand our attention, we choose to stay focused on the task at hand. When in the midst of the busyness of rush hour traffic, we find peace by anchoring our awareness in our breath and body with a sense of interest and care. When we are eating, we choose to really savor the food. When we are with someone we love, we make an active choice to really be present to and with that person. These are further examples of the awareness available to all of us in any moment.

How can the word *mindfulness* encapsulate this myriad of meanings? Has the word become so diffuse and overused that its meaning has become muddied (Hefferrnan, 2015)? Or is mindfulness like a diamond with many facets that can capture Mohammed's, Ling's, Sam's, and Sophia's experiences? The rest of this chapter unpacks the word *mindfulness*. We look in turn at the different facets of the diamond and consider both ancient and modern definitions (see Table 1.1). We outline some of the most illustrative similes, metaphors, and imagery used to define mindfulness (see Table 1.2) and consider the functions of mindfulness. By considering each of these facets and functions in turn, we outline the myriad perspectives that together represent the idea or construct of "mindfulness." We also touch on some of the most common misunderstandings and misrepresentations. The chapter concludes by offering a synopsis and working definition of mindfulness. Unpacking mindfulness in this way is the foundation for the rest of the book, sketching a map of how mindfulness helps us to navigate life's difficulties and joys.

One of the challenges we faced is the way terms and language are used differently in psychology and Buddhist psychology. To provide a middle way, we offer some operational definitions of key terms in Appendix 1. With the proliferation of mindfulness approaches and programs, we also offer an operational definition of mindfulness training and mindfulness-based programs in Appendix 2.

TABLE 1.1. Definitions of Mindfulness

"The clear and single-minded awareness of what actually happens to us and in us at successive moments of perception" (Nyanaponika Thera, 1962, p. 32).

"Mirror-like thought. Mindfulness reflects only what is presently happening and in exactly the way it is happening. There are no biases" (Gunaratana, 2002, p. 139).

"Present-moment awareness, presence of mind, wakefulness" (Goldstein, 2013, p. 13).

Ellen Langer (1989) has a somewhat different definition and refers to four interrelated dimensions of mindfulness: (1) novelty seeking, (2) engagement, (3) novelty producing, and (4) flexibility.

Self-regulation of attention (skills of sustained attention, switching, inhibition of secondary elaborative processing) and orientation to experience (curiosity, experiential openness, and acceptance; Bishop et al., 2006).

Perhaps the most often quoted definition of mindfulness is Jon Kabat-Zinn's definition, which has appeared in a number of his articles and books: "A way of being in a wise and purposeful relationship with one's experience, both inwardly and outwardly. It is cultivated by systematically exercising one's capacity for paying attention, on purpose, in the present moment and non-judgmentally."

He has also emphasized seven principles of mindfulness: acceptance, nonjudging, nonstriving, beginner's mind, letting go, patience, and trust (Kabat-Zinn, 1990, 2006; Mindfulness All-Party Parliamentary Group, 2015).

The cognitive scientist John Teasdale has described the essence of mindfulness as full awareness of our experience in each moment, equally open to whatever it has to offer and free of the domination of habitual, automatic, cognitive routines that are often goal oriented and, in one form or another, related to wanting things to be other than they are (Teasdale & Chaskalson, 2011a, 2011b).

Shauna Shapiro (2009) has defined mindfulness as the awareness that arises out of intentionally attending, in an open and discerning way, to whatever is arising in the present moment. She emphasizes attention, intention, and attitude (openness and nonjudgment).

TABLE 1.2. Metaphors of Mindfulness

Simple knowing

Simple knowing or awareness is likened to standing on an elevated platform or tower, surveying the surrounding landscape. There is no agenda but to see, and our attention and awareness are intentional, receptive, and relaxed. We have a perspective that does not overly identify with the particulars of the terrain, which is the first step in dis-identifying or decentering.

The flashlight beam of attention can be intentionally moved around different objects. The focus, size, and tonal quality of the beam can be altered.

Protective awareness

Protective mindfulness is like a town's wise gatekeeper who is able to recognize and admit the genuine citizens of the town, and to decide who is to be admitted entry and who should not be admitted. Each of the *sense doors* has a guardian who watches what experiences come to the door and actively allows, or does not allow them entry, discerning whether they will bring beneficial outcomes or bring harm. A more contemporary example might be a security guard.

A cow herder initially had to closely watch over his or her cows to prevent them from straying into growing fields. However, once the crop had been harvested, the cow herder was able to relax beneath a tree and simply watch the cows from a distance. This conveys how mindfulness training can be used for protective awareness (before the crops are harvested) and then shift to a broader choiceless awareness after the crop has been harvested.

A person at a bus stop waits for buses to come and chooses whether to get on or not. Occasionally, the person might get on a bus on automatic pilot only to realize some time later that he or she has been carried somewhere unintended—in that moment of waking up, the person can choose to get off the bus. Mindfulness is the capacity to notice buses coming and going, and then making the active choice whether to get on or off them.

Investigative awareness

Investigative mindfulness is likened to a surgeon operating on a person who has been wounded by an arrow. Rather than forcefully pulling out the arrow, a skillful surgeon would probe around the wound to determine its nature. He or she would be able to ascertain the nature of the injury, make a diagnosis, determine the most beneficial way of removing the arrow, and prescribe a course of treatment.

Reframing perception and views

Like someone driving a stick shift, we are able to voluntarily shift our minds from automatic, impulsive, and reactive modes to a mode of intentionality, discernment, and choice.

A musician can play the same piece of music in different keys. How we hear and experience music is changed fundamentally by the key it is played in, and whether it is played on acoustic or electric instruments. Mindfulness enables an intentional choice of key or mode that can transform our experience.

(continued)

TABLE 1.2. *(continued)*

The view of Earth from space is a reframed view. Astronauts have commented that when viewed from space, divisions of peoples, nations, and cultures can seem arbitrary. A view on the galaxy provides an even larger sense of perspective and scale.

<u>Bringing it all together</u>

A careful charioteer guides a chariot through a crowded street. Mindfulness has the ability to carefully direct attention, thought, and action.

A trained elephant whose power and impulses have been tamed can now help with transport and heavy lifting. Rather than a danger to the village, the elephant (the mind) has become a great friend and resource.

A horse and rider work in harmony. The rider understands the horse and their union enables great speed, endurance, and power. The horse (the mind) has become a great asset.

A kayaker's skill enables him or her to navigate every state of a river safely, skillfully, and intentionally.

Ancient and Contemporary Definitions of Mindfulness

One of the most ancient descriptions of mindfulness is of villagers taming a wild elephant. An untrained elephant is driven by impulse and can rampage when it feels threatened, leaving destruction in its wake. But when it is trained, the power of the elephant becomes a great asset to the villagers. The mind is like an elephant: it can be destructive if it is rampaging, and impulsive and an extraordinary force for good if well trained.

Ever since Buddhist psychology was introduced into Western contexts, teachers and students have grappled with how best to define mindfulness. The first Buddhist scholars, translating the Pali and Sanskrit texts in the 19th century, faced a similar challenge. Finding other terms inadequate, they borrowed the word *mindfulness* from the Christian gospels (Gethin, 2011).

It was Rhys Davids (1881) who first translated what was a Buddhist technical term in the Pali language, *sati,* as mindfulness. *Sati,* translated literally, is *remembering.* This does not mean remembering historical events or data, but rather remembering to come back to the lucid awareness of present-moment experience. It suggests that the mind is established in the present moment rather than lost in distractedness, or in thoughts of the past or future.

Mindfulness encourages a more unified way of being. Bodily sensations, feelings, mental states, and present-moment experience are perceived and held in awareness where they can be explored with attitudes of curiosity, patience,

> ## BOX 1.2. **Mindfulness Practice: Pausing to Attend to Experience**
>
> A simple exercise is to pause for a moment just now and sense what is happening in your body and mind—what is happening around you. Attending to your body experience, you sense how your body feels touching the chair, the sensations of the air on your skin, any tension in your shoulders. You might begin to sense what your mood is: Tired or energized? Restless or steady? Anxious or calm? The background whisper of thoughts becomes discernible. You may discover yourself becoming sensitized to the sights and sounds of the moment. Let the torch beam of your attention move around these experiences. Allow yourself to attend to the immediacy of these experiences that make up our moment, without adding narrative or speculation. Simply know what is present just now, in this moment.

and kindness. This type of awareness sounds remarkably simple, until we try it (see Box 1.2). We can read about how to ride a horse, but try then getting onto a horse and seeing if the written instructions are enough, especially if the horse is a bit flighty. Learning about mindfulness is much the same—it is a practice largely learned experientially.

When we try to bring awareness to our direct experience in the moment, we typically find that our mind has a strong inclination and habit to move away from the present moment. Our minds can be forgetful and distracted, easily pulled in different directions, often without us even being aware of it. Our negative thoughts, pain, or cravings powerfully draw us into a vortex of reactivity.

Mindfulness training, however, involves repeatedly coming back to our experience in this moment, a process that develops the capacity to sustain attention, to understand our present-moment experience and calm our usual reactive patterns. It can be used to respond (or not respond) to the seemingly trivial cues like phone notifications, and also to clearly nontrivial experiences, like Sam's destructive cravings in full-blown addiction.

As mindfulness becomes more established in mainstream culture, the quest goes on to find a good definition. Table 1.1 provides some illustrative definitions from Buddhist texts (Nyanaponika Thera, 1962), Buddhist scholars (Gunaratana, 2002), first-generation Western teachers of Buddhist psychology (Goldstein, 2013), and contemporary mindfulness scientists (Bishop et al., 2006; Langer, 1989; Shapiro, 2009). Rather than reflect on each of the definitions in this table, we draw out some of the commonalities and themes among ancient and modern definitions of mindfulness.

First, we can describe mindfulness as a state, process, and faculty:

- A state of *being present* (e.g., of openness, allowing, inclusive). It is an abiding way of being present in our lives that is embodied and experiential. In this sense it is the antidote to *forgetfulness*, which is the habitual inclination of the mind to be lost in preoccupation, thought, memory, and anticipation, divorced from the body and present-moment experience;
- A *process* of unfolding moment-to-moment experience; and
- A *faculty*. This is key because it connotes that mindfulness is a trainable quality that can be cultivated and applied in our lives.

Second, mindfulness has, at its core, *an intentionality in how attention and awareness are deployed*—that is, mindfulness involves deploying attention like a flashlight beam, *choosing* where to shine the light and what to leave in darkness. More than this, we can choose to *play with attention*, making the focus of attention narrow or broad, sharp or dim, energetic or more passive. We can choose deliberately, with awareness, to focus attention or allow a broader awareness. When our attention is broad, there is no single point of attention. Instead, whatever appears *on the workbench of attention* is attended to, but crucially with intentionality.

Children learning mindfulness can relate to the flashlight analogy.[8] Asking them to play with a flashlight can be a precursor to asking them to play with attention. The flashlight can be shone in different directions, and on some flashlights the beam and lens can be altered. With attention, they can *play with* what is foregrounded and backgrounded in their awareness.

Attention can also be intentionally placed in different sense modalities, including hearing, seeing, bodily sensing, tasting, and smelling. Each modality can be the primary window through which we pay attention to our experience. Attention can also be placed in the realm of thoughts, images, and moods—we choose which of these becomes the object of our attention.

Mindfulness trainings typically start with focal attention, so people can learn to stabilize and deploy their attention in the ways we have outlined above. Once this is established as a base, they are invited to broaden awareness so that their experience can be seen in a wider and more expansive way, sometimes called "open monitoring" (Lutz, Slagter, Dunne, & Davidson, 2008).

Third, attention and awareness are imbued with certain *attitudinal qualities*. Perhaps most fundamentally, we can develop an attitude of attention that is open, allowing, and inclusive, whether the experience is positive, negative, or neutral. Further attitudinal qualities include curiosity, perseverance, patience, friendliness, care, trust, and equanimity. The landscape of attention and awareness is not, we must point out, attitudinally neutral—mindfulness is not cold or mechanical. Rather, attention is imbued with a sense of purpose, interest, warmth, and energy.

Fourth, mindfulness training and mindfulness programs involve *effort*. A student of mindfulness learns about sustained effort—that is, what is too much, what is too little? This is not a striving effort, rather it is an effort that has warmth of feeling, compassion for any struggle encountered, and a sense of measured enthusiasm or dedication. Over time, a sense of trust in the ability to turn toward experience, however difficult, emerges. An analogy that is sometimes used is that the right amount of effort is like tuning a guitar string, not too tight so the note is too high in pitch, not too loose so the note is too low in pitch.

Fifth, mindfulness has an *ethical dimension*. It is deployed and trained in the service of understanding, lessening suffering, enhancing joy, increasing compassion, and providing greater opportunities to lead a mindful life. The mind can learn greater clarity, responsiveness, and calm in the present moment of experience, where distress is lessened or even ended. At the heart of this ethical dimension is figuring out what, in our experience, is wholesome, so that we can turn toward what is likely to lead to good outcomes. As we turn toward what is wholesome, we can then choose to let go of patterns and tendencies that do not enhance the well-being of others or ourselves. For example, in the face of suffering, we can bring an inclination toward compassion and let go of an inclination toward harshness.

> *To summarize, mindfulness is like a diamond with many facets. It is a state, process, and faculty; it has at its core intentionality; it is imbued with certain attitudes (curiosity, friendliness, patience, and care); it requires effort; and it is intrinsically ethical. These facets of mindfulness have sometimes been summarized into the what and how of mindfulness. The what is attentional focus and broader awareness. The how is an attitude of turning toward experience, with curiosity and care, to every aspect of experience. We would add the why of mindfulness—namely, a clear intentionality guided by ethics and a map of where we are trying to go.*

The Function of Mindfulness

The function of mindfulness is to help us shift from automatic reactivity to responsiveness, and from avoidance patterns to a genuine willingness to meet present-moment experience as it is. Classically, mindfulness helps us shift from unconsciousness to awareness, from impulsiveness to an intentional way of being. Faced with threat, adversity, and pain, our first response is to flee, dissociate, and either lean backward into the past or forward into the future. Threat and pain become triggers for rumination, anxiety, obsession, and bewilderment. We become preoccupied with *fixing* distress rather than understanding it. The habitual pattern of the mind to flinch and flee in the face of discomfort and pain can become lifelong patterns of avoidance and agitation. Caught in the avoidance mechanisms that can govern our mind and life, our capacities for resilience, tolerance, and equilibrium are undermined. When Sam was caught in the throes of addiction, his cravings and self-destructive behavior ran his entire life. To a lesser degree, this can be true for all of us. We all can go through a whole day without many spaces of lucid awareness, of being truly awake and alive.

Mindfulness reverses these habitual tendencies. It can help us cultivate the capacity to know, understand, and inhabit the present moment. As the Buddhist teachings put it: "Suffering is to be understood." Flight and abandonment do little but deepen our sense of fear and helplessness in the face of pain, hindering our ability to respond with skillfulness. Our willingness to turn toward the moment, rather than away from our present experience, is the beginning of a journey toward greater confidence, commitment, and understanding. Mindfulness can only be cultivated in the *real-life* classroom of our lives, with all the joys and sorrows that are part of every human experience. Understanding distress and its origins is the only curriculum. It is here that we learn the lessons of healing and transformation.

Many of the patterns that create distress for us have long histories, not only our particular learning histories but also in the evolutionary history of the human species. We inherited these habits of mind because they have served a function for our species. Yet the mind is malleable and capable of tremendous change. Mindfulness training is intended to help us first see, then know these patterns of mind and then start to change them. In remarkably short periods of time, such as during an 8-week mindfulness program, participants can make significant life-changing shifts in how they relate to present-moment experience (Allen, Bromley, Kuyken, & Sonnenberg, 2009). These changes are even more marked in long-term mindfulness practitioners who have engaged in sustained training over many thousands of hours (Lazar et al., 2005; Lutz, Slagter, et al., 2008). There is growing scientific evidence that these changes are mirrored in our brain structure and function, our nervous system, bodily responses to stress, and even our genomes (e.g., Goleman & Davidson, 2017; Luders, Cherbuin, & Gaser, 2016; Luders, Toga, Lepore, & Gaser, 2009; Lutz, Brefczynski-Lewis, Johnstone, & Davidson, 2008; Schutte & Malouff, 2014).

Traditionally, mindfulness has been described as having four primary functions.

Simple Knowing and Awareness

Establishing simple knowing and awareness is the starting point of any mindfulness training. Learning to shine the light of clear, sustained attention upon present-moment experience—without bias or preference—is the point where we begin to distinguish the experience itself from our capacity to be aware of the contents of experience. Awareness taps into our feelings, sensory impression, moods, and thoughts. Aspects of our experience that have been unconscious, habitual, or shrouded in confusion can be recognized and, in time, seen with clarity. In mindfulness practices, we may be invited to move the flashlight beam of attention around the entirety of our experience, highlighting present-moment sensations, thoughts, and feelings, so that we can become familiar with the nuances of the moment.

Simple knowing and awareness is likened to a person standing on an elevated platform or tower surveying the surrounding landscape—there is no agenda but to see, the awareness is receptive, relaxed, and intentional. We have a perspective that does not overly identify with the particulars of the terrain.

All of the main mindfulness practices used in mindfulness-based programs cultivate this first function of mindfulness: simple knowing. For example, in intentional walking practice, people are invited to choose a path and commit to walking that path, focusing only on the direct sensory experience of walking. The practice reveals the difference between habitual, automatic modes of walking and mindful walking. When lost in thought, dullness, or preoccupation, we could spend 20 minutes walking on a path only to realize we have seen nothing, been touched by nothing—the world has been only a backdrop to the swirl of mental activity. When we walk that same path in an intentional way—returning our attention over and over to what it is just to walk, to inhabit the body and the moment—we sense how mindfulness illuminates the world. The sights and sounds touch us; the body is a fluid changing experience. It is a clear moment of wakefulness; we remember to come back to the present moment over and over again.

The cultivation of this simple awareness, learning to sustain it in every moment of experience, initiates a profound shift in consciousness. Simple knowing is a way of attending where no judgment or narrative is added to the experience of the moment. A thought is a thought, a sensation is a sensation, a sound is a sound, and a feeling is a feeling. Historical association is released, future dreads and anticipations are released, and we establish the capacity to know the moment just as it is. We may be acutely aware of the pull of habitual patterns to interpret, evaluate, speculate, and ruminate. Yet those patterns are also known in the light of simple awareness—habit as habit, reactivity as reactivity.

> Sam's recovery from addiction had involved attending 12-step meetings. One evening after a meeting he felt agitated, impulsive, and on the verge of relapsing. Every fiber in his body wanted to act out, to phone his dealer to score a hit. He phoned his 12-step program sponsor, who agreed to meet him on the beach for a walk. While Sam waited for his sponsor, he walked on the beach. As he walked, he became acutely aware of the intensity of his agitation, how every fiber in his body wanted oblivion. The compulsion gripped him like a vice; he experienced it as a powerful impulse to act out. This was the first of many instances in which Sam closely observed his mind and body states without acting them out, each time with greater clarity. Over time, he came to see them as waves he could anticipate and surf. Sam's experience is an extreme example of a common experience—namely, the arising and falling away of cravings.

If Sam's addiction seems extreme, consider that the impulse to reach for our phone to check for notifications is much the same, as is the impulse to eat even when we are not hungry, as is the impulse to check our favorite websites rather than do something we need but don't want to do. They are all habitual forms of avoidance and escape.

The cultivation of simple awareness is a form of fasting that cuts off the reinforcement of the patterns and habit that lead to distress through thought and speculation. Central in the development of mindfulness is training the capacity to be steadfast in our attention in the face of all experience, whether pleasant or unpleasant, without pushing it away and becoming lost in the contents of experience or ruminating. Cultivating simple knowing is not easy. It is an intentional way of being present that requires a surprising amount of effort. We begin with applying our intention to be here, only to find that our attention is hijacked by more habitual modes of forgetfulness and distractedness. As we learn to apply and reapply the intention, our capacity to sustain attention begins to grow. There is a simple formula underlying this process: where there is interest, intention follows; where there is intention, attention follows.

Protective Awareness

The second function of mindfulness is protective awareness. Mindfulness teaches us a way of being that clearly recognizes the potentially destructive power of some of the habit patterns and moods that assail the mind and then acts to protect the mind. Mindfulness reveals the way that rumination, anxiety, aversion, dissociation, and identification serve to create distress, diminished capacity, and negative self-view. Through simple awareness, we explore the landscape of our mind, becoming intimate with the familiar and repetitive habits that undermine well-being so that we can begin to use our attention to choose what we allow into awareness and what we keep out of awareness. This is not easy: there is a curious tension of wanting these habits to end, yet also being enchanted by or almost addicted to them.

There is an ancient simile of the gatekeeper of a city, whose job it is to meet all visitors. The gatekeeper recognizes and welcomes the visitors to the city who are helpful and beneficial, and turns away those who mean the city harm.

> The gatekeeper would be wise, competent, and intelligent, one who keeps out strangers and admits acquaintances. While he is walking along the path that encircles the city he could not see a cleft or an opening in the walls big enough for a cat to slip through. He might think, "Whatever large creatures enter or leave this city, all enter and leave through this one gate." (Bhikkhu Bodhi, 2005)

Protective awareness requires discernment, of knowing who the residents of the city are, who are visitors, who intend benefit, and who intend harm. This can seem to be at odds with mainstream mindfulness-based applications that so strongly emphasize the nonjudgmental and inclusive nature of mindfulness. In Buddhist psychology, a judging mind inevitably creates struggle and distress. Judging and *discernment*, however, are two different processes. Mindfulness, in Buddhist psychology, emphasizes developing and strengthening our capacity for discernment as the basis of an ethical life and the bridge to skillful responsiveness.

Discernment is not concerned primarily with worse and better, right and wrong, good and bad, worthy or unworthy, but rather is supported by simple awareness. For example, if we walked down the street and witnessed a vulnerable person fall down, simple knowing would enable us to clearly perceive the event. Merely observing his or her plight would not, of course, help the injured person. Remember Mohammed, the man living with chronic pain. If he sees the sensations of pain clearly in his awareness but has no sense of agency or choice, then this is of little help. Discernment registers the pain *and* leads us to make skillful choices, to address our own and other people's distress. The moment when Sam knows he is on the point of relapse and phones his sponsor is a moment of discernment. The moment Mohammed sees his pain spiraling into a sense of catastrophizing and hopelessness is a moment of discernment. Mindfulness is thus dynamic, engaging with experience in ways that are rooted in knowing what leads to distress and what leads to the end of distress.

Discernment can be learned. When we are engaged in cultivating mindfulness of the body, we might feel the familiar pull of habits (such as aversion, rumination, and shame). Instead of letting our attention become lost in our negative patterns, we can return to a place of knowing the body as the body, a thought as a thought. This is the function of protective awareness. Protective awareness is different from avoidance or suppression, which are patterns rooted in aversion, avoidance, or fear. Instead of turning away and dissociating from difficult experiences, protective awareness helps us fully know present-moment experience, so that we can choose not to engage in patterns that create and re-create distress. The moment Mohammed acknowledges an awareness of his painful sensations by applying some well-chosen stretches will provide some quick relief from the stabbing, searing sensations. This is an alternative to the well-worn ruts of physical contraction, hopelessness, and catastrophizing.

The tendency of the human mind to blame, shame, judge, ruminate, and/or simply want things to be different from what they are, is powerful, repetitive, personal, and universal with predictable painful outcomes. These tendencies or habits can directly contribute to mental ill health. There is even evidence that anxiety and depression, and the tendency to worry and ruminate, can be passed from generation to generation (Ziegert & Kistner, 2002). There may be much we are asked to understand about these distress patterns, yet that understanding is rarely borne of more rumination. Protective mindfulness is not a process of pushing away the unwelcome, but simply learning that we do not need to live in a way in which we are repetitively overwhelmed by it. It also may help us end the cycle of unhelpful thought patterns that are passed down from generation to generation.

Investigative Awareness

The third function of mindfulness is investigative awareness. The analogy used to describe this element of mindfulness is that of a surgeon operating on a person wounded by an arrow. Rather than yanking out the arrow, a skillful surgeon would first assess the wound to determine its nature. After assessing the nature of the injury, the surgeon would then make a diagnosis, determine the most beneficial way of removing the arrow, establish a prognosis, and prescribe a course of treatment. Investigative mindfulness is centrally about understanding and insight. It is the window of mindfulness through which understanding emerges that can radically change the shape of our experience and in time, the mind. Investigation ties mindfulness to the core of teachings of mindfulness training and mindfulness programs—to know that there is distress, to know that there are origins to distress, to know that distress can come to an end, and that there is a pathway to the end of distress (Teasdale & Chaskalson, 2011a).

Investigative awareness is both experiential and conceptual. Through formal mindfulness practices, psychoeducation, and in-group inquiry, we have a growing understanding of the mind, the ways in which it creates our internal experience, and also shapes and is shaped by our external world. On the simplest level, Mohammed becomes aware of painful sensations in his back, but with mindfulness he also knows that aversion and resistance will compound the sensations. He really looks into the sensations, seeing them as they are—"searing" and "stabbing." He learns to meet pain with a caring attention and understands that he does not need to be defined by pain, that there are other things that define him, such as being a good father. Mindfulness does not always mean the sensations will disappear, but we can radically shift how we relate to the sensations and how we allow them to impact our consciousness. Investigative awareness provides discernment and choices. For example, there are many activities that are immersive, distracting, and enjoyable but we have discernment and we choose to do them (such as knitting, gardening, watching television, talking to a friend, listening to podcasts). The key in investigative awareness is intentionality and choice.

Reframing Perception and View

The fourth function of mindfulness, clearly interwoven with the previous three, is a conscious reframing of perception and view. In Buddhist psychology, this function is taught by consciously cultivating an attitude of kindness and friendliness toward ourselves, others, and all events and experiences. Kindness and friendliness are embedded in all mindfulness teaching. Aversion, on the other hand, forces us to turn away from ourselves, others, and the events of our lives. When we feel aversion, we fear the unwelcome, engage in judgment and blame, and far too often spend our lives in a state of agitated avoidance. When our awareness turns toward all experience with curiosity and friendliness, our view of others as enemies or threats begins to soften. We begin to see that we are not the broken, imperfect person we can believe ourselves to be. We allow ourselves to see that pain arises and changes; bleakness is not a constant. We can challenge our self-descriptions of unworthiness in the light of a new perception. The life we may have perceived as threatening, gray, or meaningless can be seen in new ways. We realize that we have choices that can change our thinking and our lives.

The cultivation of all four functions of mindfulness constitutes what in Buddhist psychology is referred to as wise or skillful mindfulness, dedicated to liberating the mind from distress and embodied in a mindful way of living. To bring these four functions to life, we revisit Ling, the 44-year-old court magistrate and single mother of two teenage children. Ling had a history of depression that started when she herself was a teenager. After participating in an MBCT program 2 years ago, she learned new skills to stay well in the long term. She found the program helpful and continued a mindfulness practice to sustain herself. Below we see an example of how mindfulness fulfills these four functions for Ling.

For no obvious reason, Ling woke at 3:00 A.M. with a sense of foreboding. Almost as soon as she was awake, every conditioned pathway in her mind pulled her toward a sense of worry and agitation. There was a familiar sense of knowing the day would be marred by tiredness, fertile ground that could trigger her depression (*simple knowing and awareness*). She was aware of a plummeting feeling. It was a familiar, scary place. For Ling, this recognition was the first step. With courage and firmness, she said to herself: "This is my black dog; this is depression."

The next step was a subtle but profound shift in orientation of mind (*protective mindfulness*) to one of friendly allowing: "Here you are again, familiar old friend, it's OK, I know you well." Ling is meeting the plummeting feeling with friendliness, open to investigating what she is experiencing in her mind and body. The next deliberate step was a steadying of her breath and body, intentionally bringing her attention to her belly, placing her hand on her belly and feeling the movement of her belly as her breath moved in through an in-breath and out through an out-breath. One breath, two breaths, deliberately slowing and steadying the breath. Inevitably, it seemed her mind pulled her back toward worry. Firmly, gently back to the belly, breathing (*protective awareness*). Ling is steadying herself with her attention.

After 10 minutes of steadying her attention with her breath, Ling felt she had an active choice. She could stay in bed and use a practice she knew might help her sleep or she could get up, have a cup of coffee, and get on with her day knowing she'd probably sleep well the following night (*investigative awareness*). She chose to get up, to really savor a cup of coffee (before her family woke), and get on with something she had been putting off for some time: writing a reference for one of her former colleagues. An hour later, as she printed out the letter, she stopped to read it with a sense of appreciation that she had been able to help her colleague. It brought a smile to her face to know that her reference would help her friend get a good job. It brought to mind her teenage children, sleeping upstairs. She poured herself another cup of coffee. As she sat drinking it, she stopped to really savor the coffee and bring to mind her family. The shift in mind Ling was able to make that morning was transformative and empowering, changing the trajectory of her day. Her black dog was still there, but she had been able to meet it with mindfulness (*reframing perception and view*).

We can see these different facets and functions of mindfulness in action for Ling in the course of her early morning. In the past, it is likely this moment would have spiraled into an episode of depression; her sense of foreboding would have consumed her experience, plummeting in a downward spiral. However, she recognized this and was able to *steady her attention*, bringing *qualities of friendliness and patience* to her experience. She *practiced mindfulness* of breath and body to further *steady her attention* (*protective awareness*). The foreboding was labeled as "the black dog" (*insight, reframing perception and view*) and related to with attitudes of *friendliness, equanimity*, and *patience* ("Here you are again, familiar old friend, it's OK, I know you well"). She started to feel she had an *active choice* and she chose to get up and *do something constructive*, showing *discernment* and *resilience* in the face of the early warning signs of depression. She *savored* her coffee and stopped to *appreciate* the colleague she had helped and her family asleep upstairs (*awareness of positive experience*). All of these actions of mind and body were on the tip of intention—namely, to be free of the grip of depression and enjoy better *mental health* and *well-being*, both for her benefit and for all the people whose lives she affected (her children, friends, and colleagues). These shifts in mind enabled Ling to change the trajectory of her day and over time build her *capacity* for leading a mindful life.

> **The key insight is that mindfulness has four functions: (1) simple knowing and awareness, (2) protective awareness, (3) investigative awareness, and (4) reframing perception and view.**

Metaphors of Mindfulness

Throughout Buddhist psychology and contemporary accounts of mindfulness, similes, metaphors, and imagery are used to connote mindfulness. We have already used some in defining mindfulness and summarize some of the most helpful in Table 1.2. These metaphors capture the myriad facets of mindfulness in ways that sometimes narrative text cannot: they bring a richness and texture to our understanding.

One powerful metaphor, learned from a participant in a mindfulness program, was of a kayaker navigating a turbulent river upstream from Niagara Falls, New York. The participant explained that without mindfulness a kayaker can easily be swept downriver at the whim of the river's currents and into danger. Without awareness, a kayaker is vulnerable to being dragged toward and over Niagara Falls, an experience she compared to being dragged into a depressive relapse. A skilled kayaker, on the other hand, can navigate the river, making skillful choices as she travels downriver. For example, even in a turbulent river, a skilled kayaker can find an eddy where the kayak can rest in safety and the kayaker can pick out a skillful route downriver. She compared this to seeing the early warning signs of depression, anchoring awareness and choosing to respond in ways that prevent depression and support recovery and well-being.

What Mindfulness Is *Not*

As we noted at the start of the chapter, mindfulness encapsulates myriad meanings. As such it is prone to misunderstanding, becoming clichéd or even parodied. We address some of the most common misunderstandings in turn.

Mindfulness is neither *relaxation* nor *in the service of becoming relaxed*. While relaxation may be a positive outcome of some mindfulness practices, mindfulness is about attending to and being aware of our experiences, whether they are positive, negative, or neutral. Mindfulness is not about zoning out. In fact, it is referred to in classical teachings as *waking up* to our experiences and lives.

Mindfulness is neither a *quick fix* nor *simple*. Even though one dimension of mindfulness is *simply knowing,* this does not mean that mindfulness or mindfulness practices are simple or lead to easy, quick changes. Anyone who sits down to practice mindfulness learns this soon enough, and when we stop and examine it the mind presents the texture, richness, and depth of our experience, both the pleasant and the unpleasant.

Mindfulness is not about *emptying the mind, not thinking,* or *turning away from experience*. Rather, it is about turning toward experience and being with and alongside whatever is found in our experience. What is intended is that mindfulness enables choices and clearer thinking. Some advanced practitioners of mindfulness have described states of mind that can be described as spacious, where the endless stream of thinking ceases for a while. But this is neither common nor a goal of mindfulness-based programs.

Mindfulness is not about *dismantling the self.* Instead, mindfulness is about creating conditions whereby we can learn firsthand and experientially about our minds. It is true that this learning often leads to shifts in perspective. Ling, for example, gained the understanding that experiences shift and change, they are impermanent. When she became aware of her thoughts and feelings, she was able to shift her thinking ("I am not my negative thoughts") and make positive choices, instead of spiraling into old patterns. Mohammed also experienced an important shift when he came to realize I am not my pain. Sam too saw he was not his craving, even when the cravings were so powerful. He developed a faith in his capacity to know and manage powerful mind states through many years of learning to ride the waves of these sensations. This was not so much a dismantling of the self as a new way of being and knowing. We learn that we can choose to make these shifts—like driving and selecting different gears, we can see mind states and select different gears.

Mindfulness and meditation are not one and the same. Meditation practices are found in almost every contemplative tradition and serve a variety of purposes. They can train attention, develop different types of awareness, cultivate attitudes of mind, and develop a sense of intentionality and ethics. Mindfulness, on the other hand, is a state, process, and capacity that we all have and can be trained and cultivated through these meditation practices. In mindfulness-based programs, the practices have a particular intention— namely, to better understand the mind and then to train it in the service of living with less suffering and greater joy and ease. See Appendix 2 for a fuller description of mindfulness training and mindfulness-based programs.

Mindfulness practice can evoke a range of experiences that are unfamiliar, unknown, and even frightening. These include involuntary body movements, seeing lights or hearing sounds, states such as dissociation, or an exacerbation of anxiety or low mood. This is, of course, not the intention of mindfulness practice. It is imperative that mindfulness teachers are appropriately trained. In the same way that an engineer or a doctor should only undertake work they are qualified to do, mindfulness teachers need to be well trained to do the work they are doing—they are working with an organ of extraordinary complexity and power: the human mind (Baer & Kuyken, 2016).

Finally, mindfulness is not attentional training that can be used for ethically questionable practice. If snipers train their attention so they can better kill people, this is attentional training, not mindfulness. If an organization uses certain meditation practices to bring its members into acquiescence, this is not mindfulness, it is brainwashing. Mindfulness is intrinsically ethical. In mindfulness training, everything rests on the *tip of intention*—namely, to support people to suffer less and lead meaningful and rewarding lives.

SYNOPSIS

In many ways, we are living at a time of extraordinary potential in the contemporary world. More of the world's population is living longer, in better economic security, with less risk of violence, and with improved education and opportunity. Yet we continue to see a lot of human suffering of various forms, much of it originating in the human mind and heart. We outlined how mindfulness is a confluence of ancient understandings and practices from Buddhist psychology and modern psychological science. We suggested that mindfulness and mindfulness training can provide a way to understand and then transform this suffering, and suggested that it might provide a pathway to living with greater understanding, compassion, and responsiveness. But first, we need to define mindfulness, to sketch its myriad meanings.

Mindfulness is a state, process, and faculty that can be trained. It involves awareness imbued with a clear intentionality and a particular set of attitudes—turning toward experience with interest and care. Mindfulness is *part of an extended family of qualities* that work together to produce its effects. These qualities include ethics, energy, and discernment. They operate together to develop the understanding and core psychological shifts that liberate the mind from suffering and create insight, understanding, and the possibility of a mindful life characterized by psychological well-being, satisfying relationships, reduction in anxiety and depression, freedom from addictive behavior, and a sense that life is fulfilling and meaningful, even in the midst of pain and inevitable difficulties. This ripples outward into relationships, families, communities, organizations, and the wider world.

Mindfulness has several key functions:

- Simple knowing and awareness;
- Protective awareness;
- Investigative awareness; and
- Reframing perception and views.

The following working definition includes the elements and functions of mindfulness listed above. It is intended to capture the key dimensions of mindfulness that might be helpful to those learning and teaching it.
Mindfulness:

- *Is a natural, trainable human capacity.*
- *Helps bring attention and awareness to all experiences.*
- *Is equally open to whatever is present in a given moment.*
- *Conveys attitudes of curiosity, friendliness, and compassion.*
- *Is discernment.*
- *Is in the service of suffering less, enjoying greater well-being, and leading a meaningful, rewarding life.*

CHAPTER 2

A Map of the Mind

ATTENTION, PERCEPTION, AND THE JUDGING MIND

All experience is preceded by mind
Led by mind
Shaped by mind
—ACHARYA BUDDHARAKKHITA
(1996)

Fascinating studies have asked what happens when people are dropped into deserts or wilderness locations and instructed to find their way out. It was discovered that without a map and a reference point to guide them, people were prone to walk in circles, ending in the same spot they began (Souman, Frissen, Sreenivasa, & Ernst, 2009). This parallels the story of when Siddhartha Gautama (the Buddha) left the protective fortress of his family home and spent several years on a voyage of discovery that started with several paths that he rejected as circular or dead ends. Over many years, he sketched a map of how his mind maintained distress and created suffering. He used this map to navigate his life.

A maxim in psychology is "There is nothing as practical as a good theory" (Lewin, 1951). Psychological theories are like maps: they help us understand the terrain of the mind and how to navigate it.[1] Psychological science has done much to create detailed maps of particular domains of the mind (e.g., attention, perception). Many specific mental health problems now have theories that explain what maintains and perpetuates them, including anxiety disorders, depression, addiction, obsessive–compulsive disorder, and psychosis. For example, careful psychological study has shown how selective processes like attention, catastrophizing, repetitive thought, and exclusion of disconfirming evidence are key features that maintain particular mental health problems in specific ways (Beck, 2005; Watkins, 2008). People with health anxiety are prone to being hypervigilant to bodily sensations and prone to interpret benign sensations as serious health conditions (Rode, Salkovskis, & Jack, 2001). Another example is people with a long history of depression who typically experience a normal emotion like sadness differently; when they experience sadness it can trigger a flurry of negative thoughts and memories that can escalate normal sadness into depression (Farb et al., 2010; Segal et al., 2006). These disorder-specific psychological maps (theories) help us describe and understand how these conditions come about and crucially how they are maintained. This has enabled psychologists to develop bespoke psychological treatments based on these models—by targeting these specific processes people are able to recover their mental health (Beck & Dozois, 2011; Beck & Haigh, 2014).

These maps can also be used to create *individually tailored conceptualizations* (Kuyken, Padesky, & Dudley, 2009)—that is, client and therapist together can create a map of how that person came to experience his or her particular difficulty, at this particular time, whether health anxiety, depression, or some other presentation. They can examine the beliefs and patterns of reactivity idiosyncratic to that person that maintain his or her difficulties. This is not an academic exercise; it is in the service of finding a path toward health and well-being.

Each level of map—universal, population specific, and individualized—is helpful in navigation.

Maps from Buddhist and Modern Psychology

The maps developed in Buddhist and modern psychology overlap a great deal. It is instructive to overlay them to see how some ancient insights are being corroborated and refined by modern science, and also where modern science can be corroborated and refined by Buddhist psychology. More than this, Buddhist psychology can help us identify terrain that psychological science has barely started to explore and can articulate hypotheses for psychological science to test.

We chose the analogy of a map to integrate scientific and contemplative perspectives because a map is neutral—there is no need to side with one view or the other. We use maps in pragmatic ways to describe the landscape and to help us get from A to B. In the same way, we're mapping the mind to help us live better lives. In this and the next chapters we begin to describe these maps. We start with descriptive maps of the mind from the perspective of psychological science (this chapter and Chapter 3) and then progress to maps from Buddhist psychology (Chapter 4). Chapter 5 weaves together the themes from Buddhist psychology and modern psychological science. Readers least familiar with psychological science might find this chapter and the next most instructive, while readers least familiar with Buddhist psychology might find Chapter 4 most instructive. For the integration of Buddhist and modern psychology, Chapter 5 is most instructive.

It would be hubris to claim that either psychological science or Buddhist psychology has a definitive map of the mind. It would be further hubris to pretend that we could represent these ancient and contemporary traditions in full here or that we have found a seamless synthesis. Instead, these maps are offered as sketches of the landscape of the mind. How far these ideas resonate when subject to the empiricism of either science or mindfulness practice is the real test of their validity and utility.

Coming to Our Senses

Many mindfulness-based programs introduce mindfulness by asking participants to bring full awareness to an everyday activity that we tend to do on automatic pilot. They are asked to relate to an object intentionally, with interest, equally open to whatever is present, whether it is pleasant, unpleasant, or neutral through all five senses in turn. This exercise typically uses a raisin, and each person is asked to bring his or her full awareness and all five senses to eating a single raisin. The mindfulness teacher asks people to relate to the raisin intentionally, slowing the process down, bringing attention to the raisin in turn through the attentional gateways of first seeing, then smelling, touching, listening, and only finally, tasting. This exercise is intended to begin to illuminate the processes of perception and attention, to literally help people "come to their senses" (Kabat-Zinn, 2005). Below are some typical responses from participants that came up in the teacher-led inquiry following the exercise (adapted from Kuyken & Evans, 2014):

TEACHER: What did you notice? What sensations?

LING: I noticed I had a clump of raisins, not just one . . . and I immediately found myself planning various baking projects . . . and then I was reminded of being at my grandmother's house as a child . . . I also noticed I was not really listening and I ended up eating the raisins long before you said to. (*Smiles apologetically.*)

TEACHER: Gosh, such a lot going on, good noticing of your thoughts. What did others notice?

MOHAMMED: The raisin looks like the moon, craters, ridges, but soft, shiny surfaces as well.

TEACHER: So, really seeing it and seeing similarities with the moon, but also some different features; lovely description, thank you. What about other people?

SOPHIA: My mind didn't wander, but I didn't like it. I noticed the texture, the stickiness, it was kind of yucky. It made me want to throw it away.

LING: (*in response to Sophia*) I had a kind of different experience. The smell was so strong, sweet, and warm. It flared up everything, all my senses.

TEACHER: . . . and how was that?

LING: The smell brought me out of my daydreaming and I had a slight sense of anxiety, but then it became a nice feeling—the smell was strong, sweet, and warm, it made my mouth start to water and look forward to eating it.

TEACHER: How interesting, Ling, thank you. And Sophia, your experience was of your mind not liking the texture and saying, "yucky" and wanting to throw it away, thank you.

SAM: I noticed when you asked us to put it in our mouths, that until I bit into the raisin, it was hard and tasteless. It was only when you said to bite into it that the taste was released, a real moment of taste buds firing off, like Ling said. I also had this strong urge to swallow it and have another one (*smiling*).

TEACHER: (*also smiling*) Interesting.

SAM: Yes.

TEACHER: There is a lot going on here for people in just a few minutes. Other experiences anyone?

SAM: . . . the main thing here for me was the slowing down. I wanted to swallow it quickly; if I were at home, I would grab a handful and eat them quickly. When I slowed down, I noticed so much more. It became a three-course meal (*laughing*).

TEACHER: A few other people are nodding here as well. Did anyone have a different or challenging experience?

SOPHIA: I arrived at the class today after a stressful morning. The car wouldn't start, I was late getting out of bed, and I am worried I haven't remembered the homework forms you asked us to do, which I completed late last night. (*Seems close to tears at this point.*) I have had to take time off work to come to these mindfulness classes and

I am worried about falling behind with my work and wasting this opportunity, about not doing it right. My mind was preoccupied with all of that, and I was barely able to follow your instructions.

TEACHER: Gosh, you have had a really full morning, Sophia, no wonder your mind was preoccupied. (*Pauses to take a breath, inviting the group to do the same while keeping steady attention on Sophia and the group.*) The mind is good at attending to things that need attending to. How was it for you when I kept inviting you to attend to different aspects of the raisin, to come back each time?

SOPHIA: It was like my mind was like Velcro—you kept asking me to unstick it from the worries, but each time it got stuck back again. (*Half smiles.*)

TEACHER: What a great way of describing it. Yes, worry is like Velcro, isn't it? I see other people nodding. What we'll do in the classes is develop another analogy. The mind is like Velcro, but it is also a bit like a puppy that can be trained—we have it on a long lead, and each time it does something uninvited we call it, rein it back in with the lead, gently but firmly, being affirming each time it comes back, and patient each time it bounds off, reining it back in and so on . . . until we have trained the puppy. It takes time and patience, but like investing in training a puppy, it pays off later. What we also see with this eating practice is that when we really attend to the raisin we see things we don't normally see, the sensations you described, of smelling it, really seeing it, the taste buds firing off—so much to explore. Also, when we slow things down it also shows us what the mind is up to—liking, not liking, making associations, getting stuck like Velcro. As we learn to steady the mind, we'll learn more. Thank you.

Mindfulness-based programs start with this exercise because it introduces so much of what is learned in the program through an everyday activity, such as eating, that we can all relate to. It illustrates, experientially, the way the mind shapes our reality, often without us even being aware of how it is doing this. It introduces the idea that by stepping out of automatic pilot and bringing awareness to each moment, we can illuminate and, in time, transform the mind. We return to the raisin exercise throughout the chapter because it illustrates some of the key psychological science that is vital to understanding mindfulness and mindfulness practices.

In the rest of this chapter, we cover aspects of psychology that help illuminate mindfulness. We overview:

- Automatic pilot;
- Perceptual processes;
- Attention as the gateway for experience (including sections on alerting attention, orienting attention, executive attention, and attention while multitasking and task switching);
- Distinguishing sensations, emotions, cognitions, and behavioral impulses;
- The dynamic, ever-changing nature of the mind; and
- The discrepancy monitor that drives the judging mind.[2]

Automatic Pilot

Airline pilots can engage automatic pilot to maintain a plane's particular altitude, bearing, and speed. Our minds can also engage in a form of automatic pilot. Let's revisit the raisin-eating exercise above. People have been eating all their lives and most have eaten raisins many times. It is no longer novel. We know what to expect and how to do it, so it is natural to eat raisins on automatic pilot. But what this exercise demonstrates is that when we step out of automatic pilot, we come to our senses, both literally and metaphorically. Of course, without this ability to automate much of what we do regularly, everything we do would need to be relearned each time we do it. For example, the first time a child walks without help, rides a bike, or ties his or her shoelaces, it is a deliberate trial-and-error learning process. Over time, however, it becomes automatic and natural—it can be done *without thinking about it.* Automatic pilot enables the mind to carry out everyday, routine tasks, without our deliberate, intentional attention, using established learned ways of thinking and acting. The mind's ability to do much of its work automatically is an extraordinary strength, enabling a huge array of everyday tasks to be learned and then carried out unconsciously so that we can focus on other things, especially new situations and challenging situations.

Eating, walking, riding a bike, and tying our shoelaces are just a few of the many actions that we can do on automatic pilot. Others include recognizing faces, detecting other people's emotional states, gauging the emotional climate of a social encounter, and understanding spoken or written language. For example, automatic pilot is quick, involuntary, and outside our control in understanding words or simple sentences.

When can automatic pilot become problematic? In the second week of the mindfulness program, Sam reported back on his homework, which included eating one meal a day mindfully. He described how he had eaten a particular meal each day for lunch for years, a ramen noodle pot, with a flavor packet to which he added hot water. He described how bringing full awareness to adding boiling water to the plastic container and eating the meal made him realize how "chemically" it smelled and tasted. To his surprise, he realized he did not like the smell, taste, or texture. He had been eating something for lunch every day for years on automatic pilot that he did not actually enjoy! He changed his lunch choices as a result. Just as importantly with mindfulness, a *negative experience* can evolve into something else. It is not unusual for someone to say something like "When we started the mindful eating exercise, I thought 'oh no, I don't like raisins.' But when I smelled it, it smelled different to how I expected, sweeter actually, and I have a sweet tooth. When I moved it around my mouth, it was pretty neutral and a bit tasteless, and I thought, 'ah yes, this is why I don't like raisins.' But then when I bit into it, the sweetness sort of exploded in my mouth in a way that pleasantly surprised me. A single raisin is really sweet and full of taste! I'm not saying I now like raisins, but there is more to the experience than I realized." By exploding an experience into its five senses a richness is revealed that had been obscured by automaticity.

Sometimes things that we have done on automatic pilot—that may have been functional before—no longer serve a purpose. A trivial example is leaving for work on the usual route, but forgetting that this morning we needed to do another errand first. We have to overrule automatic pilot and find a route to our errand and then on to work. A less trivial example is how automatic ways of thinking perpetuate common mental health problems. Psychologists have identified the scripts that run automatically and feed and maintain anxiety (typically, hypersensitivity to threat) and depression (typically, negative beliefs about the self, others, and the world; Beck, 1976). This negative thinking happens on automatic pilot and maintains mental ill health, like a program running biased, prejudiced, negative propaganda. This form of automaticity may have been useful at one point, but is now a dysfunctional habit. Ling is an example of this:

Ling's childhood years were challenging and she had to find ways to survive. As a young child, she remembered her father regularly beating her mother, sexually abusing her cousin, and then, when Ling was around the age of 8, he started to sexually abuse her. Ling was eventually taken out of the home when she was 12 and lived much of her teenage years in residential care. There, living with other teenagers, most of them also from abusive families, she learned to survive by developing excellent antennae for rejection and social exclusion. To be the outcast in the residential home was a disaster—there was nowhere to escape. Ling learned how to avoid rejection at all costs by being able to detect the smallest signs of rejection, and having an array of chameleon-like disguises to hide any vulnerability that might solicit bullying or rejection. Underneath, the beliefs she developed—about being unlovable, when she felt her mother rejected her and her father abused her—became more and more embedded and diffuse, permeating the way she saw herself, others, and the world. All of this was an understandable survival strategy for the situation Ling found herself in as a child and adolescent. When she became an adult with good friends and two children whom she loved, however, it was no longer functional. In fact, this sensitivity and belief system was highly dysfunctional in meeting the challenges of parenting two teenagers. In her job as a court magistrate, her beliefs about vulnerability were forever being triggered by family cases of abuse, and she'd come home in the evening disturbed by what she'd heard all day. Crucially, until she started a mindfulness training program, Ling was largely unaware of how pervasive this negative thinking was, or how damaging to her life. It tended to occur as a preprogrammed script, almost beyond awareness, like the color of the wall paint in her living room that she had stopped noticing years ago.

Automatic pilot also means we sometimes miss the richness of life and wonderful experiences, like eating, being with loved ones, making love, laughing, and enjoying art, music, or nature. Because everything runs routinely, we may neglect to see the nuances, the fullness of our experience and life. We can find ourselves with someone we care about, but daydreaming, not fully present, perhaps not even hearing what the person is saying. One of us (WK) experienced this one evening after a busy day at work: I was reading a bedtime story to one of my daughters—she was probably 4 or 5 at the time. At the end of the story, she wanted to talk about the story before I said goodnight and turned out the light. I realized with horror that I had read the whole story on automatic pilot, not taking it in, while my mind was ruminating about work.

Mindfulness exercises, like eating the raisin, provide the opportunity to see automatic pilot and to step back and fully experience our thoughts, feelings, sensations, and actions. Mindfulness can also reveal when automatic pilot is helpful or unhelpful. Crucially, when we become aware of how much time we spend on automatic pilot another possibility reveals itself: to be more awake to our lives and ourselves. Automatic pilot relies on a supporting cast of perception, attention, and evaluation, as well as an extensive learning history and bank of memories, topics to which we turn next.

> *The key insight from psychological science is that we can navigate the complexities of life by switching on automatic pilot to do things that are familiar. However, it can sometimes take us down old pathways that are less helpful and can mean that we are not fully awake to the richness of our lives.*

Perceptual Processes

The mindful eating exercise above illustrates, first, that we are often not actually aware of what our senses are picking up. We may even, in our minds, be transported to a different place altogether. The raisin, for example, triggered a memory for Ling of her grandmother's house. People report that they normally eat raisins by the handful, without really tasting them at all. Second, the mindful eating exercise teaches us that when we do *tune in*, the senses are illuminated. We notice smell as "strong, sweet, and warm," seeing "soft, shiny surfaces" and "taste buds firing off." Third, when perception is slowed down, we see the detail and intricacies of what is being attended to in the present moment.

Our perception can also sometimes play tricks on us. The mindful seeing exercise in Box 2.1 illuminates our perceptual processes. Take a moment to try this exercise.

For most people, this exercise shows that when we intentionally attend to seeing, we become aware of some of what is involved in perception. The automaticity of perception is key to being able to quickly understand and navigate the world. But we can also miss the richness of perception. By slowing it down, we can open to color, shape, and brightness, and really pay attention to these facets of seeing. We can learn to come closer to the point at which we make contact with a sense so that we can observe firsthand how experience unfolds in ways we are not normally aware of. For example, when we fixate our sight on a focal point, seeing tends to include peripheral objects and tries to draw

---

BOX 2.1. Mindfulness Practice: Seeing Exercise

If there is a window, find an object through the window you can attend to. If not, find an object near to where you are to which you can attend. It doesn't really matter what the object is, anything will do, but choose a point in the object and steady your attention on that object. As best you can, see the object in terms of colors, shape, shade, patterns, and movement. Bring curiosity and a beginner's mind to the object—a bit like a baby in its crib who has never seen this object before. What exactly is the color as you see it? Is the color steady or does it change and morph? What is the shape of the object? If you find your mind wandering, gently but firmly bring it back. Crucially, your mind will almost certainly *rush ahead* and try to summarize the experience—this is *x* or *y*, or I know what this is. Gently and firmly note this and bring yourself back, as best you can, to just seeing. Perhaps end the exercise with expanding the seeing to include the space around the object. As you expand your seeing, bring awareness to what is in the frame: objects, colors, textures, and edges.

them into *seeing*, a phenomenon that has been called "covert attention" (Posner, 1980; Posner, Snyder, & Davidson, 1980). This illustrates how the brain operates like a digital image enhancement system, illuminating the focal area, adding information, *touching up* the image. . . . Seeing is not, as was once thought, a mechanical translation of light picked up in the eye to an image represented in the mind. Perception is a much more creative and constructive process. One of the most influential perception theorists and researchers called his seminal book *The Intelligent Eye* (Gregory, 1970), to communicate this idea of seeing as a constructive process.

The earliest philosophers identified the now well-known five senses of seeing, hearing, tasting, smelling, and touching. Psychological science has added others to the list, including senses for temperature, time, hunger/thirst, and balance. Other useful further distinctions include how we perceive the outside world (e.g., seeing), how we perceive our internal world (e.g., bodily sensations, pain, hunger), and how we sense our place in space, including perception of movement. We can learn to see these different perceptual processes by bringing awareness to them. Mindfulness practices can help us explore all of these senses and even be playful with the different aspects of perception. We can learn to slow down and really see how we perceive the world from the first point of contact through the sense organs, through to how the experience comes to be represented in our mind. For example, consider the text on this page. It starts as light and lines, but is turned into language and becomes comprehension. The seeing exercise above illustrates how sensations of light, color, and pattern are in a continual dance with the brain in the service of seeing and making sense of the world.

All of the senses work in broadly similar ways—namely, a receptor picks up the raw data and transforms it into something the brain can work with. The brain then makes sense and meaning out of the information, integrating it into a whole, and that whole becomes our experience. To know and understand that perception is a constructive process is a key feature in any map of the mind. Understanding perception is important in mindfulness and mindfulness-based programs because all of our experience starts from perception.

It is worth pausing to consider the term *making sense*. We create meaning from our sense impressions. To *see* any object, our minds have to translate information, filling in gaps, drawing on prior knowledge—it is a process of construction that creates what we consider to be our reality. William James (1890), one of the first *modern* psychologists, put it this way: "The mind works on data it receives as a sculptor on a block of stone." This is illustrated with the expression "I see," which is often used to mean "I understand."

Without mindfulness, it is almost impossible to step back from and slow down the processes of attention and perception enough to illuminate our experience. The mind has learned to see, categorize, and label our experience quickly so that we can act on it efficiently. For example, on a sidewalk in a big city, perception necessarily breaks down the many things we are attending to and perceiving (e.g., a road with moving cars we need to avoid), a pleasant smell perhaps we want to pursue (e.g., a nice café), and background noise we can safely ignore (e.g., an airplane flying high overhead) so that we can make sense of it all. What the seeing exercise above does is intentionally stabilize attention and slow perception down so we can see something of the processes of perception. The eye, nervous system, and brain take patterns of color, light, and shape, and transform them into seeing. The example of the busy cityscape shows how much is going on in the background, without us being aware of it. What is learned in mindfulness programs is that we can always choose to slow down and bring awareness to how we experience the world through our senses, not just in mindful eating or with a seeing exercise but also in a busy everyday city environment.

This *stabilizing* and *slowing down* enables us to more fully appreciate the richness of life—it is no coincidence that poetry and art often choose to depict the realm of the senses. It can be awe inspiring when we see how extraordinarily well engineered our minds are to do this work and what can be revealed when we look at our experience with curiosity and care. Mindfulness brings renewed interest and awe to each of our different senses, illuminating the process of perception so that we can see more clearly when it serves us well, and also when it doesn't.

The key insight from psychological science is that while perception starts in our sense organs, it is largely a constructive and creative process. Mindfulness enables us to really see this process, which helps us "come to our senses."

Attention as the Gateway for Experience

Attention is our capacity to choose what we focus on; it is our ability to discern signal from noise. James (1890) defined attention as "taking possession of the mind, in clear and vivid form, of one out of what seem several simultaneously possible objects or trains of thoughts." Attention is a natural human capacity made up of several key qualities and dimensions.

In the previous chapter, we introduced the metaphor of mindfulness as a protective gatekeeper who greeted all visitors and then exercised discernment about who to allow in and who to exclude. Any effective gatekeeper or security guard needs to be skillfully attentive. Sensations, thoughts, and images are met at the gateway of attention so that a decision can be made about whether to allow or deny entry into awareness.

In all mindfulness practices, participants are asked, as best they can, to maintain their attention on their moment-by-moment experience. In the mindful eating exercise, for example, participants are invited to take possession of their sensory experience (e.g., touching, seeing, smelling, and tasting). However, sometimes sensory experiences trigger memories (Ling: "I was reminded of being at my grandmother's house as a child") or thoughts and associations (Mohammed: "The raisin looks like the moon, craters, ridges, but soft, shiny surfaces as well"). Attentional training is intended to help people learn first to see this happening and then to choose what to attend to and what to let go of. James (1890) included this last point in his definition when he elaborated that attention "implies withdrawal from some things in order to deal effectively with others."

There is now a large body of theoretical and experimental literature on attention, and typically psychologists single out three dimensions of attention (Baddeley, 1996, 2012; Mirsky & Duncan, 2001; Posner, 1980): alerting, orienting, and executive attention.

Alerting Attention

The mind is continually scanning a huge amount of information and one of the main functions of attention is to alert us to anything that needs consideration. Our *modus operandum* is to scan everything just long enough to establish whether it is familiar or novel, and to evaluate whether it is safe or poses a threat (Phelps & LeDoux, 2005). We are primed to become alert and take speedy action to deal with certain types of information (e.g., something new or threatening).

Alerting attention is a bit like a security guard continually scanning the environment. It is akin to arousal or vigilance. If something is detected, a "cognitive/neural alarm" is sounded. The mind has a predilection to turn to issues and problems that are novel, require attention, or that we somehow judge as requiring our attention. Examples of this automatic aspect of alerting attention are physical pain (e.g., when we touch something sharp or hot), immediate external threats (e.g., we are cycling and a car pulls out of a side street in front of us), or social cues that demand attention (e.g., our boss or partner gives us a disapproving look). Alerting attention tends to be automatic and fast, largely beyond our voluntary control. It is hard-wired in primitive parts of the brain and associated with neuroendocrine functions associated with alertness and arousal (Phelps, Delgado, Nearing, & LeDoux, 2004; Phelps & LeDoux, 2005). It involves cognitive processes that involve "deep" brain structures (Rogan, Staubli, & LeDoux, 1997)—brain structures we have in common with many other species. This makes evolutionary sense—threat can be detected quickly and responded to in ways that enhance our chances of survival. Detecting and responding well to these threats means that we survive and our genes are replicated into the next generation.

Orienting Attention

Orienting attention is the turning of attention to something to enable us to examine it further. This can be what happens immediately after alerting attention. What is this threatening or novel situation? Attention turns toward it automatically to investigate and try to make sense of the situation. Here, orienting attention runs off fast with established ways of exploring things. Is it moving toward or away from me? Is it hot or cold? Is it intensifying or lessening? Once we have oriented attention, this can be followed by the question "What now? Do I sustain attention and extract sensory details or move on?" This question suggests an analytical approach, but it is often a fast and efficient analysis.

In this way, orienting attention can be intentional. In the raisin exercise, people are asked to intentionally orient their attention to each of their senses in turn, including sight ("The raisin looks like the moon, craters, ridges, but soft, shiny surfaces as well"), smell ("The smell was so strong, sweet, and warm"), touch ("I noticed the texture, the stickiness, it was kind of yucky"), and taste ("It was only when you said to bite into it that the taste was released, a real moment of taste buds firing off"). The eating exercise is a practice in stepping out of habit and automaticity and staying with particular senses and extracting more sensory detail. When orienting attention is within our intentional voluntary control, it relies on our executive attention.

Executive Attention

Executive attention involves us using certain functions to manage the demands on our attention. To best plan and reason, we must choose what to bring to the forefront of our awareness (from the many stimuli that our minds process at any one time), as well as decide how long to stay with a task, and how to manage information on the "workbench" of working memory. In this metaphor, attention is like a workbench where we choose what to place on the workbench and then which tools we use to work on it. So we can, for example, choose to bring the sensations in the nostrils into awareness and watch them change moment by moment as we breathe in and out, and as other thoughts, images, and sensations come to mind we choose to note them, and come back to the sensations in the nostrils. Adele Diamond (2013), a contemporary cognitive scientist, summarized executive functions this way: they "make possible mentally playing with ideas; taking the time to think before acting; meeting novel, unanticipated challenges; resisting temptations; and staying focused." (p. 135)

A key feature of executive attention is that we have a certain capacity to process only so much information at any one time. While the allocation of attention is often automatic, it is to a degree under voluntary control, depending on our disposition, intentions in a given moment, the demands of a situation, and the context of the moment. If, for example, we read this in a quiet setting with no distractions, then there is less demand on our executive attention. Conversely, if there is background music, people talking, and mobile devices sending alerts, then there are more demands on our attention—the limited bandwidth is being used up and may even be exceeded, which can make it difficult for us to maintain our attention on reading.

With the mindful eating exercise, the teacher asked people to bring their direct experiences of the raisin to the center of their attention. This is not always easy and in Sophia's case, her attention was divided as her mind pulled toward what it judged to be more pressing issues. She moved in and out of being able to bring her attention to the eating exercise. As we will see a bit later, the mind is adept at dividing its attention in particular ways, and at any one time many overlearned and automatic tasks go on in the background while something is attended to in the foreground. For example, although you are reading this text, just off the edge of the radar of awareness your mind is busy doing a whole range of other things, such as holding your posture, regulating your temperature, and continually monitoring your body and the external environment.

There is considerable debate about how selective attention involves both automatic, rapid processes, and more controlled, considered processes. As we make sense of our world, there is almost always both bottom-up, sensorial input and some degree of top-down *meaning making*. For example, Ling described how when she was asked to place the raisin near her nostrils and attend to the smell, it "brought me out of my daydreaming and I had a slight sense of anxiety, but then it became a nice feeling—the smell was strong, sweet, and warm, it made my mouth start to water and look forward to eating it." In these few moments, we see automatic processes that can go on in the background (e.g., daydreaming). Then when Ling intentionally orients her attention to her sense of smell, a series of sensorial impressions and bodily reactions unfold in a mixture of controlled and automatic ways. In 1890, James wrote, "My experience is what I agree to attend to. Only those items which I notice shape my mind—without selective interest, experience is utter chaos." What we now also know is that in every moment, there is much we don't notice that is being automatically processed and that is also shaping our minds. Executive attention is the set of cognitive functions we use to make order out of chaos.

Executive attention takes up cognitive resources, which as we've already noted, are limited. It requires working memory to hold and process information. Working memory is a workspace within our mental architecture where we place and work with information (Teasdale & Chaskalson, 2011a). This limited capacity of working memory deserves more discussion as it is pivotal in our day-to-day life and is something that mindfulness training can help us with. For example, when we are anxious or tired, our working memory resources are depleted, which affects our ability to pay attention. In the example above, Sophia really struggled to bring her attention to the eating exercise as she had had a poor night's sleep and her mind was preoccupied with worry about all that happened that morning. The tiredness and preoccupation depleted the cognitive resources available to her. Similarly, our working memory capacity can be overwhelmed by too many competing demands. Many things we do are adversely affected when working memory is compromised or overwhelmed, such as driving, reading, following a conversation, and decision making.

Attention While Multitasking and Task Switching

We live in a world with many competing demands on our attention and there is a belief that being able to multitask is a valued skill to which we should aspire. Young people are often in an actual or virtual social group, subjected to information coming in from several social media streams in parallel, often while listening to music as well. When asked to do one thing at a time they might say, "Why, when I can multitask?" At work we can have a primary task (say, writing a report), but have our attention pulled away by e-mail, social media, and text messages. Consider the exercise in Box 2.2.

What the exercise in Box 2.2 illustrates is that while much information can be processed in parallel and automatically, it is something of a myth that we can easily multitask, especially with tasks that require attentional control and make demands on working memory (Gopher, Armony, & Greenshpan, 2000). These are two different cognitive demands, and we don't actually do them in parallel—we need to switch between them to be able to do them at the same time—and this can take extra time and cognitive resources. Doing more than one task at a time, especially if it is complex or new, takes attention and energy because multitasking actually normally means *task switching* to be able to perform the tasks in parallel (Yeung & Monsell, 2003). The mind and brain struggle to manage some of the complex multitasking we demand of them in our frantic and busy world. Instead, what we are normally doing

---

BOX 2.2. Exercise: Task Switching or Multitasking?: An Illustration

Take the phrase "Attention is the gateway to experience." In your mind, count the number of letters in this phrase. How many seconds does this take you?

There are 33 letters and it normally takes people 20 seconds or so to count them.

Now spell the phrase out in your mind, letter by letter ("*a, t, t, . . .*"). How long does this take you? This usually takes people a few seconds less, but still a fair bit of time.

Now spell it out in your mind and count at the same time. This usually takes people quite a bit longer, certainly not the same amount of time. If the popular myths about multitasking are true, we should be able to do both in the same or less time, but this fundamentally misunderstands attention and working memory.

Spelling, counting, and reading require executive attention, and doing them at the same time pushes our cognitive capacity to its limits. Reading, naming letters, and counting place demands on many of the same but also some different parts of the cognitive system. We cannot easily do all of this in parallel—instead, the cognitive system has to switch between reading, naming letters, and counting, which is why it takes longer.

We can do tasks in parallel only if they are overlearned or automatic, and use different parts of the cognitive system. Tasks that require the same systems or are less well learned need to be done more intentionally and serially, that is to say, in turn.

---

when we *multitask* is rapid *task switching*, which enables us to at least try to do various things in parallel. And we don't or can't always do this.

A now classic experiment asked people to watch a short film showing two teams passing basketballs, one wearing white shirts, the other wearing black shirts. Viewers were instructed to count the number of passes made by the team in white shirts and ignore the number of passes made by the team in black shirts. This requires perception of the whole visual field but a lot of orienting attention, inhibition of irrelevant information, and executive control, which takes up a lot of working memory. Halfway through the film, a woman in a gorilla suit appears in the video, thumps her chest and walks off again. The gorilla is in the shot for 9 seconds. About half of the people watching this video do not see the gorilla, and cannot afterward believe it was there. This experiment demonstrates vividly how attention is the gateway to experience: in this example, something as striking as a person in a gorilla suit in the midst of a basketball game does not get through the attentional gate to awareness, even though the eye will have registered it. In the experiment, people are following the instruction to orient their attention to the number of passes made by the team in white shirts (Chabris & Simons, 2010). The mind *decides* not to orient and elaborate attention to the gorilla because it is prioritizing the counting task.

In our daily lives, we have to contend with many pulls on our attention, including managing all the demands at home and work, family demands, e-mails, social media streams, texts, and so forth. We have to pick and choose where to place our attention. The mind has to *switch between tasks*, and even when we decide to switch it involves the activation of a new set of rules and procedures. This takes up cognitive resources (Ophir, Nass, & Wagner, 2009).

Mindfulness practices and programs are intended to illuminate these processes of attention. As James (1890) learned through his introspective empiricism, we too learn "the faculty of voluntarily bringing back our wandering attention, over and over again, is the very root of judgment, character, and will. No one is compos sui if he have it not."

It turns out that James's (1890) observation at the turn of the 20th century was prescient. An important body of research work has explored how attention is a key part of self-regulation and self-control (Diamond, 2013; Gopher et al., 2000; Hofmann, Schmeichel, & Baddeley, 2012). There is now an intriguing body of research suggesting that self-regulation predicts the trajectories of people's lives. One striking example is an influential study carried out in Dunedin, New Zealand, that recruited 1,000 people at birth and is following them throughout life. They are currently in their 40s (Moffitt et al., 2011). The research team measured self-control and a range of outcomes. Measurements were taken at birth and then at regular intervals (ages 3, 5, 7, 9, 11, 13, 15, and 18 years and into adulthood). Self-control was assessed by observations of the children and by ratings of parents and teachers and, when they were older, by the children's self-report. Self-control measured in childhood and adolescence was associated with wealth, health, substance misuse, and criminality in adulthood—that is, people who had greater self-control as children went on to do better in many aspects of their lives.

Furthermore, researchers were able to show that self-control was not always stable and could change over time. Certain *snares* can change the trajectory of young people's lives, such as substance misuse and teenage pregnancy (Fergusson & Lynskey, 1996; Lippold, Powers, Syvertsen, Feinberg, & Greenberg, 2013; Moffitt et al., 2011; Reinherz et al., 1993). Interestingly, when self-control was seen to change in childhood and adolescence, adult outcomes changed correspondingly. For example, when children who had poor self-control learned self-control in adolescence, they had better outcomes in adulthood. The findings of the Dunedin study make sense. Being able to manage our attention shapes what we say and do, which in turn shapes our lives and the lives of those around us.

Sarah-Jayne Blakemore, professor of cognitive neuroscience, studies the adolescent brain. Her research program has challenged and reformulated received wisdom that the brain is largely fully formed by late childhood. Research is beginning to show that during adolescence, neural circuitry is developing that enables adolescents to learn how to make good decisions in a range of situations and contexts (Blakemore & Robbins, 2012). Blakemore (2018) provides a review of this fascinating body of work in her book *Inventing Ourselves: The Secret Life of the Teenage Brain*.

The Dunedin findings taken together with Blakemore's work raises the intriguing possibility that training attention in childhood and adolescence could change the trajectories of people's lives, a question we are addressing in our current ongoing research (Kuyken et al., 2017).

To summarize what we have said so far about attention:

- Attention is the doorway for experience;
- There are different types of attention—alerting, orienting, and executive attention; and
- Attentional control is a key feature of self-control that is learned throughout life.

Conditions like depression and chronic pain hijack attention, drawing attention in with a proliferation of understandably negative thinking (e.g., "This is unbearable, how will I cope?"). Seeing this process, stepping back from it, and allowing other experiences into the landscape of our experience is how we re-create our worlds. Mindfulness training can enhance attentional control in brief 8-week programs, but even more reliable effects are seen in longer, more sustained mindfulness trainings (Jha, Krompinger, & Baime, 2007; Lutz et al., 2009; MacLean et al., 2010; Morrison, Goolsarran, Rogers, & Jha, 2014; Mrazek, Franklin, Phillips, Baird, & Schooler, 2013).

The key insight from psychological science is that attention is the gateway to experience. To a significant degree, attention is something we can both control and train.

Distinguishing Sensations, Emotions, Cognitions, and Behavioral Impulses

Many of us go through our days without being aware of the richness of our experience, without pausing to ask, "What is my experience just now?" The simplest psychological model helps us take any experience in a given moment and differentiate it with several essential elements:

1. Bodily sensations
2. Emotions
3. Thoughts, images, remembering, planning, reverie, and appraisal
4. Behavioral impulses and behaviors

The context or given situation is the fifth element—namely, the preconditions for each particular moment. This five-part model is widely used in cognitive therapy (see Table 2.1). People find it very helpful because it is a key part of understanding our mind's reactivity (Kuyken et al., 2009; Padesky & Mooney, 1990).

The five-part model enables us to separate experience into component elements in any context or situation. For example, we can parse Ling's experience with the raisin exercise into bodily sensations, thoughts, emotions, and behavior (see Figure 2.1). We can see that she had some mind wandering

TABLE 2.1. Different Elements of Experience

Element	Description
Bodily sensations	Bodily sensations are experienced initially as sense impressions in their own right, but the mind very quickly moves to label and classify thoughts and feelings about the sensations. So, a direct experience of *tightness* in the shoulders may become *back pain* or *stress tension*.
Emotion	Classically, several emotions are seen as (1) basic (e.g., happiness, anger, surprise, sadness, disgust, fear), (2) more nuanced states that are combinations of emotions (e.g., pride), or (3) emotions that include appraisal and elaboration (e.g., gratitude, disappointment).
Thoughts, images, and appraisals	This is the cognitive domain and refers to thinking. It includes thoughts, images, appraisals, memories, planning, imagination, mind wandering, daydreaming, reverie, and so on.
Behavioral impulses and behaviors	Behavioral impulses can be differentiated into basic states (e.g., arousal and excitation) and into more elaborated impulses or actual behaviors (e.g., to seek out a sense of mastery, a movement toward compassion or reconciliation). At the very basic level, the level of arousal and energy can determine whether we are inclined to action or not. Basic emotions like fear and anger are often very directly associated with action tendencies, such as the impulse to fight, freeze, or flee.

Note. The fifth element is the context of the moment in which an experience unfolds. Each moment comprises an ever-shifting dynamic of bodily sensations, emotions, thoughts, and behaviors.

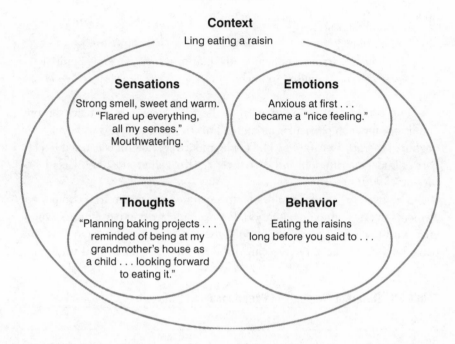

FIGURE 2.1. Ling's experience of the raisin.

as the raisins triggered plans (baking projects), memories (her grandmother's house), and anticipations (of eating the raisin). This was associated with emotions (a "nice" feeling) and bodily sensations linked to senses of smell and taste ("sweet and warm"), which elicited a bodily salivary response. This initiated the action of eating the raisin.

In any given situation, there are myriad bodily sensations potentially available to awareness. Thoughts or images can arise, often automatically and without us being fully aware of them. They are often closely linked with emotions and bodily sensations. There may be connected action impulses or behaviors. All of this arises within a context of the situation we are in and of our preexisting state of mind. As we bring greater attention to our experience, we can begin to focus on these different elements and see how experience is created and elaborated. For example, imagery often shapes emotion directly (Holmes & Mathews, 2010), whereas language can be equally powerful but often more subtle or indirect in its effects on emotion.

"Bring someone to mind who has helped or looked out for you, a teacher or a mentor, someone with whom you had a positive relationship. Really imagine the person, perhaps remembering a specific time he or she was kind and helpful to you. Sharpen the image so you can see the picture of him or her in your mind and what was happening at this moment of that person looking out for you. What feelings arise as you do this?"

Imagery can be evocative—when we bring a benefactor to mind like this the associated feelings often arise automatically.

It can be novel and interesting when we first begin to recognize and then separate our bodily sensations, emotions, thoughts, and behaviors. It is the first step of mapping the mind, illuminating our experience with greater clarity. This simple five-part model is offered as a way for us to break down our experience so we can begin to relate differently to it. It can turn experiences that are a fused, blended, and even a *soupy mess* into something more nuanced, differentiated, and clearer. It has universality, because all of our experience is part of the human condition, and specificity, because we all have somewhat idiosyncratic ways of experiencing.

As we learn to differentiate between the different elements of experience, we start to see the connections between body states, emotions, thoughts, and behavior (see Figure 2.2).[3] We can see how our thoughts shape our emotions and bodily sensations; we can see how our bodily states, particularly fatigue, shape our thinking and emotions; we can see how behavioral impulses are associated with emotion and body states; we can see how emotion shapes our thoughts and behavior. The double-headed arrows in Figure 2.2 communicate these relationships. This is both normalizing ("I'd always treated my thoughts as facts; I didn't realize I was more prone to think negatively when I was tired") and empowering ("I've learned I have choices. If I am tired, I need to take care of myself and cut myself some slack").

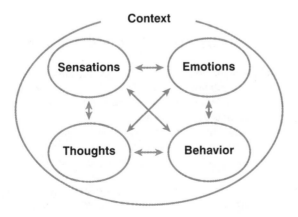

FIGURE 2.2. Differentiating our experience: The five-part model.

The key insight from psychological science is that in any given moment our experience can be separated into discrete elements (i.e., bodily sensations, emotions, thoughts, and behavior). We learn how these arise and influence one another; crucially, we can choose how we relate to our sensations, thoughts, emotions, and impulses.

The Dynamic, Ever-Changing Nature of the Mind

Mindfulness practices reveal how dynamic the mind is. When we practice, we can see more clearly the unfolding of moment-to-moment experience. Nothing is permanent or static. Even as our minds create feelings, bodily sensations, and behavioral impulses, they continuously change. In Ling's case, while she was attending to the raisin she noticed she was in a reverie (planning and remembering), and as she brought her attention to the smell of the raisin, she first experienced a pang of anxiety that morphed into "a nice feeling" as she intentionally brought her senses of smell and taste into the foreground. She became aware of her mouth watering and a behavioral impulse to eat the raisin (see Figure 2.1). However, it is likely that if she had stopped to inquire into the "pang of anxiety," it, too, would comprise thoughts and images, emotions, bodily sensations, and behavioral elements. As Ling followed the teacher's invitation to attend to smelling the raisin, this created a new set of thoughts, feelings, sensations, and behavioral impulses. Mind states and the elements that comprise them are in a continual state of change and flux. Each moment is a context that shapes the next. Bringing attention and awareness to our experience reveals this dynamic flux.

BOX 2.3. Exercise: Walking Down the Street

Take a moment to imagine yourself walking down the street. Consider what is going on in your body and how you feel. Take a moment to connect with your breath. Track the full duration of this in-breath and this out-breath. Maybe do this for a few breaths, until you feel steady.

Now imagine yourself walking along the street and visualize someone coming toward you on the other side of the street. It is someone you know. Imagine yourself waving to the person, smiling. He or she walks past without acknowledging you.

Stop to consider: What bodily sensations are around, maybe in your face, chest, shoulders? What do you feel? What thoughts or imagery are around you? What do you feel like doing?

The example in Box 2.3 is used in both cognitive-behavioral therapy and mindfulness-based programs to illustrate this point. It is likely that this exercise triggered a set of bodily sensations, emotions, thoughts, and action tendencies. For people who have experienced depression, these are most typically feelings of sadness, perhaps embarrassment or fear; bodily sensations, perhaps a sinking feeling, contraction in the belly and chest, heat in the face; and behaviorally, an urge to withdraw and hide. Ling had experienced much adversity in her life and during one phase while she was living in residential care, the other children would exclude and bully her. In this exercise, her thoughts and appraisals arose out of her earlier learning, along the lines of "The person is ignoring me because they don't like me," or "I have done something to upset them and they are going to exclude me." This is illustrated in Figure 2.3, where the five-part model is used to differentiate the experience of this moment for Ling.

Other people can have more neutral emotional and bodily reactions to this same imagined scenario. Here the appraisal is more typically "They are busy and preoccupied and didn't see me." The content of people's appraisals in this exercise is not the point; what the exercise illustrates is the dynamic,

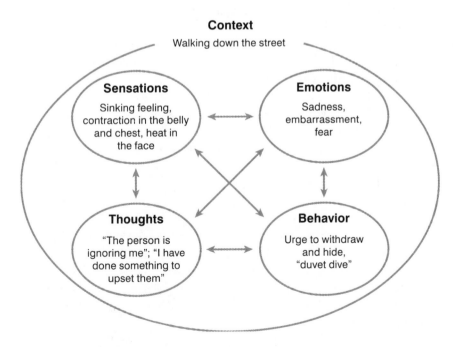

FIGURE 2.3. Ling's experience of the "walking down the street exercise" differentiated into the five-part model.

changing nature of the mind, and how we appraise situations shapes our experience in that moment.

> *The key insight from psychological science is that our experience is dynamic, continually unfolding and changing, driven in part by our appraisals and judgments, and colored by our situation, learning history, and current state of mind.*

The Discrepancy Monitor That Drives the Judging Mind

There is a strong evaluative component at every level of the mind. This evaluation is at two levels. The first is the simple evaluation of whether an experience is pleasant, unpleasant, or neutral. This is sometimes referred to as primary appraisal (Lazarus, 1993). In Buddhist psychology, it is *vedenā* or feeling tone (Bhikkhu Analāyo, 2003). The second, more elaborated appraisal is how this experience compares with how it should be, how we'd like it to be, how it was in the past, and so on. This is sometimes referred to as *discrepancy thinking*, the tendency to monitor how we think things are and compare them to how we think things should be (Higgins, 1987; Masicampo & Baumeister, 2007; Williams, 2008).

Mindfulness practices reveal this all-prevailing judging mind and how it automatically and quickly inclines toward certain types of experiences and turns away from others. With the raisin exercise, the invitation is to relate to the raisin with a *beginner's mind* as if the object has never been seen, smelled, or tasted before. This is difficult because automatically the mind fills a void with labels ("Ah, this is a raisin") and then just as quickly forms a judgment of whether the raisin is "nice" (Ling) or "yucky" (Sophia). This judging mind, of how things are compared with how we would like them to be, is a continuous background process in our experience.

When Siddhartha Gautama (the Buddha) came out of his closeted life and saw firsthand and up close sickness, old age, and death, he experienced distress because it exposed the discrepancy between how he had thought life was (safe and predictable in the closeted world of his father's overprotection) and the realities of suffering and dying. Our minds do this all the time at all levels of experience, from the larger existential questions of illness, old age, and death that Siddhartha faced to more mundane questions, such as "Is the raisin 'nice' or 'yucky'?"

Our judging is largely automatic and associative (Bargh, Chen, & Burrows, 1996), taking place at preconscious levels without our full awareness. As we have already seen, alerting and orienting attention have biases built in

(Friedman & Forster, 2010). Our minds continuously monitor all incoming information from a range of sources (sensory inputs, such as hearing and seeing, and body states), asking questions such as "Is this as expected? Is this safe? Is this threatening? Do I need to attend to this experience?" This appraisal often requires no intentional conscious effort on our parts and is based on myriad associations we have learned during our lives (De Houwer, Thomas, & Baeyens, 2001; McLaren & Mackintosh, 2000; Paivio, 1969) while using the mind and body structures evolved to support the survival of our species (Barnard, Duke, Byrne, & Davidson, 2007).

We are a social species, and our survival would have depended on the safety and advantages conferred by being part of a social group (Darwin, 1871). Our minds are therefore attuned to social cues about affiliation, because to be able to detect threats to the group would have been selected for in our evolutionary lineage. Alerting attention and the myriad positive and negative associations the mind makes are the architecture on which our judging minds rest. An important feature of this learning is habituation. When we have learned something is safe, we classify it as familiar and our attention glosses over it. This makes sense because it is efficient, but it also means we stop fully paying attention to a whole swath of our experience, both relatively trivial (e.g., our food) but sometimes also important, such as the people we love with whom we spend a lot of time (e.g., our partners or children). Associations, habituation, discrepancy monitoring, and judging are supported by neural circuitry designed to support us in processing information efficiently (Barnard & Teasdale, 1991).

Ling's life had made her sensitive to being excluded. In the "walking down the street" exercise (Figure 2.3), this earlier learning quickly coalesced into emotions and thoughts about not being liked and excluded. In the exercise, she was struck by how associative and fast her mind created these thoughts. She noted almost immediate bodily sensations of contraction and a strong urge to withdraw and do what she referred to as a "duvet dive," to escape the fear and plummeting feeling in the safety of her bed. To be able to begin to know her mind in this way, it was helpful to Ling to see with some degree of decentered distance the processes of attention, making meaning, and judging. It gave her first an understanding and, second, a sense of choice and possibility when she realized "It might be possible to learn to respond in different ways."

As we discussed, mindfulness training can enable us to see our experiences more clearly, and to notice when we react automatically to them. It can teach us to respond in more flexible ways. This is illustrated in Box 2.4, where we learn about Matthieu Ricard, an experienced mindfulness practitioner who is able to see his mind reacting to a highly alarming stimulus (the sound of a gun) and modulate his response so he returns to a resting state.

BOX 2.4. The Cognitive Neuroscience of the Startle Response and Discrepancy Monitoring

Richard Davidson, an eminent neuroscientist, has dedicated his career to developing the subdiscipline of contemplative neuroscience. He has researched very experienced mindfulness practitioners to try to understand how mindfulness training affects our brains and bodies. We have known for some time that as accomplished musicians' expertise develops over time, they show changes in the structure and function of the brain associated with the sensory and motor cortices used when playing their instruments. This is referred to as neuroplasticity, the brain's structure and function adapting to new environments, experiences, and learning (Davidson & Irwin, 1999).

It turns out that very experienced mindfulness practitioners also demonstrate changes in the structure and function of the brain associated with focusing attention, managing distraction, reorienting processes, and sustaining focus (Davidson et al., 2003; Goleman & Davidson, 2017)—that is, when the brains of very experienced mindfulness practitioners are studied we see that how they manage their attention, the degree of executive control they can exercise, and the way they choose to modulate different mind states is mirrored in the activation and deactivation of brain circuits. Moreover, structurally there are observable differences in brain structures associated with these functions. For example, one of Davidson's most important collaborators is Matthieu Ricard, a scientist who became a monk, and who has over many years engaged with extensive meditative practice (more than 20,000 hours!). Ricard has trained his mind in the same way a musician trains to play his or her instrument.

There are now numerous experiments where scientists have studied how Ricard's mind, brain, and body responded to a range of situations. One illustrative study involved asking Ricard to enter different meditative states (focused and open awareness) and then seeing how he responded to the loud sound of a starter gun, which reliably and understandably alerts attention and elicits a significant startle response (Levenson, Ekman, & Ricard, 2012). His startle response was no different from that of control individuals, who were men matched on key features like age and education. However, during open awareness, Ricard's extensive meditative training showed that although the gun shot elicited a startle in terms of his body (this is a deep brain stem response), he was able to modulate his response to bring himself back to a resting state. His subjective experience was that the more his mind was present to his experience as the gun went off, the more he could accommodate the loud noise into the dynamic landscape of his experience. In contrast, if his mind was wandering, his startle response was stronger. His training had made him highly attuned to his experience and able to modulate his experience. Presumably, he was able to choose to orient his attention to particular aspects of his experience in helpful ways.

Our learned patterns, associations, and appraisals can also create and maintain mental health conditions. People with phobias are prone to have associations to their feared object triggered relatively easily. I (WK) was raised in Africa and there were many snakes, including in our garden, some of which were dangerous. I developed what I consider a reasonable fear of snakes. One day after we moved to England, I was walking in the woods as a young boy and I stood on a stick that moved as I stepped on it. Instantly, my mind, alerting me to what it saw as a threat, created a snake out of the stick. In that moment, the stick was a moving dangerous snake that was about to bite me. Equally instantaneously, my mind and body were seized by fear and I leaped backward, much to the amusement of my friends. There is a large body of research showing that such fast, automatic processing is wired into the mind and body, is learned associatively, and has obvious evolutionary advantages (LeDoux, 2000; Phelps & LeDoux, 2005; Rogan et al., 1997).[4]

People with anxiety disorders are prone to be overly alert to and oriented to threat, and have exaggerated patterns of thinking, such as "I will fail in my exams," "Everyone can see how nervous I am," or "Something bad is going to happen" (Beck, Hollon, Young, Bedrosian, & Budenz, 1985). People who are depressed are prone to judgments about themselves that can be overly negative and harsh (e.g., "I am worthless and unlovable"; "People don't like me"). They often have a large bank of negative memories that are all too readily available (Beck, Rush, Shaw, & Emery, 1979) or, worse still, schematic overgeneralized memories linked to these meanings (e.g., "All of my friendships end in rejection"; Williams et al., 2007). Executive attention can get overwhelmed when trying to inhibit these aversive thoughts and memories from dominating awareness. At one level, this judging mind is simply a normal characteristic of the mind. However, it can also act like quicksand that sucks people into anxiety and depression.

A growing body of evidence is finding that these key aspects of the mind (e.g., stabilizing attention) can be trained. Physical exercise shapes the cardiovascular system and tones and strengthens the muscular body. In the same way, mindfulness exercises affect the structure and function of the mind and body—the structures and functions of the brain have "neuroplasticity" (Davidson & McEwen, 2012; Garland et al., 2010; Goleman & Davidson, 2017). One of the first stages of mindfulness practice is to help people better know and understand their minds, and to see as best they can this judging experience for what it is—namely, meaning making—all the time. This understanding develops over time so that in very experienced mindfulness practitioners, challenging mind and body states can be worked with, as we saw with Ricard down-regulating the arousal triggered by a gunshot (see Box 2.4). We all, through our learning history, developed habitual patterns of mind that were functional at one time, but can now lock us into unhelpful reactivity, patterns of which we often are not even aware. The path of mindfulness practice is intended and structured to reveal and then transform these patterns and habits.

> *The key insight from psychological science is that at every level of the mind we are continually judging our experience: "Is this new or familiar?"; "Safe or threatening?"; "Does it require my consideration or action?" This is driven by a discrepancy monitor: "How are things?; How should they be?" Our sense of contentment or distress is a function of these discrepancies when we judge that things are not as they should be. These patterns can be known and changed.*

SYNOPSIS

In the last hundred or so years, psychological science has mapped the mind in important and instructive ways. In this chapter, we outlined a working map of the mind by choosing from basic psychological science some of the most helpful elements that support mindfulness—namely, that:

- Our mind spends much of the time on automatic pilot, which has many advantages but also some costs;
- While perception starts in our sense organs, it is a constructive and creative process;
- The kind of attention we pay actually alters our experience of the world (i.e., we actively create our experience);
- Our experience can be separated into bodily sensations, emotions, thoughts, and behavior;
- The mind is dynamic and ever changing;
- Appraisal, judgment, and discrepancy monitoring are present at every level of perception and attention, powerfully shaping our experience; and
- The mind can be trained and transformed through mindfulness practice.

In the next chapter, we build on these ideas to explore how the mind pulls all of this together to make sense of the world.

CHAPTER 3

A Map of the Mind

BEING AND KNOWING

When asked what consciousness is, we have no better
answer than Louis Armstrong's when a reporter asked him
what jazz is: "Lady, if you have to ask, you'll never know."
—STEPHEN PINKER (1997)[1]

Psychological science has transformed many mysterious aspects of the mind
into testable theoretical ideas. Like Louis Armstrong's response, we all know
what it is to be conscious—the embrace of someone we love, the taste of
food we like and don't like, the experience of a throbbing toothache, and
the beauty of the natural world. The simple invitation in mindfulness practice is to open to this knowing. This chapter builds on the basic psychological science in Chapter 2 to outline how our mind binds together the myriad
changing perceptions, sensations, emotions, thoughts, and action tendencies
in each unfolding moment. How our minds construct a narrative structure, so
we can make sense of our experience. We review:

- How a wandering mind is an unhappy mind;
- Different ways of knowing and being; and
- How we make sense of the world.

A Wandering Mind Is an Unhappy Mind

One of the first things we discover when we start a mindfulness practice is
how much our minds wander. When asked to bring our attention to the body
or breath, we quickly discover that our minds wander to remembering the

past, planning the future, commenting on our experience, inferring other people's intentions, daydreaming, and so on. People say things like my mind is "like a toddler, just running off in all directions." They often worry that they are doing something wrong, saying things like "Surely mindfulness practice is about steadying attention, emptying the mind; I'm getting this all wrong." As we saw in Chapter 1, the Buddha described the mind as being like an untrained elephant following its impulses, for better (e.g., foraging in the forest for food) or worse (e.g., creating havoc and destruction when surprised by a loud noise while walking through a plantation). Mind wandering is a universal experience. Our minds are inclined to wander—it's what they do.

In a now classic psychology experiment, 2,250 adults were asked to record three data points on repeated occasions over several weeks: (1) whether their mind was wandering, (2) how happy they were, and (3) what they were doing (Killingsworth & Gilbert, 2010). The three questions were repeated at random times over a period of weeks, providing a large database. This seminal study yielded several key insights. First, the study showed that people reported that their minds were wandering about half the time. Second, that mind wandering tended to be associated with unhappiness, regardless of what people were doing. Finally, whether the mind was present or wandering was a better predictor of happiness than what people were actually doing. The study's title, "A Wandering Mind Is an Unhappy Mind," gave away its main finding.

In a parallel program of work, neuroscientists were trying to establish paradigms for examining the neural correlates of various cognitive functions, such as attention, perception, planning, and so on—that is, "Which brain structures and networks are involved in these functions?" The neural correlates of mind wandering were discovered by chance. When experimenters asked people to simply do nothing while awaiting the *actual* experimental task, they found participants' brains were not only active but active in particular ways—that is, doing nothing while waiting for the experiment to start was associated with the activation of particular brain networks that neuroscientists named the default mode network, on the presumption that the mind defaults to this state when we are at rest (Raichle, MacLeod, Snyder, Powers, Gusnard, et al., 2001). What we've learned is that the default mode comes online when we take time out from intentional activity. Both science and mindfulness practice have discovered that our default mode is mind wandering.

Leading researchers (Smallwood & Schooler, 2015) have made important distinctions between (1) mind wandering when you are trying to focus on something (e.g., in mindfulness practice); (2) mind wandering when we are "at rest"; and (3) free association, perhaps even intentional mind wandering that can characterize reverie or creativity. For example, we might choose to attend to issues we're worried about, plans we need make, projects we're working on, or mulling over pressing problems (Hasenkamp, Wilson-Mendenhall, Duncan, & Barsalou, 2012).

Mind wandering is often concerned with creating the narrative of our lives. More recent work has looked at mind wandering in particular groups of people. As we'd predict, in people prone to depression, when their mind wanders they engage in particularly circular, negative forms of rumination (Hamilton et al., 2011).

> Ling described how sometimes her morning involves having a shower, doing her makeup, and getting dressed, and not once being present because she is worried about the day ahead, rehearsing problems from the day before, and so on. When she started a mindfulness program and she came up close to her wandering mind, she judged herself for this, too, which triggered further rumination along the lines of "I am useless, this just proves it, I can't even do this mindfulness practice."

This is consistent with the theoretical accounts within cognitive therapy that have long hypothesized that for people prone to depression, there is an underlying tendency to think negatively about the self, the future, and the world (Beck et al., 1979). These tendencies tend to lie dormant until they're triggered by, for example, low mood (Segal, Williams, Teasdale, & Gemar, 1996).

There are individual differences in people's ability to see these processes unfold in the mind and show flexibility in how they respond (Diamond, 2013). Crucially, mindfulness programs are designed to support this flexibility. There are now some compelling studies showing that mindfulness programs not only facilitate greater mindfulness but that when participants learn mindfulness skills it is associated with positive outcomes (Alsubaie et al., 2017; Bieling et al., 2012). How specifically might that happen?

Mindfulness training helps people notice mind wandering and learn to intentionally bring their minds back to the present moment. As we'd predict, mindfulness training is associated with reduced mind wandering and reduced activation of the default mode network, an effect that is markedly more pronounced in advanced mindfulness practitioners (Brewer et al., 2011; Farb et al., 2007; Morrison, Goolsarran, Rogers, & Jha, 2014). The more we practice mindfulness, the better we are able to recognize mind wandering, steady the mind, and choose how and where to deploy our attention.

Try the mindful pause exercise in Box 3.1. Most mindfulness instructions include the instruction to notice mind wandering and bring the mind

BOX 3.1. Mindfulness Exercise:
Mindful Pause, Noticing Mind Wandering, and Coming Back

Take a moment now to pause and notice your mind, and perhaps use a word to note the state of your mind. Is it sharp, dull, alert, tired? Now do the same with your emotional state, noting your emotional state just now. Are you content, discontent, curious, bored? Scan your body, noticing whatever sensations are present, such as ease, contraction, coolness, warmth.

Now, very deliberately, focus your attention on your breath, the sensations of breathing in your belly. The simple invitation is to shine the beam of your attention onto your breath as you experience it in your belly, right now, as you breathe in and breathe out, noticing this in-breath, this out-breath. Sensing into the direct sensations as they are in the belly, allowing them to fill your awareness. Allow any thoughts, feelings, and bodily sensations to be there in the broader field of awareness, but foregrounding your breath in your belly, this breath. Not looking to change anything, just be with the sensations of your breathing in your belly, exactly as it is, intentionally, with full presence, curiosity, and patience.

Inevitably, the mind will wander. This is both normal and part of the practice. Each time you notice the mind wandering, include this as part of the practice ("Ah, this is mind wandering"), perhaps noting where the mind wandered to (planning, memories, judgments, etc.), and then, with care and firmness, bring the attention back to the breath.

Continue on for a few minutes with the practice of attending to the breath, noting mind wandering, escorting the attention back to the breath.

back each time to whatever is the focus of present-moment awareness. This brief mindfulness exercise is a way of stepping out of automatic pilot at any time, by first noting the state of our minds and bodies (i.e., where we're at), and then intentionally gathering our attention to the breath, using a focus on the breath to stabilize and anchor attention. We learn that mind wandering is both a part of our everyday experience and our mindfulness practice. We learn to recognize mind wandering and to train attention by coming back to the breath each time. This capacity to manage our attention opens a doorway to different ways of being in and knowing the world.

The key insight from psychological science is that the mind is inclined to wander. Mind wandering can be associated with unhappiness, especially in people prone to common mental health challenges like depression. Mindfulness training enables us to first recognize mind wandering and in time to know when it is helpful and when it is not.

Ways of Being in and Knowing the World

There are different ways of being in and knowing the world. We sense, perceive, attend to, and make sense of the world, using this to navigate our way through life as best we can. But like the musical notes, keys, and instruments that make up music, our senses, perceptions, and awareness can be configured into different ways of being and knowing. Like music, consciousness can take many forms and be experienced in many different ways. Jazz, soul, rap, classical—these are all different forms of music. So, too, the mind can take different forms.

Psychological science has started to explore these ways of being and knowing. Several psychologists over some 30 years have been instrumental in this important shifting emphasis in psychology, notably among them Phil Barnard, Daniel Kahneman, Iain McGilchrist, Zindel Segal, John Teasdale, Francisco Varela, and Mark Williams.[2] A key theoretical foundation of mindfulness-based programs is that while conceptual ways of understanding and being in the world are important, present-moment, experiential ways of being and knowing are also important (Kabat-Zinn, 1990; Segal, Williams, & Teasdale, 2013). Moreover, mindfulness-based programs train this direct, experiential way of being as well as helping people learn how to switch modes and deploy modes in the service of greater understanding, compassion, and skillful action (Crane et al., 2017).

The first mode of mind people learn about in mindfulness programs is automatic pilot (as described in Chapter 2). Note that the moment of recognizing automatic pilot is a moment in which we start to understand the mind and begin to exercise intentional choices. When Ling recognized that her morning routine was carried out on automatic pilot while she ruminated about the day ahead, she saw how this veiled her experience and could set her up to have a bad day.

Next, we map out two modes of mind in greater detail: the experiential and the conceptual. We then go on to outline how we can shift between these modes in ways that are both helpful and unhelpful.

The Experiential Mode of Mind

The experiential mode of mind is direct, present-moment awareness of our ever-changing experience, and involves seeing, hearing, bodily awareness, emotion, behavioral impulses, and so on. Psychological science has tended to focus on what is unique to the human mind, neglecting the fact that there is likely more overlap than difference with other species. Experiential knowing is something we share with many other species.

Herd animals, such as gazelles, for example, have a behavioral impulse to eat driven by a need for satiety. They also graze alongside their herd on the pasture, perceiving the rest of the herd together as a group, and knowing when they are safe and when there is a threat to the group's safety. When the herd senses a threat, the attention shifts away from grazing and orients toward the threat in preparation for an appropriate response that gets it and the herd to safety. As soon as the threat passes, the gazelle shifts back to a mode characterized by safety, group cohesion, and a drive for satiety. The animals return to grazing. The threat system down regulates and the contented state is reestablished. There are familiar states, conditioned through associative learning. All the external and internal stimuli are processed alongside one another to form an integrated meaning that enables an appropriate response. These ways of perceiving and understanding the world are common to much of the animal kingdom, including us, Homo sapiens (Sapolsky, 2004).

The experiential mode is powerful and useful. It allows "things to be present to us in all their embodied particularity, with all their changeability and impermanence, and their interconnections, as part of a whole which is forever in flux" (McGilchrist, 2009, p. 93).

The experiential mode brings into awareness the full bandwidth of our experience in any given moment, including our body sensations, emotions, thoughts, and behavioral impulses. Information from all these sources is brought online and we have an *embodied* experience that enables us to more fully tune in to how things are (see Table 3.1). The embodied quality of the experiential mode is a unification in moment-to-moment awareness of bodily sensations, emotions, thoughts, and action tendencies, held with the attitudinal dimensions of nonjudging, patience, trust, and equanimity.

As we discussed in Chapter 2, stimuli are first registered through one of the main senses—seeing, hearing, and other bodily sensations. Experiential knowing involves integrating all of the information from these systems so that we can make sense of the world (Teasdale & Barnard, 1993). It helps us figure out whether a situation is safe or a threat, familiar or novel, and how we can

TABLE 3.1. Experiential Being and Conceptual Mode of Mind

Conceptual mode	Experiential mode
Abstract, with conceptual representation and narrative	Direct experience, with all its particularity, bandwidth, and dynamics
Judging and analyzing	Allowing
Thoughts and images understood as realities	Thoughts and images experienced as mental events
Past and future focused, mental time travel	Present-moment focus

get our basic needs met (e.g., warmth, satiety). We are social animals, and like all social animals, group cohesion and dynamics are key. We need to know where our family is: Is it intact and OK?; What is our place in the structure? The mind is in constant dynamic flux as we perceive and reperceive, as we update all the changes in our internal and external worlds.

Experiential knowledge has been integrated through associative learning. For example, we may have learned that this way of doing things works well, this setting is generally safe, this is my kin. . . . This integrative learning enables the selection of an appropriate response in any given moment, and these responses are subject to continuous learning (Glockner & Witteman, 2010; Kahneman, 2011).

The Conceptual Mode of Mind

As Homo sapiens, we are also able to envision a future where we plan, create, remember the past, and learn, so that we can know the world *conceptually*. In a conceptual mode of mind, we can stand back from our experience, reflect on what it means, and have gratitude, pride, aspirations, regrets, and so on . . . We have created mental narratives for our lives, stories with us as the actors. This mode evolved to help us get what we want in goal-directed action by using planning, creativity, and language. Moreover, we can use our high-level language abilities to describe and communicate our experience to ourselves and to others. The ability to reflect on and communicate our experience— the conceptual world—is more uniquely human.

> This world is explicit, abstracted, compartmentalized, fragmented, static (though its bits can be set in motion like a machine), essentially lifeless. From this world we feel detached. But in relation to it powerful. (McGilchrist, 2009, p. 93)

The conceptual mode of mind is an extraordinary human capacity. It is something of a miracle and includes our abilities to:

- Have abstract thought;
- Re-create the world in imagination;
- Be intentionally creative;
- Plan; and
- Have a database of rich autobiographical memories.

It is what enables us to navigate our complex lives. It is what has enabled our species to learn to farm, invent, find ways to live in challenging climates, create art and write symphonies, send astronauts into space, wage wars, design electronics, build incredible buildings, and create international structures that support world stability. In evolutionary terms, this language-based conceptual mode of mind is a relatively recent development. It is likely that spoken language evolved as recently as 100,000 years ago (Dunbar, 2003; Dunbar & Shultz, 2007). Moreover, to the degree human beings have uniquely developed language, this conceptual mode is relatively unique to our species.

The distinction between these two modes of mind is summarized in Table 3.1.

Shifting between Modes of Mind

When are these modes of mind helpful and unhelpful? When is it skillful to intentionally change modes? Although they are extraordinary capacities, these ways to be and know the world can also present problems. The first problem that we have already noted is our *tendency to become dissociated from the richness and potentiality of our direct experience, to live much of life on automatic pilot.* The continual *busyness* of many people's lives compounds this problem. The more we rush from experience to experience—busy doing, doing, doing—the more the experiential mode becomes inaccessible to us. The eating exercise that introduced the previous chapter illustrates how when Ling slowed down and brought awareness to her experience she literally came to her senses: "The smell brought me out of my daydreaming and I had a slight sense of anxiety, but then it became a nice feeling—the smell was strong, sweet, and warm, it made my mouth start to water and look forward to eating it."

The second problem is more subtle. Conceptual knowing divides everything into ideas (concepts) in ways that do not always *map onto the actual landscape of experience.* We turn experiences into separate entities with enduring characteristics and labels that take on a life of their own. These ideas can be highly abstract and totally disconnected from our current sensory reality. As Wittgenstein (2009) put it: "Words deliver us a picture and the picture holds us captive." Of course, we need to be able to quickly categorize our world: this is a member of my family, this is a stranger, this is a dog, this is a chair. But these concepts can also constrain our experience and "hold us captive." The moment an experience becomes a concept, our thinking tends to close to other ways of construing the experience.

In mindfulness practice, people are invited, as best they can, to explore sensations directly, and the experiential mode supports this exploration. This is a key point both for those teaching and learning mindfulness. We're invited to ask questions like "Where exactly is the sensation?"; "Where does it start and end?"; "Is it dull or sharp?"; "Does it pulse or is it steady?"; "Where are the edges?"; and "How does it change from moment to moment?" We're invited to move beyond concepts to direct experiences, and to see what this can teach us.

The third problem is that *there is a fundamental mismatch between the conceptual world of separate, isolated things* and the sensory world of interrelated, interdependent, constantly shifting dynamic patterns. When we stop to examine the landscape of our mind, the mismatch between knowing things experientially and conceptually becomes apparent. It is sometimes difficult to integrate concepts with more direct experiential knowing. So we default to automaticity (automatic pilot) and a primary conceptual mode. We neglect the richness of experiential knowledge and the understanding it can offer us to better navigate our lives.

The fourth problem is the discrepancy monitor we introduced in Chapter 2. The reliance on concepts and language, combined with our natural inclination to judge our experience, creates a powerful discrepancy monitor. We find ourselves asking, "How are things?" followed immediately by "How should things be?" (Higgins, 1987, 1996; Higgins, Bond, Klein, & Strauman, 1986). This drives compulsive efforts to change our experience to match how we believe our experience *should* be. Our goals and discrepancy thinking powerfully shape our experience, in subtle, preconscious ways in which information is registered and appraised (bad, good, escape, cling to), through to more elaborate ruminative thoughts (e.g., "Oh no, why do I feel this way again? What have I done to deserve this?").

From an early age people develop views of what they should be like, what others should be like, and what the world should be like. These views take us away from our direct experience. Instead of experiencing the world, our conceptual mode of mind continually notes discrepancies and tries to fix them with questions like "Why has this happened and how can I fix it?" When our conceptual mode of mind becomes driven by discrepancy thinking, it can create the conditions for compulsive *striving*, where we continually try to fix our experience and situation.

What does shifting modes look like for Mohammed?

For Mohammed, mindfulness practices enabled him to know his "pain" in a different way: it was "stabbing," and "pulsed," but was also fairly consistently in a particular part of his body. The sensations were still unpleasant, but he discovered that in each moment they had a "particularity" and it changed from moment to moment. Through the body scan he had an extraordinary insight— "In most moments there is more right with my body than wrong." Mohammed was also able to relate to his thoughts about his pain experientially. In the same way that he felt the sensations more directly, he could see the thoughts like bubbles rising in a boiling pot of water. He no longer identified with the thoughts about pain (e.g., "This is unbearable")—the thoughts became experiences that could be held in awareness.

We are not suggesting that automatic pilot, conceptual mode, or experiential mode is more or less, right or wrong, or better or worse. Each has its function and its time. What is important is knowing that each mode is available to us. We learn that we can choose to shift gears in and out of automatic pilot and in and out of experiential and conceptual modes. Mindfulness practice reveals this understanding. Over time the learning broadens and deepens, and there is a growing sense of confidence and capacity: "Ah yes, I recognize this; I have a deep confidence that I know what I need to do here."

The key insight from psychological science is that we have this extraordinary capacity to be in and know the world in these different ways. Automatic pilot enables us to navigate familiar territory and enormous complexity using learned patterns of reacting and behaving. We can recognize automatic pilot and recognize when it does, and does not, serve us. We can choose to engage experiential and conceptual modes of mind. Mindfulness practice enables us first to see and know these modes of mind and then, in time, learn to move between them in ways that serve our deeper intentions.

Constructing Meaning of the World

There is a similar deep structure in all natural systems: simpler patterns are bound together to create more complex patterns, which are then bound together to make even more complex patterns. In the mind, simple patterns of information are bound into more complex, coherent patterns of information by establishing connections of relatedness.
—JOHN TEASDALE (2016)

Our minds see patterns and create meaning, largely automatically, in both the experiential and conceptual modes. What we see, hear, and feel coalesce into patterns as we appraise information, draw on memories, and use language, imagery, and associations (Bargh et al., 1996; Cesario, Plaks, Hagiwara, Navarrete, & Higgins, 2010). Being able to quickly make meaning out of a set of circumstances enables decisions such as safe or not safe, belonging or not belonging, approach or avoid. Such decisions involve binding together many elements, perception, attention, and memory (Barnard et al., 2007).

Humans have evolved language into the mind's architecture and language is a powerful way to construct meaning. Here is an experiment to illustrate the compelling associative power of language (Kahneman, 2011). Take a moment to read the two words below and see what happens for you.

Banana   *Vomit*

In simply reading these words, the mind is likely to make quick, associative, powerful leaps, and most interestingly, just from these words may well construct a narrative story with bodily associations. Consider how much you feel like eating a banana right now. Just reading these words can for a short while create a story in which bananas have become aversive. In this example, all we have done is read two words. Actually, all we have done is turn our eyes to patterns of light and color on the page and everything else has unfolded from there. The mind is inclined to create meaning and stories; it doesn't like a vacuum of meaning, and the conceptual mind prefers a narrative structure, with a beginning, middle, and end, and a clear role for the main actor—me, myself, and I.

In Box 3.2, we consider one more example used in mindfulness-based cognitive therapy (MBCT) to illustrate how the mind constructs meanings and narratives (Segal et al., 2013). Even with limited information, the mind creates a story or narrative, and new information is used to update the narrative. As we begin to read Box 3.2, most of us naturally consider that John is a student and so populate the story with a boy of a certain age, perhaps with an image of how he is dressed, the surroundings shaped by our memories and circumstances. The second step introduces that John is "worried," and emotion shapes our thinking here; perhaps it adds some urgency. What might

---

BOX 3.2. Exercise: John Was on His Way to School

Read the following four statements in turn, allowing your mind to make sense of the information in each statement, perhaps allowing imagery to be conjured up, before moving to the next statement.

1. John was on his way to school. (*Pause, allow your mind to make sense of this information.*)
2. He was worried about the math lesson. (*Pause, allow your mind to make sense of this information.*)
3. He was not sure he could control the class today. (*Pause, allow your mind to make sense of this information.*)
4. It was not part of the janitor's duties. (*Pause, allow your mind to make sense of this information.*)

Note. Adapted from Segal, Williams, and Teasdale (2013, p. 299).

he be worried about? Again, we draw on our bank of associations and may add appraisals to the narrative such as "perhaps he is worried about an exam, situation with his friends, or he is being bullied—maybe he is a bully and has been reported?" The third step is ambiguous and provides latitude for the mind to go in all sorts of directions with its narrative. The final step for most people changes the actor in the story, so the mind has to completely update.[3]

In some ways, how we construct meaning is commonplace; we do this continually, all the time. In other ways, the world our minds create is wondrous. McGilchrist (2009) summarized the key insight this way:

> The broader field of attention, open to whatever may be, and coupled with greater integration over time and space, is what makes possible the recognition of broad or complex patterns of attention, the perception of the thing as a whole, seeing the wood for the trees. (p. 43)

Context Is Key

Context powerfully shapes our experience. How we make sense of information and/or situations is affected by the context in which it is presented, what came before, our prior learning, our current state of mind, and how information is framed. For example, if we like or don't like bananas, this will affect the associative experiment above with the words *banana* and *vomit*. In the exercise with John on his way to school, when we learn that John is a janitor we have to recalibrate our entire understanding. This change of context changes everything. Our experiences at school, or that of our children or grandchildren in school, will also likely shape our appraisals.

Let's consider again the "walking down the street exercise" we introduced in Chapter 2, where we wave to a friend on the other side of the street. Read the scenario in Box 3.3 and see how context affects your responses.

One of the key learning points in mindfulness programs is that our current mental and emotional states heavily influence how the mind makes meaning in any given situation. First of all, the *workbench* of working memory has limited capacity, and that capacity is taken up by any current online emotional state. When our attentional resources are consumed by processing emotions, it limits their availability for other executive functions (Baddeley, 1996; Diamond, 2013; Hofmann et al., 2012).

More than this, our emotional climate primes the way we construe and make sense of the world (see Fox, 2008). Our state of mind and thought patterns are colored by our predominant mood. Excitement and fear, for example, impact our thinking, our bodies, and our behavior, and are associated with a

BOX 3.3. Exercise: Revisiting the Walking Down the Street Exercise, but in Two Frames of Mind

You see a friend walking on the other side of the street. You wave but he or she doesn't wave back and passes by without reciprocating your greeting.

First, consider how this scenario might play out in your mind on a day you are feeling well rested, happy, content, and hopeful. In this state, how might you interpret the person on the other side of the street who does not respond to your hello and wave?

Take a moment to consider how your bodily sensations, emotions, and thoughts unfold as you imagine the scenario in a contented frame of mind.

* * *

Now consider a day you are feeling a bit low, tired, and worried. How would this mental state affect how you would interpret the person on the other side of the street who does not respond to your hello and wave?

Take a moment to consider how your bodily sensations, emotions, and thoughts unfold as you imagine the scenario in a low, tired, or worried frame of mind.

highly selective attention. In classic experiments when people are presented with situations where their safety is threatened, they only attend to and remember the aspects of the situation directly relevant to the threat; all the peripheral information is barely registered, let alone remembered (Loftus & Palmer, 1996). We can see how emotion can incline the mind to attend to things selectively, but also to create a mental world that focuses on ourselves and our needs, and selectively attends to only parts of the landscape.

Emotions like sadness and shame are the same, but shape the mind in different ways, placing the self front and center, and generally in a negative light. Sad states make negative memories more accessible, predispose us to see ourselves more negatively, and see others as viewing us negatively. It is emotion that *colors* our experience. Shame shrinks our attention to what we think we have done wrong—it is a *contracting* emotion. Anxious or worried states predispose us to interpret the world as more threatening. They are *captivating* emotions, driving us toward threat.

Other mental states—such as joy, gratitude, care, compassion, and playfulness—create a more spacious, receptive, inclusive attention. This enables us to understand the world with a greater orientation to how others think and feel, creates the conditions for connection, and provides the conditions for creativity (Fredrickson & Losada, 2005; Garland et al., 2010).

The music directors for films are responsible for creating the atmosphere of a film through the soundtrack. They know that music powerfully frames our mental state and this in turn frames how we experience the film as a whole. Political campaigners understand this too, infusing political messages with either fear or hope.[4]

The key insight from psychological science is that out of our perceptions and sensations we construct meaning. We create a narrative structure and try to make sense of things, even if we're presented with only partial information. Context is absolutely key. Everything around and within us shapes how we make sense and construct meaning.

SYNOPSIS

The richness of our dynamic, unfolding experience can easily be lost when we live a life of automaticity and busyness. Mindfulness programs invite us to wake up to life and to living.

This chapter suggested that:

- Our minds wander much of the time and an untrained wandering mind tends to be an unhappy mind.
- We have different ways of knowing and being in the world, and we highlighted two: experiential and conceptual modes of mind. They serve us in different ways at different times.
- Our minds are continuously *constructing meaning* out of our moment-to-moment experience. They are inclined to look for patterns. Context is important—both the context outside us and the internal context of our current state of mind. These contexts shape how we make sense of our experience.

Like stepwise improvements in telescopes, developments in psychological science enable us to have an overview of the mind as well as to see ever more detail (Glasser, Coalson, Robinson, Hacker, Harwell, et al., 2016). Psychological science is still young and there is much we don't yet know about the mind. In the next chapter, we turn to ancient Buddhist psychology. Its ideas were constructed through a different form of discovery: the experience of examining and training the mind through mindfulness practice. We suggest that there is much that psychologists can learn from Buddhist psychology and vice versa.

CHAPTER 4

A Buddhist Psychology Map

FROM SUFFERING TO FLOURISHING

There is a direct path for the surmounting of sorrow
and lamentation, for the ending of pain and struggle,
for the realization of peace and freedom—namely
the four ways of establishing mindfulness.
—BHIKKHU NANAMOLI AND BHIKKHU BODHI
(1995)

We yearn to be happy, but are bewildered when lasting happiness eludes us. We yearn for peace, yet struggle and confusion are persistent visitors. We yearn to live caring and compassionate lives, yet our present moment can be filled with shame and blame. We yearn for connectedness and a sense of being fully alive, yet are so easily forgetful and distracted. Throughout our lives, we will all have our own measure of joy and sorrow, encounters with both the lovely and the unlovely, and experience events that delight or sadden us. Buddhist psychology consistently teaches that although our lives include difficult conditions and challenges, both true joy and deep distress are created in our own minds, arising out of understanding or confusion. There is little in the world that can gladden a discontented mind. At the same time, there is little in the world that can distress a mind characterized by balance and joy.

In Chapters 2 and 3, we considered the map of the mind offered by modern psychological science. In this chapter, we look at the map of the mind offered by the ancient teachings of Buddhism, and specifically Buddhist psychology. The last part of the chapter relates these teachings to the key elements within mindfulness-based programs. Chapters 5 and 6 go on to elaborate how this map is used to help people move from suffering to flourishing through mindfulness training.

Specifically, we discuss:

- The Story of the Two Arrows;
- The three domains of distress (the pain of pain, impermanence and change, and what fuels distress); and
- The four ways of establishing mindfulness (mindfulness of the body, feeling tone, mental states and mood, and our experiences of the world).

Buddhist psychology emphasizes that for us to understand distress, we must first understand the world our minds construct in every moment. By tracking psychological processes through the lens of mindfulness, we begin to discover the route out of distress and toward understanding, compassion, and joy.

Life can be truly difficult, although it is often no one's fault. Our difficulties, however, can be met with familiar avoidance strategies (dissociation, emotional suppression, and denial) or with mindfulness, compassion, and understanding. The Buddha was a radical in his time. Seeing the ineffectiveness of avoidance and the impossibility of transcending the world, he was unique in proposing the possibility of finding peace and well-being in the midst of this chaotic life, with all its unpredictability, distress, ill health, and the inevitable effects of aging. In pursuit of that possibility, he began to be deeply interested in mapping the mind. He presented a deceptively simple but profound map of distress. It encompassed the minor irritations and vexations we encounter routinely and the serious challenges in life, such as chronic pain, illness, and death itself. There is no one word in English that can adequately describe this range of distress. Kabat-Zinn (1990) used the phrase "full-catastrophe living" to capture the spectrum of challenges we have to meet as human beings. When we find ourselves beset with pain or discontent, we often don't see the patterns that create torment. Instead, we resort to strategies that inadvertently maintain and exacerbate it.

The Story of the Two Arrows

A lucid illustration of how we compound distress is the Story of the Two Arrows. It is a teaching that links the ancient teachings with mainstream mindfulness, making this central teaching relevant to mindfulness practitioners and teachers. It first introduces the idea of being struck by two arrows:

If an arrow pierces an untaught person, they first experience physical pain. They then may experience fear and worry, and become distraught. They thus experience two kinds of feeling, a bodily feeling and a mental feeling. It is as if the person were pierced by one arrow and, following the first piercing, they are hit by a second arrow.

As we can see, that person will experience feelings caused by two arrows: physical pain and the pain of his or her reactivity to the pain. The story then goes on to describe how mindfulness enables a person to avoid the second arrow.

> . . . in the case of a well-taught person, when they are pierced by an arrow they will experience a painful feeling, but they will not worry nor grieve and lament, they will not beat their breast or weep, nor will they be distraught. It is one kind of feeling they experience, a bodily one, but not a mental feeling. It is as if a person was pierced by an arrow but not hit by a second arrow following the first. So this person experiences feelings caused by a single arrow only. (Thanissaro Bhikkhu, 2017)

This ancient story is just as relevant for contemporary mindfulness-based programs as it was when it was first articulated more than 2,500 years ago.

The key insight is that pain (the first arrow) is part of the fabric of life. But the compounding of pain with worry, resistance, avoidance, and catastrophizing (the second arrow) is optional.

The Three Domains of Distress

Buddhist psychology offers a comprehensive way of mapping distress and suffering along three distinct domains or dimensions.
—"Teachings of the Buddha" (Nanamoli & Bodhi, 2009)

The Pain of Pain

The first domain of distress is referred to as the pain of pain. It describes the afflictions of mind and body that many of us have experienced. Examples may include not enough food and we are hungry, a demanding physical working life and our back hurts, a toothache, and bitter cold and our hands and feet are numb. Hunger, pain, and cold are experienced in the body. None of this has anything to do with how mindful or unmindful we are. It is the nature of the body. Aging holds its own measure of pain, illness, vulnerability, and frailty. The body will inevitably die and the process of dying is typically painful and difficult. This is the pain of pain, or the first arrow. In Buddhist psychology, a whole range of distressing emotions was recognized as both a personal and universal experience that is simply painful. Grief, sadness, despair, and fear are painful. The pain of pain is no one's fault—it is the nature of all bodies and the potential of all minds to register and process this pain.

Pain can be met with resistance, fear, or denial. It can also be met with care, compassion, and understanding. In the face of the pain of pain, we can try to dissociate from the body or we can learn instead to inhabit the body with mindfulness. We can blame ourselves for experiencing difficult emotions or we can learn to meet them with compassion.

Much of the early work developing mindfulness programs explored how people could work with pain associated with long-term, chronic conditions (Kabat-Zinn, 1982). There was no expectation that mindfulness was going to heal damaged spines or bring chronic illness to an end. These are the first arrows. Yet mindfulness clearly affected how pain was experienced and the impact it had on the person's life. These are the second, optional arrows.

Everything Changes, Nothing Stays the Same: Impermanence and Instability

The second domain of the human condition describes the simple, unarguable fact that each of us lives in a world of conditions that are forever changing, unreliable, and unpredictable. It is not a negative or a positive truth, but simply the unarguable nature of all things. We cannot demand that the sun shines more than the sky pours with rain. We cannot determine that we will have only lovely, pleasant events, sensations, and people in our lives. We cannot command that the trains run on time and that our plans always succeed. Health turns to illness, people we love change in ways not always easy to accept, our views and passions alter, and in the end, we face our own mortality and the mortality of all we know. Sometimes we welcome change when it serves us well—the ending of tooth pain, or when a difficult neighbor moves away. Other times we despair, fear, and flee from the changes that we perceive as threatening to our expectations and cravings for stability. Rather than placing a value judgment of good or bad, we have the alternative choice to see and understand the world as it is, constantly in a state of flux. The conditions we live in cannot deliver limitless safety, certainty, and lasting happiness. Buddhist psychology points out that it makes no sense for us, as constantly changing beings, to try to seek outward stability in that which is constantly changing and unstable.

Deep understanding of impermanence and the innate instability of our condition is described in Buddhist psychology as one of the most liberating of all understandings. It has the power to bring much of the painful reactivity we experience to an end. Intellectually, of course, we nod our heads wisely, sure that no one truly believes that anything is permanent or eternally stable.

Experientially, though, change can be a powerful trigger for waves of struggle and distress. Mindfulness practice invites us to embody our understanding of impermanence in the face of all change, learning to release the habits of grasping that foster distress.

Mindfulness illuminates all experience so that we see directly the passing thoughts, the moods that alter, the views that shift, the body sensations that intensify and ebb. It opens the door to the profound understanding that we are, in actuality, a process, rather than static. We are dynamic, unfolding beings living in a dynamic world that changes in every moment. As we learn to stop fighting the reality of change and instability, we become more able to glimpse peace, calm, courageous acceptance, and equilibrium. Over time, the glimpse becomes more than that—an enduring understanding in which we have unshakable confidence.

Resistance, Denial, Aversion, and Craving All Fuel Distress

The third domain of the human condition is our resistance to pain and denial of change. Resistance and denial create and re-create the very torment we try to avoid. We end up compounding our struggles and distress. Craving and aversion drive our rejection of our changing moment-to-moment experience. We try to fix what we feel we cannot bear. In the Story of the Two Arrows, these processes invite the second arrow.

When Mohammed suffered with back pain, he was overwhelmed with thoughts such as "This is 24/7, if I have to live with this pain for the rest of my life, it would be unbearable." Occasionally, he even had the thought, "Perhaps I would be better off dead." He worried that the pain prevented him from caring for his family, and worse still that he would be a burden to them in the future. The jobs he could take on as a plumber were very limited by his condition.

The physical sensations of pain and the limitation on Mohammed's ability to work are real and are the first arrows of distress. And although his worries about the future and catastrophizing thoughts are understandable, they are the second arrows, compounding his distress and triggering waves of anxiety and reactivity. He cannot know how the future will turn out. Rather than allowing the second arrow to pierce us, as Mohammed automatically did, we can choose instead to meet it with curiosity, patience, equanimity, and kindness. We do that through a process of training the mind, based on mindfulness practice.

Mohammed completed an 8-week mindfulness-based program that taught him to observe how his mind could construct realities and imagine futures in which he was useless and dependent on others. During a mindfulness class, he relayed how during the week he had watched his young son constructing elaborate figures and structures out of Lego blocks. He described how he had seen a parallel in his mindfulness practice, where his mind also created structures through forecasting the future and catastrophizing whole scenes where he had become dependent, relying on the care of others. Crucially, he began to see that he had a choice: at any moment he could recognize and step back from this destructive process, and instead create a new, more positive structure of thinking and feeling.

Mohammed's experience illustrates how over time the second arrow of reactivity compounds distress, and how mindfulness training enables a powerful alternative process of knowing and transforming the mind. With the deepening of mindfulness, the second arrow becomes optional. Although difficulties and affliction are of course unavoidable, we can learn to respond to them skillfully, rather than compounding the pain and unpleasantness with aversion, fear, self-blame, shame, judgment, worry, and agitation.

The Story of the Two Arrows is deceptively simple, but its nuances require a lifetime of learning. Sophia's story reveals how hard it can be for us to identify what the second arrows are.

Sophia's first child had been stillborn, an experience that had haunted her on an almost daily basis for decades. Losing a child was a terrible loss. She misunderstood the Story of the Two Arrows. She identified the death of her child as the first arrow and her grief as the second arrow. She believed both were stifling her capacity to recover and live her life fully. She had come to be ashamed of her ongoing grieving, as if it was a choice, a weakness, or a personal flaw. She talked about her inability to engage with either mindfulness practice or her life. She lived with her grief and a layer of self-judgment. Losing a child was bad enough. Compounding it with feeling bad about grieving was another layer of suffering. In exploring this more fully through her mindfulness practice, Sophia came to understand this was part of a larger fabric of self-blame, a tendency toward judging herself harshly. Grieving was the first arrow—and as deserving of compassion and care as the terrible experience of losing her child. In time she became increasingly able to meet her tendency to judge herself harshly with the same compassion.

In the face of loss and unwelcome change, we may well tell ourselves, "I don't want this to be happening, I can't bear this"; "Life is unfair"; and "I am a failure." We shoot a volley of second arrows that compound the initial pain. To differentiate the first arrow, the pain of pain, from the second arrows, over which we have a choice, requires a framework of attention and awareness, understanding, and compassion.

The key insight is that nothing is permanent; everything changes and mental and physical pain and ill health come and go—this is part of life. When we meet pain with denial and aversion, this tends to fuel distress and suffering.

The Four Foundations of Mindfulness

There is one discourse in Buddhist psychology that sets out more or less the whole route map from suffering to flourishing: the *satipatthana* discourse (Nanamoli & Bodhi, 1995). For millennia it has served as a guide for people on a path of developing mindfulness. It provides a practical framework for establishing mindfulness in every aspect of our present-moment experience. This framework is as relevant today as it was 2,500 years ago.[1]

The beginning of the *satipatthana* discourse suggests that mindfulness practice offers a direct path to overcoming distress, for the ending of suffering, and discovering an enduring peacefulness. Establishing mindfulness begins exactly where we are right now—in what are described as the Four Foundations of Mindfulness:

1. Mindfulness of the body (i.e., somatic experience).
2. Mindfulness of feeling tone (i.e., the primary appraisal of experience as pleasant, unpleasant, or neutral).
3. Mindfulness of mental states and mood (i.e., the cognitive and affective realm of experience).
4. Mindfulness of our experience of the world (i.e., the cognitive, discursive aspect of our experience, including what supports well-being and the factors that obstruct well-being).

The four ways of establishing mindfulness are intended for our everyday lives as living practice. They suggest that we have everything we need, in every moment, to deepen our capacity for awareness and understanding. Although we explore each of these four ways of establishing mindfulness separately, it is essential to bear in mind that they are interactive elements of experience, shaping and informing one another.

The First Way of Establishing Mindfulness: Mindfulness of the Body

Cultivating mindfulness of the body is the basis for much of the experiential learning in mindfulness practice. The teaching encourages us—whether sitting, standing, walking, or lying down—to know the body as the body, to contemplate the changing nature of the body, to consider the body free from the wish for it to be different from what it is, and to contemplate the common humanity and universal story of all bodies. In this sense, bringing awareness to the body is an experiential lesson in our minds.

This instruction can be challenging because we have a paradoxical relationship to the body where we are prone to both overly identify with it and dissociate from it. Both patterns hold within them the potential for causing distress and also the potential for learning. In the midst of the myriad forms of distress, however, it is always possible to bring attention back to the body—one mindfulness teacher puts it this way: peace is always just one breath away (Thich Nhat Hanh, 1975). In other words, at any moment, we can anchor our attention in the breath to help us step out of the patterns of mind and body that cause distress and suffering.

There is no singular way of bringing awareness to the body. Within mindfulness-based applications, a primary practice is the body scan, a guided practice that intentionally moves the attention throughout the body from the toes to the crown of the head. This generally takes about 40 minutes to do in mindfulness-based programs. As awareness sweeps through the body during the body scan, no preference is given to highlighting or fixating on any single sensation, event, or part of the body. All are treated the same. Mindful movement and mindful walking are introduced as further practices to bring awareness to the body, with the main difference being that now the body is moving and we can attend to the sensations associated with movement. A significant and radical shift is made in these practices from being preoccupied with the contents of experience (e.g., bodily sensations, emotions, thoughts, impulses) to inhabiting a quality of awareness that holds these experiences with curiosity and stable attention. Students of mindfulness dedicate considerable time learning to bring awareness to the body.

Mindfulness of the body is always a present-moment practice. We do not have yesterday's toothache or tomorrow's back pain. We only have the here and now. What we come to notice is that apart from moments of physical distress or great pleasure, we rarely pay true attention to our body. Instead, we choose to live primarily in our thoughts. As a result, it is unusual for us to know what it means to be an embodied human being, yet this is the essence of mindfulness and a key to bringing distress to an end.

We rarely attend to certain aspects of our body, yet other aspects seem to draw our attention. In mindfulness practices, people are invited to bring attention to different parts of their bodies equally, with an attitude of curiosity and befriending, whether it is the toes, the abdomen, the face, or indeed a broader awareness of the body as a whole. It is instructive to see what experiences there are to be had in different parts of the body, and how they unfold.

Ling's introduction to mindfulness practice was the body scan. She soon discovered a lot of resistance in her mind, which she experienced as fidgeting and resistance to turning toward her bodily experiences. Her resistance was exacerbated by thoughts such as "This is so difficult. I am never going to be able to do this; this is going to be yet another thing I fail at."

With gentle perseverance and support from the mindfulness teacher, Ling's concentration stabilized long enough for her to attend to at least some parts of her body to note sensations. For example, she began to notice the contour of her toes, their shape, the air on her feet, the contact points of her feet with the floor, and the slight sense of stretch and pull in the ligaments and muscles of the ankles as they supported the weight of her feet. Her mind would often be carried away (e.g., with thoughts of all the things to do at work) or react to the scan itself (e.g., "OK, I am getting this now, but it won't be long before I lose it"), but she followed the firm invitation to note when the mind is carried away and bring it back to the body. This recognizing and returning was part of the mindfulness practice.

Ling had suffered various forms of abuse growing up and when she attended to certain parts of her body, she felt "numbed out," or was bombarded with upsetting imagery accompanied by strong associated bodily sensations. Before starting the practice, the mindfulness teacher had worked carefully with Ling to anticipate this and supported her in trusting herself to know when to turn toward experience and when to back away. They worked together so Ling could make wise choices about working with trauma-related experiences.

Scanning through her body involved the whole spectrum of experiences. For example, after one practice, Ling described to the mindfulness teacher, "I was really able to notice lots of things about my toes that were surprising—the shape, the feeling, the air—but I zoned out completely from other parts of my body. I don't remember where my mind was when we were invited to attend to the pelvis; the movement of my abdomen with each breath was steady, like lying on a floating air mattress in the sea, but when we got to my neck and face, it felt contracted and tense. I kept coming back to my breath in my belly as an anchor, and that helped. Sometimes my breath was steady and other times shallower and faster, but it was always there."

There are many challenges that stop us from truly inhabiting our bodies. All too often, we slip into the habit of being lost in thought, preoccupied with the past and future, and giving primary attention to our emotional and psychological life over the somatic experience of the moment. Experiences of pain or illness are challenging to meet; it can seem more comforting or safe to flee from the body. Past experience of abuse leads us to see body dissociation as a means of self-protection. While self-protection may have worked at one time in our past, it no longer serves us well. Cultural values that associate beauty, youth, strength, or sporting prowess with worthiness can be translated into an unarticulated but lived disdain for the body. Fears of aging and vulnerability are translated into the ongoing pursuit of distractedness that camouflages the reality of the body of the moment. Cultivating mindfulness of the body is at times described as swimming against the tide of habitual patterns that lead to dissociation rather than embodiment.

People have contemplated the body throughout their lives, often through the lens of fear, aversion, and expectation. We look into the mirror in the morning with a critical eye, wondering when we began to resemble our mother or father. As we contemplate the body through the lens of mindfulness, though, we can appropriately ask ourselves "What are the lessons to be learned?" and "What are the cognitive shifts that occur that can help us radically reshape our relationship to our body?"

As we establish mindfulness in the present-moment experience of our body, we begin to inhabit our life as it is rather than how we believe it should be. The mechanisms of avoidance, aversion, and distractedness may still operate because we are human, but they have less power to create and perpetuate distress. As we begin to unify our body, mind, and life in a present-moment recollectedness, we open the door to some of the primary insights and cognitive and behavioral shifts that help end distress.

Mindfulness of the body offers a number of insights, including:

1. Knowing the body as the body, without creating a whole narrative, is a lesson for our life. Sensation is seen as sensation—not who I am. The unpleasant, the pleasant, and the neutral are all seen through the lens of mindfulness, without the reactivity of fear, anxiety, and judgment that spirals into distress.

2. Seeing the body as a process, we see it changing moment to moment, rather than something fixed or static that we fear or dismiss. Rather than "My knee," "My back," or "My illness"—with all the past and future associations attached to those phrases—we begin to discern the fluid nature of all sensation, ebbing and waning moment to moment, and discover the mind can be fluid in its perception of and responsiveness to those changes.

3. Training ourselves to be present in an intentional way, we have the choice to not engage with the impulsiveness and reactivity that govern our minds and lives all too often. The possibility of intentionally inhabiting the body rather than being diverted by passing thoughts, images, and judgments is a powerful building block in meeting the moment as it is and calming the pattern of dissociation.

4. Discerning the difference between the present-moment actuality of the body and our narrative about it is something we can learn. The sensation in our body and the reaction in our mind are not the same. The sensation in our body may be pleasant or unpleasant (the first arrow). Our reaction to it and our narrative about the body is separate and we can see that it is the reaction that frequently brings much greater distress (i.e., the second arrow). We

can learn that no matter how diverting, charged, or entrancing our narratives and judgments are, we have the tools to see this happening and to simply return to the body and present-moment collectedness.

5. Staying present with the body as it is helps us begin to sever the link between the unpleasant and painful and our underlying emotional patterns of aversion and fear. Similarly, we see the link between the pleasant and lovely and underlying tendency to grasp and hang on to these experiences. When we release the grip of aversion and attachment, we can see the painful fading and allow moments of appreciation, joy, and gratitude to arise and pass away. This is a powerful shift that allows a more steady and balanced way of being present in the body and the whole of our lives.

6. Viewing our body in a sustained way helps reveal how intertwined our mind and body are. Bodily pain is experienced in the mind in immediate and direct ways—"ouch, aargh." Likewise, the mind shapes experience in the body. When our mind is appreciative and joyful, our body is much more likely to be experienced as at ease, calm, and light. The mind and the body work in unison.[2]

7. Exploring the body with mindfulness uncovers the ways in which historical emotional patterns and trauma become unconsciously embedded in the body, registering in numbness or areas of pain that seem to have little to do with present illness or trauma. Probing these areas with a kindly attention, they begin to come to life and loosen. The process is instructive, part of the classroom of mindfulness practice.

8. Committing our attention to attending to the body with care and compassion helps us learn that these attitudes are an antidote to the automatic reactions of aversion and agitation. Care and compassion, we discover, have a way of melting the ice structures of aversion and judgment. "I am failing at this" and "I am a loser" melts as we meet it with "This is part of my experience, part of the human condition—I am as deserving of care and compassion as the loved ones to whom I show unhesitating care."

Breathing is an anchor to the body. Mindfulness of the body begins with the moment-to-moment experience of breathing. We establish a simple knowing of the breath just as it is, whether deep or shallow. The intention underpinning mindfulness of breathing is to calm agitation and tension within the body. Within mindfulness of breathing, we establish a moment-to-moment sensitivity and attention.[3]

The invitation to notice mind wandering and come back again and again supports the development of sustained awareness. It requires great patience and effort to bring the mind back to the breath and the body each time it wanders and to meet the breath and body as they are, whether the breath is short or long, shallow or deep, the body calm or agitated. We learn to know our experience somatically, as it is.

As we practice, we come to see directly that it is the nature of our body and all bodies to change, and that sensations arise and pass away moment to moment. In this sustained contemplation, we understand that we are not in control of the landscape of arising and passing sensation. We become more acutely aware of the fluid nature of somatic experience, learning that our body is not a fixed thing but is a process. We learn to establish mindfulness within the actual somatic experience of the moment rather than in our story about it or our reactivity to it. We begin to soften the tendency to be so closely identified with the body as who we are.

As we become more skilled at observing our breath and body, some insights are offered. We can observe and hold experiences in our awareness; experiences come and go; thoughts too can be seen as experiences, not facts; and what we considered to be our pain is part of a wider human experience of anyone who inhabits a body—there is a freedom that comes from seeing experiences in this way. Try the mindfulness exercise in Box 4.1. It is a simple invitation to inhabit our body.

BOX 4.1. Mindfulness Exercise: Inhabiting the Body

Take a moment to be still and simply turn your attention to your body in this moment. If it helps, close your eyes and begin by sensing the posture of your body and how your feet are touching the ground. Sensitize yourself to how the air and your clothing are touching your skin, the sounds you are hearing. Sense the posture of your spine, the expression on your face, the placing of your hands. Take a moment to adjust your posture to one that communicates to you a sense of dignity, ease, and presence. Now take a moment or two to sense your body breathing—notice the beginning and ending of a single breath and how your body responds to each in- and out-breath. Intentionally settle your attention into the body and allow the thoughts and images to simply sit in the background of your attention.

Sense with mindfulness the landscape of sensation within your body in this moment—whether pleasant or unpleasant—and the more muted sensations present in every part of your body. Be mindful of how sensations change moment to moment, ebbing and fading. Explore what it is to steady the attention within your body—standing or sitting—as your body senses, breathes, and listens. When your attention is drawn elsewhere, bring the same simple knowing—a thought as a thought, an image as an image—and return once more to an awareness of the body of the moment, just as it is, without demand or expectation.

Over time, Ling learned to steady her attention enough for her to begin to see the body scan not only as a useful way of stabilizing her mind but also as a teacher. She learned that she could bring attention to all of her body, even those parts associated with trauma and abuse. She learned that she could always anchor her attention in her breath. The patterns and processes associated with trauma, while much more conditioned and intense, were the same here as for other experiences and she could transfer the learning from one to another. "When I was first doing the practices, I would get really impatient ("I have so much to do, I don't have time for this") and I'd feel myself getting wound up. I let it all just be there. I treated feelings and dark thoughts like my black dog, like we talked about. My mind got stronger, not quite a six-pack, but it's still good to know I can choose what I pay attention to, what I don't have to pay attention to (laughing). There are parts of my body that I really don't like and which bring back horrible memories. My breath is always there, I loved what you said once about peace is just one breath away. When I feel anchored to the parts of my body I don't like, or I am scared, where bad feelings and memories come up, I try to see them like the black dog, as best I can."

Ling became able to choose with discernment when to turn toward experiences, when to stay with them, and when to let them go. Developing her attentional muscles was key, but so was the attitude she learned to bring to her practice, including those key attitudes of curiosity ("I wonder what I'll find"), patience ("Staying with this, whatever comes up, with steadiness and perseverance"), courage, and kindness ("It's OK, let me feel this; it's OK"). By the end of 2 months of a daily practice, Ling described the practice and coming back to her body as a "refuge."

The Second Way of Establishing Mindfulness: Mindfulness of Feeling Tone

The second domain of mindfulness cultivation is the feeling tone of experience, sometimes described as the primary texture of experience. Every sensory impression has a feeling tone that is pleasant, unpleasant, or neutral. Pleasant and unpleasant sights, sounds, tastes, physical sensations, scents, and thoughts are all part of our experience. Feeling tone is present in every moment of perception. Moreover, the direct sensing of pleasant, unpleasant, or neutral is common to all living organisms. Plant life can detect light and water and move toward it, and also detect darkness and cold, and contract.

Feeling tone is intrinsic to sensory impression. There are some universal, objective felt experiences. If any of us were cold, hungry, or stubbed our toe, it would be felt as unpleasant, independent of the degree of mindfulness or mindlessness present. But much of the feeling tone of sensory experience is subjective and directly related to our learning history. The bird lover delights in the sound of the dawn chorus; the insomniac finds it deeply unpleasant. The sight of a sunset delights one person, while the same sight triggers sadness in another. The sound of the bell at the end of a meditation session is the most pleasant sound in the world to someone sitting with an aching back. To another person, deeply contented in the moment, it is an unpleasant intrusion. Crucially, feeling tone is preconceptual: it is an automatic and immediate tagging of experience as pleasant, unpleasant, or neutral. It is an important link in the chain of experiencing.

Pleasant and unpleasant sensory impressions flood our consciousness. Many simply pass through, barely noticed. Yet there are other sensory impressions where a feeling tone tagged as pleasant or unpleasant has the power to trigger underlying cognitive patterns and tendencies, sending the mind into a tailspin of rumination, anxiety, aversion, and obsession. Lurking in our consciousness is a primary tendency of aversion that associates itself with the unpleasant sensory impression registered in our body and/or mind. *Aversion* is a spectrum word that covers a range of reactivity that we address more fully in other chapters. It is one of the main saboteurs of mindfulness and well-being, and can include judgment, anxiety, resistance, blame, shame, and defensiveness.

Pleasant sensory experiences of body and mind can also trigger potentially overwhelming surges of craving, grasping, and clinging. The onset of craving and aversion sets in motion the construction of a world characterized by agitation, the centralization of self-view, and behavioral patterns of pursuing the pleasant and avoiding the unpleasant.

Heroic efforts to sustain the pleasant and avoid the unpleasant can govern our minds and lives. Part of this is understandable, since we want to feel good and don't want to feel bad. What is not taken into account, in our efforts to only ever feel good and never bad, is that we simply are not in control of the myriad conditions that affect our life in every moment. Feeling tone and the triggering of aversion and craving are automatic. They are patterns of reactivity of thought and behavior beyond our volitional control, and often beyond full awareness. Resilience, compassion, confidence, and courage are too often the casualties of the embedded disinclination to meet each moment as it is. In the clutch of reactivity, choice and responsiveness are beyond reach.

Feeling tone is a subtle element early in the chain of our moment-to-moment construction of experience, easily overlooked and dismissed as unimportant. But in Buddhist psychology, feeling tone is said to rule or govern consciousness. It is the start of an experience unfolding. It has been described as a "master key" because if it is unlocked, then reactivity is stemmed at its source (Goldstein, 2013). Feeling tone is the first link in the chain of reactivity. If this link is broken, the chain of reactivity is broken.

Mindfulness helps us better understand the moment-to-moment feeling tone of our experience. We learn to see the pleasant as pleasant and the unpleasant as unpleasant, freeing our sensory impressions from the optional layers of reactivity, speculation, habit, and identification. It allows us to attend to sensations and experiences as they come online, revealing how feeling tone links to aversion (turning away) and craving (pulled toward), triggering those habitual patterns into motion. At a deeper level, this link between feeling tone and reactivity is seen to be the crucial point where conditioning and patterns of the mind arise in the present and set the stage for their rearising in the future. Mindfulness practice reveals these links and provides the potential to break them. It is a key insight and empowering moment in mindfulness practice.

For Ling, fragments of experience, such as memories, feelings of sadness, or shame could easily trigger aversion and a downward spiral into depression and conflict. This is true for many people prone to depression. Ling had developed a range of strategies to dissociate or avoid these experiences. Although these strategies were functional when they were first learned and in the short term, they tended to store problems for the future. Many fragments of sensory experience that had an unpleasant feeling tone could trigger aversion and dissociation and, if this failed, rumination and proliferation. For example, the moment of waking up and sensing "grunginess," the fragment of the thought "They are excluding me," the beginning of sensations of sadness, or the physical sensations of tiredness—each of these moments could easily cascade. For Ling, all these momentary experiences, labeled unpleasant, were links in a chain potentially leading toward depressive relapse; although she had learned to turn away from and avoid these moments using her usual coping strategies, her mind still managed to turn them into a chain of associations. Mindfulness practice, however, provided Ling with an experiential laboratory where she could examine her usual strategies so that she could better understand when they led to good outcomes and when they led to bad. She could see that dissociation and avoidance provided short-term relief, but stored up problems for the future. Becoming aware of these early links in the chain was key to breaking the chain, something we explore more in later chapters.

While feeling tone is an important link in moment-to-moment experience, we must be careful not to confuse this basic imprint of feeling tone with emotion, a more complex construction farther down the chain. Feeling tone is much simpler—the fleeting preconceptual moment of contact, the sense impression experienced as pleasant, unpleasant, or neutral. That's all, nothing more or less.[4] Take a moment to explore this for yourself by doing the exercise in Box 4.2.

> **BOX 4.2. Mindfulness Exercise: Mindfulness of Feeling Tone**
>
> Take a few moments to be still. You might begin this practice by taking some moments to establish mindfulness within the body. Become aware of the posture of your body, the places you make contact with the ground or a seat, mindful of the body breathing. Allow your attention to settle within the body and within this moment, however it is. Begin to sense the range of sensory impressions arriving at your door in this moment—the sounds that appear, the sights, if there are smells or tastes. Sense the sensations making an impression in the body and the thoughts or images that arise in the mind. Bring a simple attention to the feeling tones carried in each sensory impression—noticing whether it is pleasant, unpleasant, or neither. Explore what it is to bring a simple mindfulness to those sensory impressions—aware if the attention begins to move toward the pleasant or away from the unpleasant, mindful of those movements, and exploring the possibility of simply knowing the pleasant as pleasant and the unpleasant as unpleasant. You might be aware of the reactions of aversion or wanting that arise, the beginnings of the narratives about the pleasant and unpleasant. It is a moment of choice and mindfulness when we can return to a simple knowing of the moment as it is, rather than becoming lost in the extra layers of impulse or story.

The Third Way of Establishing Mindfulness: Mindfulness of Mental States and Mood

The Third Foundation of Mindfulness is a deepening awareness of our present-moment mental state and mood. It includes the full array of basic emotions, such as sadness, anger, happiness, disgust, shame, and pride, as well as more complex emotions, such as contentment, awe, guilt, and envy. This foundation includes the full array of mental states, including positive states, such as joy, appreciation, love, and gratitude. Schadenfreude, for example, is a complex but easily recognizable state where someone else's failures or fall from grace elicits an array of thoughts and feelings of pleasure and delight in his or her failure, followed possibly by guilt about having these feelings. Gratitude is also a mix of thoughts, feelings, and bodily sensations that includes thankfulness, appreciation, connection, and typically a sense of openness in the chest and a half smile in the eyes and mouth. There are hundreds of words for emotions, and each one can have many variants. For example, sadness can have shades of sorrow, anguish, or dejection. Happiness variants include joy, bliss, and contentment. Anger variants include annoyed, furious, and resentful. Surprise includes amazed, shocked, and stunned.

Mindfulness of mental states also includes states of mind, such as settled, distracted, dull, alert, expansive, or contracted.[5] There are subtle differences across cultures, which suggests that our mental states are to some degree shaped by our learning and cultural context (Lomas, 2016). Importantly, there are limitations of language to fully describe experience, especially experiential ways of knowing which are by definition not based in language. Some experiences simply cannot be captured adequately by language; to describe them with language shapes and parses the experience, taking us away from the lived experience. Consider how difficult it is to fully describe your experience when you hear music that really moves you, or you see something in nature that takes your breath away, or something happens to someone you care deeply about that leaves you reeling.

Some of the main examples of mental states are:

- Basic emotions: happiness, surprise, sadness, fear, anger, disgust, shame, and pride;
- More complex emotional states: joy, appreciation, love, gratitude, interest, embarrassment, anxiety, depression, tiredness, exhaustion, boredom, schadenfreude, and resentment; and
- States of mind: settled, calm, expansive, sharp, distracted, dull or contracted, peaceful, and agitated.

There is always a mental state or mood. Many are lovely, such as calm, peaceful, contented, joyful, loving, and kind. Many, however, are difficult and repetitive, such as anxiety and agitation. Some are mixed states. In Inuit, *iktsuarpok* refers to the anticipation of waiting for someone. This has both a pleasant looking-forward-to aspect, as well as an element of anxious anticipation and potentially a certain impatience (Lomas, 2016). Some of our mental states are subdued and quiet; some are dramatic, lingering, and intense. Some of the mental states we experience are familiar companions, present so often in our lives we describe ourselves by them: "I am an optimistic person, an anxious person, a fearful person, a happy-go-lucky person, an angry type, a contented person." Some mental states are much more fleeting.

We perceive the world through the lens of our current mental state. We are prone to interpret and react to the world through this lens. The mood of the moment becomes our world of the moment. In the grip of fear, the world is seen as filled with threat and danger. When sadness reigns, the world is seen as bleak and life meaningless with little prospect of change. In the grip of an aversive mental state, we perceive only that which is irritating, wrong, and imperfect in the world and in ourselves. With a mental state of calm and spaciousness, we see the world full of generous people. Mental states, particularly unhelpful emotional states, are akin to a colored lens through which we see the moment and create a subjective world of experience. Moods create attentional biases, inhibiting our capacity to be fully mindful of any moment.

Mental states create thought processes and narratives that confirm our mental state, creating a closed feedback loop that is not always helpful. Aversive mental states, for example, rarely produce thoughts of kindness, tolerance, and acceptance. Instead they become the foundation of thoughts of judgment, comparison, and blame. A mood of sadness rarely leads to thoughts of possibility, creativity, or happiness. A single sensory impression can trigger a mental state—mental states in turn trigger ways of perceiving the world that feed and reify the mental state. If we look carefully at the mental states we experience, it becomes clear that difficult, afflictive mental states tend to produce long, obsessive, and compelling narratives. Mental states of contentment, happiness, or peace have little narrative or rumination attached to them, but instead are expansive and free flowing. They can enhance our sense of possibility, of our own resourcefulness.

Although we do not usually observe the workings of our mind, mindfulness practice allows us to first see mental states and how these affect our moment-to-moment experience. In the absence of mindfulness, closed feedback loops are created that powerfully affect our capacity to see clearly and to inhabit the moment as it is.

When we reflect on our experience in a single day, we become aware of the changing nature of the mind. The mind of anxiety at breakfast can turn to the mind of calm and appreciation by lunch, only to turn once more to a mind of heaviness by dinner. The malleability of the mind is clearly undermined by patterns of reactivity and identification. Mindfulness teaches us to replace those patterns with curiosity and kindness, allowing the mind to be a fluid, changing process.

With mindfulness we become acutely aware of the changing nature of our world of experience and the powerful impact that our mental states have upon the degree of well-being or distress that we experience in any given moment. We learn we can be aware of our mental states as they are, and in the light of that awareness, afflictive mental states lose their power to govern our lives and determine our well-being.

The clues to reading the mental state of the moment are readily accessible with mindfulness. There is a growing awareness of how mental states shape the body and we learn we can approach the imprint of sadness, anxiety, aversion, or pain in the body. We can learn to step out of the narratives that solidify the mental state. The clues to the mental state of the moment may be in the continuum of thinking that bears a repetitive emotional tone. If we see ourselves moving through the day worrying, judging, and planning, these are clues inviting us to be mindful of the underlying mental state of anxiety. We also become increasingly familiar with the body of calm, the body of ease, and the body of sensitivity.

Mindfulness of mental states is powerful because we can begin to learn what mental states tend to lead to good outcomes and what mental states tend to lead to negative outcomes. We can learn to bring discernment into this investigation of our current mental state, asking ourselves "Is this helpful or unhelpful?" and "Does this lead to distress or the end of distress?" These are not intellectual exercises. They are ways of developing an understanding that guides our response to our mental state of the moment. If we see the unhelpfulness of a mental state and clearly understand the familiar struggle and torment it produces, we may use our mindfulness to choose to take our attention elsewhere (e.g., to the bodily experience of the moment). This is not an act of avoidance or suppression but a conscious choice to follow a pathway of the moment that interrupts the closed feedback loop of distress. When we are aware of a mental state that is helpful (e.g., calm, curiosity, spacious), we can learn to explore this with mindfulness, deepening our capacity to cultivate the healing, the lovely, and the skillful.

With mindfulness, we also learn to develop an emotional vocabulary for the landscape of our mental states. Sadness is sadness, fear is fear, and a thought is a thought. It is liberating to recognize a mood as a mood, a thought as a thought. They are not self-defining or fact. When we stop identifying ourselves by our prevailing mental state, they lose their power over us. Mindfulness helps us become aware of the changing nature of our mental states, so that we notice both the difficult moments and the wholesome moments when a mood of appreciation, happiness, or contentment appear.

After a tiring day at work, Ling was eager to get home to her family, and approached the station with anticipation of a relaxing and happy evening in store—only to hear the announcement that her train was delayed. In a moment her mental state changed to irritation, she felt her shoulders tense, and a stream of annoying and blaming thoughts began. Sitting on the platform bench, Ling was joined by a stranger with a puppy, a black Labrador, tail wagging, that began to plead for her attention. She felt an inner shift—while smiling at and stroking the puppy, her body relaxed and she felt a simple pleasure and delight. Thoughts arose of how she would now have little time in the evening to enjoy her family but would need to use the limited time to catch up on household tasks. Again she felt her mood sink and resentment appear. Her body tensed up and her mind contracted.

In these few minutes Ling went through four significant shifts in mental state: eager anticipation to irritated tension to delight and to tense resentment.

Without awareness, the afflictive mental states would dominate to such an extent that the loveliest puppy in the world would not have made an impression. Instead, the thoughts and body impact of the mood would have further deepened the irritation and tension in an increasingly charged and escalating cycle. The work of mindfulness is to become more aware of shifts in mental state, aware of how the body manifests mood, and to turn toward it rather than fueling the thinking that would only solidify and perpetuate afflictive mental states. This builds a sense of capacity and confidence.[6] Take a moment to explore your current mental state by carrying out the exercise in Box 4.3.

The Fourth Way of Establishing Mindfulness: How We Experience the World

The Fourth Foundation of Mindfulness is how we experience mental patterns. This foundation includes two strands of teaching. One strand describes the psychological habits and moods that keep us ensnared in confusion. The second strand describes the qualities of mind that when cultivated, dispel that confusion. Together, they describe the challenges and the creative tensions of cultivating mindfulness—namely, making a radical shift from a habitual way of being to a more embodied, mindful, compassionate way of being.

BOX 4.3. Mindfulness Exercise: Mindfulness of Mental States

Take a few moments to settle your body into an intentional posture of wakefulness and stillness. Inhabiting the body with mindfulness; taking some moments to notice the life of the body just now—the body sensing, feeling, touching, listening, and breathing. Turn your attention to the mind of this moment—simply knowing the mood of the moment. Does the mind feel heavy or bright, restless or calm, spacious or contracted, anxious or at ease? Simply knowing, without judgment or blame. Sensing whether the mood of the moment is impacting the body in any way: Is there a body of heaviness or alertness? A body of anxiety or ease? A body of restlessness or calm? Become mindful of the thoughts and images present and how they are flavored by the mood and have the potential to intensify the mood. Exploring what it is, in the midst of whatever mood is present to sustain a bodily posture of calm, ease, and alertness—this is a home for your attention, rather than being drawn into the mood.

We long for happiness, yet it remains so elusive; we long for peace, but too often feel like Sisyphus, perpetually pushing the boulder up the hill, only to have it roll back to where we began. We long to live full, meaningful, wakeful lives, yet can feel lost and bewildered. We long for relatedness, yet too often feel estranged. The important question we must all ask ourselves is "What is frustrating us from fulfilling these core longings and how can that frustration come to an end?"

The Fourth Foundation of Mindfulness primarily addresses this question, but in a mostly experiential way. Once more our experience of distress is placed at the center of the investigation. Buddhist psychology points to five primary strands of reactivity that create mental distress.

1. We crave for things to be different and desperately seek to replace the unpleasant with a pleasant experience.
2. The mind reacts with aversion to the difficult, challenging, and unfamiliar, struggling to find the means to dissociate, get rid of, suppress, or avoid these unpleasant experiences.
3. When we are unable to avoid or get rid of what is difficult, restlessness and worry follow as we seek ways to manage or fix the world of conditions and our experience of the moment.
4. When fixing the problem is found to be impossible, we seek numbness or dissociation as a way of distancing ourselves from the reality of the moment.
5. Threaded through all of these recognizable patterns is doubt— doubting our capacity to change or our effectiveness to live the life we long for. This doubt and skepticism can be directed at ourselves (e.g., "This is a waste of my time," "I'll never master this") or it can be directed externally (e.g., "These teachings are mumbo jumbo," "I am not persuaded that these practices will create the changes the teachings claim").

If we examine carefully any experience of psychological or emotional distress, we can see the ways in which these five primary patterns are implicated. They could be described as patterns of forgetfulness that sabotage intention, aspiration, and mindfulness; forgetfulness here refers to forgetting to be aware of our experience (the first three foundations) with beginner's mind and with care.

As the holidays approached, Ling determined once more to try to relate to her teenage children with kindness and respect. Historically, holidays had degenerated into familiar family patterns of blame and negativity where Ling felt judgmental of her children. She found herself unable to contain her disapproval and criticism. The first family dinner on the holiday unfolded in familiar ways, with Ling interrogating her 16-year-old teenage daughter about her life choices, barely concealing her disapproval. Her daughter was interested in art, philosophy, and humanities, and wanted to leave school to travel the world. She'd said she could always study later. Despite Ling's intentions to remain calm and balanced, she felt herself again being overwhelmed by judgment and aversion. Agitation followed as she found herself aware of the way in which the atmosphere quickly deteriorated, and with sadness and regret, she could see her children wanted nothing more than to get away from the dinner table.

> LING: (*to her 16-year-old daughter*) You need to decide soon about what you want to do after school, whether you want to go to university and, if so, where.
>
> DAUGHTER: Yes, I know. (*Picks up her phone.*)
>
> LING: So, what are your thoughts?
>
> DAUGHTER: Don't know.
>
> LING: (*aware of rising impatience*) Well, maybe you can give it some thought now. (*adding on as an afterthought*) I'd like to help.
>
> LING'S SON: (*Chimes in, clearly wanting to be somewhere other than part of this conversation.*) Do you mind if I go to my room?
>
> LING: OK.
>
> DAUGHTER: Can I go too?
>
> LING: No, and put down your phone.

At this stage, Ling could see that the possibility of a conversation had slipped away and she found herself descending into lifetime habits of dissociation and numbness. She let both children retreat to their rooms, and after they'd gone, sought comfort in bingeing on food that offered some temporary comfort and solace, but which triggered waves of shame and self-judgment: "I am a rubbish parent," "I am not equipping my children for life."

The pattern of craving for sensual pleasure was a familiar way for Ling to seek comfort in the midst of discomfort. Many of us look to food, fantasy, and distractedness to comfort ourselves. Aversion is used to push away what we feel we cannot bear or find threatening. Agitation and restlessness trigger the compulsive doing we engage in to find solutions for discomfort. When we are unsuccessful in rearranging the conditions of the moment in ways that feel safe and pleasant, we tend to seek numbness and dissociation. All these universal patterns of reactivity interact with one another. They are not linear (e.g., self-doubt can trigger the craving to be a different kind of person, aversion can trigger restlessness), and when strategies to fix the difficult fail, we may retreat into numbness. At times, numbness and dissociation are momentarily successful in helping us to forget distress and suffering. However, as mechanisms of self-protection, they offer no lasting well-being or happiness. The failure of these patterns of defense triggers waves of doubt in our worthiness, sense of capacity, and hope for the future.

As we engage with mindfulness practice, we become increasingly aware of how these habitual patterns arise and shape our behavior. Change is not always easy, of course, and tension can arise in us as we learn to live a mindful, rather than a habitual and impulsive life. Because we so often fall into negative patterns when we try to change (e.g., craving, aversion, agitation, dissociation, and doubt), we may be tempted to see this process as completely negative. We may judge ourselves, which only compounds the tension (i.e., creating a second arrow for ourselves). With practice, though, we begin to see that it is natural for tension to be woven into the process of transformation. We come to realize that these patterns are not life sentences; they are mental states and psychological habits that can be transformed. Resilience, well-being, and compassion are not developed outside of these patterns, but within them.

Ling was able to pause the downward cycle of shame, self-doubt, and negative thinking through first recognizing what was happening and then responding with some compassion, first for herself and then to her daughter. "When I was her age, I had been in a state facility for young people for years and was about to have to live self-reliantly. It's amazing really how strong I was, but I had no idea at the time, it was day-to-day survival."

She tidied up the kitchen after dinner, taking a certain pride in looking after her children in this simple way. Outside her daughter's room, she took a three-step breathing space and then knocked on the door and, choosing to leave the earlier conversation for now, simply said, "You OK?" When her daughter looked up and nodded, Ling added "Give some thought to what you'd like to do tomorrow and we'll figure it out at breakfast; maybe we can go on a boat trip?"

She then stopped by her son's room; he was playing a computer game and she simply sat and kept him company for a bit. He seemed to be OK with that and Ling took the moments to appreciate how it was to sit with her son, allowing herself to think "This feels good to sit with him; when I was his age I was in care. I can't even remember exactly what was happening. He is safe, looks contented, and kind of cool and handsome in that hat!" A smile of appreciative joy spread through her body. "What are you smiling at?" he said. "Nothing, just happy," she replied. She allowed herself to fully drink in the moment and be present to her son in silence as he played his game. He, too, seemed contented enough to have her presence in the room.

Embedded in Buddhist psychology is the suggestion that we consciously cultivate wholesome and liberating qualities that serve to uproot habitual tendencies. This same cultivation is explored experientially in contemporary mindfulness. Mindfulness practitioners become increasingly sensitized to the arising of craving, aversion, restlessness, dissociation, and doubt, and learn to sustain the intention of mindfulness rather than become lost in forgetfulness. We learn we can approach these habits as useful objects of mindfulness, rather than becoming judgmental about them. They can be investigated, explored, and understood. Practitioners develop the interest and courage to turn toward the difficult and find resilience rather than being overwhelmed. We learn that calm and well-being are not postponed to some future moment but found through our willingness to befriend these patterns rather than avoid them. We discover it is possible to calm the waves of restlessness, aversion, and craving through no longer feeding them with narrative and reactivity. This creates a space where we can cultivate balance and a sense of inner collectedness in the midst of agitation.

When we turn our attention to our mind–body experience, we encounter the actors of craving for the pleasant experience, as well as aversion, restlessness, worry, sleepiness, numbness, and doubt. All of these can lead us into realms of confusion and dissociation. Participants in mindfulness programs are invited to navigate their way through these patterns with kindness and curiosity rather than being disheartened by their intensity. Sustaining attention in a body scan practice can trigger our old patterns into life. Many report their boredom, lack of interest, and the mind wanting to go to more pleasant fields of daydreams and reveries. This can happen, for example, when we first start to step out to meet our pain, or when difficult thoughts or emotions arise; resistance and aversion appear to be cojoined with the difficult. People report the challenge of being still when the primary impulse is to flee, and they find themselves drawn into familiar, painful patterns of rumination. The body and mind can be flooded by agitation and worry. When any of this feels overwhelming, the obvious escape route is simply to fall asleep as a mechanism of dissociating from a present that feels too much to bear. Doubt appears in our thoughts of self-judgment, unworthiness, and incapacity. We may have doubts about the practice, our ability to meet the magnitude of distress, and in our capacity to change.

Through their own practice, skilled mindfulness teachers are familiar with the territory of the patterns that create and re-create distress and have learned to navigate this territory. In teaching mindfulness, they learn to accompany their students' navigation through their own learning and experience. Participants come to understand, through the inquiry, that the sometimes challenging journey toward mindfulness is not abnormal or unusual, but what the mind does in reaction to distress and change.

LING: (*in the eighth mindfulness session of her 8-week mindfulness program, after the body scan practice*) I got so restless, I wanted to run out of the room.

TEACHER: (*noticing that Ling seems steady as she speaks*) That sounds really uncomfortable; well-done for staying with it. What supported you, what helped you work with the restlessness?

LING: I won't pretend it was easy, and my instinct was to shift and distract myself somehow, any way I could. But I said to myself, "It's OK, Ling, this is part of the practice." I noticed where the agitation was really strong, it was in my arms and legs, and I noticed the racing thoughts—"I want to get out of here"—and what these thoughts were creating: a lot of agitation. I let myself take a deeper breath, but I'd be dragged back into feeling bad—you know, agitated. I must have done this 20 times in half an hour. (*Smiles.*) I can't say it was enjoyable, but it gave me a sense of being OK to work with it. I feel pretty steady now having done that rather than run out or zone out, which was my instinct.

TEACHER: (*affirming Ling with her eyes and posture*) Good work, Ling.

As we've seen, it is a human and understandable impulse to want to distance ourselves from pain. Unfortunately, it is not effective and only compounds our difficulties. During the mindfulness class, we learn to return to the body with interest and affectionate curiosity in the face of the mind wanting to slip into distractedness, seeking to be elsewhere. In the midst of aversion, we learn via the practices to cultivate tenderness, care, and kindness. As we learn to sustain attention within the body, our body and mind begin to calm and be less drawn into patterns of agitation and rumination. Rather than simply being experienced as overwhelming cascades, we begin to see thoughts as events in the mind, which deflates their power to govern our mind. With practice, the tendency to dissociate or fall asleep weakens and we can experience a deepening sense of wakefulness and aliveness. One of the greatest benefits of the practice is experienced in a growing sense of inner capacity. We become aware of our ability to discover that we can choose what we attend to; that resilience in the face of the difficult is possible; that deeply embedded habits of blame and despair begin to weaken; and that it is possible to establish a kinder, more generous and forgiving relationship with our own mind and body. Confidence deepens through our efforts and experience, and doubt begins to wane.[7]

In Table 4.1, we map the Four Foundations of Mindfulness onto the essential elements of 8-week mindfulness-based programs (Crane et al., 2017). However, it is important to bear in mind that all Four Foundations of Mindfulness are present in most mindfulness practices and this table is indicative, not definitive.

TABLE 4.1. Four Ways of Establishing Mindfulness

Four Foundations of Mindfulness	8-week mindfulness-based program
Mindfulness of the body	• Body scan practice • Movement practice • Sitting practice • Walking practice • Mindfulness of everyday activities, including eating practice • Keeping the body in mind when listening and speaking • Three-step breathing space practice
Mindfulness of feelings: the feeling tone of experience	• Pleasant and unpleasant experiences calendar • Three-step breathing space practice
Mindfulness of mental states	• Pleasant and unpleasant experiences calendar • Thoughts and feelings exercise • Seeing/hearing practices • Three-step breathing space practice
Mindfulness of how we experience the world: the cognitive, discursive aspect of our experience	• Working with challenges and hindrances • Practices intended to illuminate stress, depression, and reactivity • Practices intended to illuminate appreciation, joy, gratitude, and responsiveness • Three-step breathing space practice

Note. The paper "What Defines Mindfulness-Based Programs?" (Crane et al., 2017) sets the essential, core elements of such programs. In this table, we refer to these essential elements rather than refer to a particular program, such as mindfulness-based stress reduction. Some of the elements are only used in some programs (e.g., three-step breathing space), but the table is intended to be illustrative of how the Four Foundations of Mindfulness are taught and learned, not a definitive index. The teachings and mindfulness practices within the 8-week mindfulness-based programs are introduced more fully in later chapters.

SYNOPSIS

Although we yearn for contentment and wakefulness, our experience can be of distress and suffering, which can cut us off from the richness of life. In this chapter, we outlined the map of the mind offered by Buddhist psychology to explain how distress and suffering are created. We also outlined how Buddhist psychology provides a route map from suffering to flourishing. This map includes:

- The two arrows: the first arrow of pain, ill health, and ultimately dying (which is part of life), and the second arrow, the compounding of pain with worry, resistance, avoidance, and catastrophizing (which is optional).
- The insight that everything changes, nothing stays the same.
- Struggle, denial, attachment, and aversion, which fuel distress and suffering.
- The four ways of establishing mindfulness, called the Four Foundations of Mindfulness.
  - Mindfulness of the body: the somatic experience.
  - Mindfulness of feeling tone: the primary appraisal of experience as pleasant, unpleasant, or neutral.
  - Mindfulness of mental states and mood: the cognitive and affective realm of experience.
  - Mindfulness of our experience of the world: the cognitive, discursive aspect of our experience, including what supports well-being and the factors that obstruct well-being.

Through mindfulness practice, a greater sense of resilience and equanimity begin to emerge as the mind steadies and calms. Toward the end of the *satipatthana* discourse, this learning is summarized (Nanamoli & Bodhi, 1995):

A person really knows, "This is suffering"; s/he really knows, "This is the origin of suffering"; s/he really knows, "This is the cessation of suffering"; s/he really knows, "This is the road leading to the cessation of suffering."

This chapter outlined the ancient Buddhist teachings that provide a map of the mind that were developed more than 2,000 years ago. In the next chapter, we consider the confluence of the ancient Buddhist teachings with modern psychological science before turning to how this map can be used to navigate from surviving to thriving (Chapter 6).

CHAPTER 5

An Integrated Map
of Distress and Suffering

The science of meditation is in its infancy. We need decades
more study. People talk about artificial intelligence and
machine learning, but we haven't scratched the surface of
what human intelligence is really all about.
                              —JON KABAT-ZINN (in Booth, 2017)

Between stimulus and response, there is a space. In that space
lies our freedom and our power to choose our response. In our
response lies our growth and our freedom.[1]

An itch becomes a scratch.
A momentary sadness develops into a "duvet dive."
Searing back pain triggers the thought "I can't bear this, and if I have to
    endure this for the rest of my life, I'd rather be dead."
A critical comment inflames a powerful inner critic.

How does Sam's itch so automatically elicit a scratch? How does Ling's
momentary sadness develop into a plummeting duvet dive, or *in extremis*, even
another full-blown episode of depression? How does Mohammed's painful
back sensations elicit such a self-destructive thought? For Sophia, how does
receiving even a small criticism elicit such a powerful wave of self-criticism?

In this chapter, we bring together the psychological science and Buddhist
psychology outlined in Chapters 2–4 to map how distress and suffering are
created and maintained. This forms the basis for a route map out of distress
and suffering toward well-being and flourishing (Chapters 6–8).

Stimulus and Reaction

We start with the simplest model, captured in the quotation that opens the chapter. In each moment, *we can open to the space between a stimulus and our reactions*; we do not have to react to all of life's difficulties.

We illustrate with examples from Sophia and Sam.

Since Sophia was a teenager her life has been marred by a harsh inner critic that is triggered when she feels she falls short of her own exacting standards. Sophia recognizes this as a long-standing problem that was probably implicated in the onset of her anxiety as a child and her depression in her 20s. It has blighted her adult life. Even in her 60s, this inner critic can flare up in any domain of her life, as a mindfulness teacher, parent, and grandparent, and as she struggles with her worsening health status with the relentless march of her Parkinson's disease. Recently she received one small negative comment on a course evaluation that flared up a blaze of self-criticism.

Sam suffers from psoriasis, a skin condition that involves itchiness, so the urge to scratch was a familiar stimulus. During a mindfulness practice Sam became aware of itchiness (which he had learned to resist because it worsened the condition), but found himself carried away in a torrent of thinking. When the mindfulness teacher asked Sam about this, he described the powerful stream of thoughts: "I hate having psoriasis, it's so unfair;" "I know if I scratch this too much, the irritated skin will get worse and I'll suffer even more later," "I wonder how visible the rash on my face is to others, do they think I am a freak?" "I am a freak, this condition has ruined my life."

Perception is a continually unfolding process where each experience evolves and cascades into the next. Stimuli produce reactions (see Chapter 3 and Figure 5.1). If we feel an itch, we have an impulse to scratch. The itch is

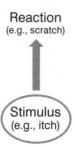

FIGURE 5.1. From stimulus to response.

the stimulus, and the impulse and behavior (scratching) is the reaction. More often than not the movement from stimulus into response happens automatically, rapidly, beyond our awareness. It can sometimes be hard to distinguish between stimulus and response. For example, Sam could not distinguish the chain of events between itch (stimulus) and scratch (response). When Sam's psoriasis flared up, he would find himself impulsively scratching. Afterward he would know scratching made things worse, and be frustrated and upset. In Sam's case, both the scratching and torrent of negative thinking were the reaction. Sophia's inner critic flared up like kindling in a fire from the slightest perceived criticism. Our reactions and the stimuli that trigger them are often fused together, as though they are a single experience.

What Is a Stimulus?

A stimulus refers to a broad array of experiences that come from our environment, as well as internal experiences in our minds and bodies. Externally, it refers to everything we can potentially perceive (e.g., shapes, light, sounds, movement, other people, situations). Internally, it includes our bodily sensations, such as itchiness, pain, discomfort, muscle relaxation and tension, warmth, coolness, all our sense impressions, sounds, and sights. In short, it includes the many bodily sensations that our minds can discern and attend to. Stimuli can also be mental states, including thoughts, images, imaginings, and remembering. Stimuli can be feelings, encompassing the whole array of emotional states (happiness, joy, sadness, fear, etc.). Finally, they can also be impulses, such as when we have the impulse to connect with someone or to escape a situation.

What Is a Reaction?

A reaction is the way we process stimuli, often automatically. In the example of an itch, the reaction is scratching. Although Ling is not fully aware of it, there is a chain of reactivity between her momentary sadness and her duvet dive. In the example of Sophia, when she reads the course evaluations, her reaction is a wave of self-criticism.

What Is the Difference between a Reaction and a Response?

There is a crucial distinction between reactivity and responsiveness (Kabat-Zinn, 1990). Reactivity is:

- Often automatic, relying on deeply ingrained, natural ways of perceiving, understanding, and behaving (e.g., if we are thirsty, we seek out water; if we are tired, we sleep);
- Learned (e.g., if we hear our name, we turn to see who said it); and
- Sometimes functional, helping us navigate the world.

Reactivity can, however, also be dysfunctional. Many psychiatric disorders can be characterized by particular reactive patterns. For example, people prone to anxiety are hypervigilant to threat. Reactivity, both functional and dysfunctional, tends to follow well-worn grooves of habit. Crucially, in reactivity there is no gap between stimulus and reaction, leaving us no space for making choices.

Responsiveness refers to more flexible ways of perceiving, understanding, and behaving. Crucially, there is a space between stimulus and response, a space where we can observe our reactions unfolding. Within this space, we have the potential to respond in flexible and creative ways. If we are able to slow down and stay steady with the sensations of an itch, resisting the temptation to scratch, we can see that usually the itch initially gets stronger, and we have a powerful and rising urge to react by scratching it. But inevitably, we notice that the sensations of the itch change, flooding and then ebbing, coming and then going. This seemingly trivial example is not trivial at all. It powerfully illustrates that all experiences come and go, even when they are accompanied by a compelling call to action. We can come to realize that sensations, and all our experience, are impermanent.

In all forms of addiction, stimuli (e.g., cues associated with the addiction) can produce powerful cravings (e.g., to take the addictive substance). There are parallels in how Sam's itchiness creates an urge and how a variety of internal and external stimuli create an urge to drink and use drugs. As we said earlier, the urge to reach for our phones when we're bored, or to eat, even if we're not hungry, have many parallels. These urges, if acted on, create temporary relief but maintain the distress and suffering. In mindfulness-based relapse prevention for people with addictions, participants learn to "ride the waves" of cravings (Marlatt & Gordon, 1985). The same is true with cravings and urges in other mindfulness trainings. We see the cravings get stronger and stronger, but if the wave can be ridden, we learn that, just as with surfing, the wave will eventually crash and disperse back into the body of the ocean.

Sam's rock bottom involved a binge of drinking and drugging that nearly killed him. It landed him in a rehab center to detox. On his discharge from rehab, he discovered that there was an endless set of people (e.g., his dealer and people he had regarded as his closest friends), places (e.g., his home, his dealer's home, the places he bought alcohol), and things (e.g., his phone) that were stimuli and triggered cravings. He used the metaphor of "riding the waves" to describe the rising of his cravings; he experienced a compelling urge to act on his cravings, to give in to the old reaction of drinking and drugging, and the various steps in the chain of reactivity that preceded drinking and drugging, such as texting his dealer. With extraordinary courage and fortitude, the support of his therapist, a 12-step program, and a 12-step sponsor, Sam learned that if he rode the wave of craving, just as assuredly as it built up, it would fall away again. In the gap between these multiple stimuli and his craving lay his recovery from addiction.

The key insight is that the mind processes the many stimuli that make up the landscape of our lives, which we then react to. The movement from stimulus to reaction can happen automatically and rapidly. We are often not even aware of it. Awareness and understanding opens up a space between stimulus and reactivity, and in that space we start to have a choice to respond more flexibly, creatively, and skillfully.

The Second Arrow(s) of Suffering

The direct path from stimulus to reaction is through a single direct arrow, where we experience the stimulus as a bodily sensation or mental state that triggers an immediate reaction. For example, we touch something hot and retract our hand, we meet suffering and extend compassion, we see something lovely and feel a sense of wonder and appreciative joy.

Our minds are primed to appraise experiences. We automatically evaluate stimuli as pleasant, unpleasant, or neutral (see Chapters 2 and 4). We evaluate each experience against how it should be, how it was in the past, and how we would like it to be in the future. Together our initial appraisal (pleasant, unpleasant, or neutral) and evaluation (how we compare it with how we think it should be) create the second arrow of suffering. The first arrow is automatic and will happen regardless; it is the pain of pain (e.g., hunger, pain, and cold) or the joy of joy. The second arrow is how our minds *react* to the experience, thus creating further distress and suffering.

The example above of Sam's psoriasis illustrates how his itchiness is the first arrow, and the volley of negative thinking and urge to scratch are the second arrows (see Figure 5.2). The unpleasantness of the itch and the strong understandable urge to be free of it is the moment at which the second arrow is discharged. The negative thinking is the second arrow, adding a second layer of suffering onto the unpleasant itchiness.

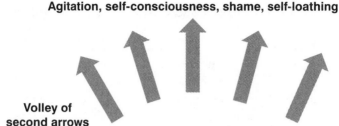

Agitation, self-consciousness, shame, self-loathing

Volley of second arrows

"I hate having psoriasis, it's so unfair."
"I know if I scratch this too much the irritated skin
will get worse, and I'll suffer even more later."
"I wonder how visible the rash on my face is to
others, do they think I am a freak?" "I am a freak,
this condition has ruined my life."

First arrow

Stimulus
(itchiness)

FIGURE 5.2. The first and second arrow of suffering: Sam's volley of second arrows.

Sophia was diagnosed with Parkinson's disease in her early 60s and suffers from tremors. These tremors can be considered the pain of pain, her first arrow of suffering. Her story is another example of how her reaction to the tremors, the second volley of arrows, compounds her suffering.

When Sophia experienced bad days, when unpleasant tremors were ever present, it was all too easy for a second volley of arrows to be dispatched. A natural reaction would be for Sophia to compare how she is now with how she was when she was well, before she was diagnosed with Parkinson's. She could also easily let her mind run into the future, envisaging all the scenarios of future degeneration when she might need a lot of help or even go into a nursing home. This could be scary. In darker moments, her mind would turn to imagining how the illness might end her life. Her lack of motivation, itself a symptom of the Parkinson's disease, pulled her toward inertia. Memories of her stillborn child were never far away. The rumination about the past and future, the inertia—these were the second arrows for Sophia, compounding the tremors with a second layer of suffering. "It's like a battle from ancient times, a whole army of archers firing arrows."

The key insight is that we can be aware of bodily sensations, emotions, and thoughts when an experience first happens (i.e., the first arrow). We react to these concerns in understandable ways—in ways that can provide short-term relief. But some of these reactions add to our suffering (second arrow of suffering).

How Are Distress and Suffering Maintained?

How do reactivity and the volley of second arrows lock the mind into a cycle of distress and suffering? To answer this, we differentiate between the *what* and the *how* of distress and suffering—that is, we first separate out the content of the mind gripped in reactivity—namely, the constituent sensations, emotions, thoughts, and impulses (the what). We then separate out the processes that fuel and maintain reactivity—namely, how we appraise and evaluate our experience and crave more of the pleasant—and turn away from and try to avoid the unpleasant (the how). We then consider how *context* powerfully shapes our experience.

The What: Sensations, Emotions, Thoughts, and Behaviors/Impulses

We experience the world as a continual unfolding of perceptions, thoughts, feelings, and impulses. We can understand our experiences better if we break them down into their constituent elements and see how they relate to one another. Cognitive therapists have helpfully developed a way of differentiating experience into several essential parts that can arise in any moment (the five-part model; Padesky & Mooney, 1990; see Chapter 2):

- Bodily sensations;
- Emotions;
- Thoughts, images, remembering, planning, reverie, appraisal;
- Behavioral impulses and behaviors; and
- Context.

We described the five-part model in Chapter 2 and provided examples of how the moment of a friend not returning our wave can be deconstructed into sensations, emotions, thoughts, and impulses (Kuyken et al., 2009).[2] As we discuss later, the context of each moment powerfully shapes our experience. For now, we use the first four parts of the model (sensations, emotions, thoughts, and impulses) to unpack the content of Sophia's inner critic.

Sophia's inner critic could be triggered in all domains of her life and had colored her entire life. A characteristic example was how Sophia reacted to a critical comment in the evaluation of an 8-week mindfulness course that she had taught. As was typical, it had gone well and she got excellent overall course evaluations. Many participants commended the course, the teaching, and Sophia as a teacher. However, among the evaluations there was one comment that the teaching had been too simple. This person wrote, "I knew it all before." This one evaluation dominated Sophia's immediate reaction to the course evaluations, triggering her inner critic. At the moment that Sophia's inner critic was triggered, her bodily sensations included a knot in her stomach, tightness through her chest, shoulders, and face, and feeling "sick to her stomach." Emotionally, there was a sense of foreboding and fear. Familiar thoughts flashed through her mind, such as "My teaching is not good enough, anyone can teach better than me . . ." A memory would often surface, unbidden, from when she taught a challenging group of students more than 30 years ago during her training as a high school teacher. She was asked to cover one of her school's most disruptive classes for a teacher who was out sick. In the memory, Sophia becomes anxious and thoughts came to mind, such as "I am losing it, this will degenerate into chaos," "I am a terrible teacher," "The principal will come in and see me losing it and realize I am a terrible teacher." As the memory played out in her mind, Sophia experienced a strong urge to withdraw. The constellation of sensations, emotions, thoughts, memories, and impulses made up the content of Sophia's reaction (see Figure 5.3).

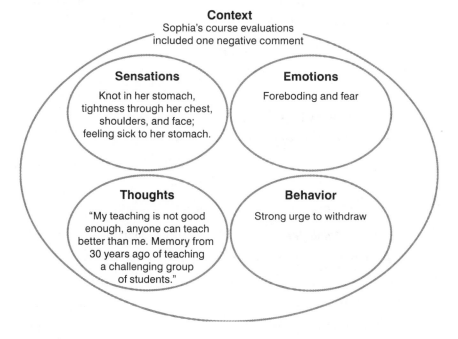

FIGURE 5.3. The five-part model: Sophia's inner critic is activated by a negative course evaluation.

Sam's addiction also shows us how sensations, emotions, thoughts, and impulses can be differentiated from one another.

Sam drove past his former drug dealer's house soon after leaving rehab (see Figure 5.4). The sight of his dealer's house was a stimulus for craving. Using this model we can parse the moment into the physical agitation (sensations), emotions (excitement and anxiety), associated thoughts ("I could so easily text him," "Why did I drive this way?"), and behavioral impulses (to text the dealer).

Addiction is on a continuum and not just the preserve of those with diagnosable substance abuse disorders. For example, we can map out for ourselves the moment we reach for our phone (the behavior), in a moment of boredom (feeling), with the thought "I wonder if there have been any texts or social media updates." When we notice this trail of sensations, emotions, feelings, and thoughts, we are also more able to notice the behavioral impulse—an underlying wish to escape the unpleasant sensations associated with boredom.

This descriptive model can be used in mindfulness-based programs to map out in any moment the *what* of the mind. It works equally well for an everyday situation, like reaching for our phone in a moment of boredom, or the moment someone in recovery from addiction, like Sam, is at risk of

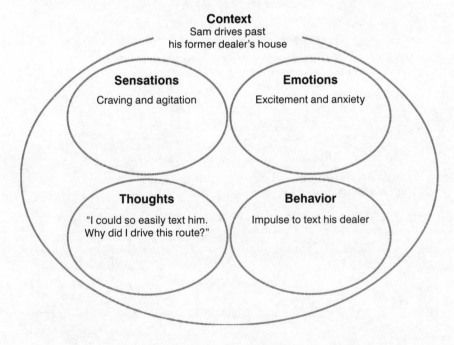

FIGURE 5.4. The five-part model: Sam drives past his former dealer's house.

relapse. It can be used equally for moments of distress, and for moments of pleasure, talking with a friend, for example, and moments that are rewarding, when something we do goes well.

The key insight is that our experience can be broken down into sensations, emotions, thoughts, and behaviors.

The How: Wanting Things to Be Other Than How They Are (Craving)

To understand how the mind gets locked into cycles of reactivity, we need to understand the unfolding process of experience, as well as what drives the process. As experiences unfold, we tend to engage in the following processes:

- Labeling our experiences as pleasant, unpleasant, or neutral;
- Evaluating our experiences and elaborating on them; and
- Craving and discrepancy monitoring.

Labeling

Our mind continually monitors our experience and categorizes it as pleasant, unpleasant, or neutral. This is the very earliest part of the unfolding of any experience. Much of this happens preconsciously, never entering awareness (see Chapters 2 and 4). However, when we pay attention, we can see the moment we label an experience as pleasant, unpleasant, or neutral. For example, a loved one's smile, the taste of good food, a moment of accomplishment, and an object of beauty are pleasant. An itch, searing painful sensations, and the smell of rotting food are unpleasant. In normal conditions, the sensations of the body in contact with the ground, the ambient temperature, and background sound are neutral. Labeling the myriad stimuli potentially available to our awareness largely happens automatically without our even knowing it. There are numerous sensations unfolding in any moment of our experience and it would be neither possible nor helpful to attend to them all. Only a fraction of our experiences surfaces into awareness and those that do are usually the ones we label as pleasant or unpleasant.

Evaluating and Elaborating

The second part of the process is where something enters awareness and we evaluate it and elaborate on it, often with a judgment, followed with an attempt to change and fix it. We may say to ourselves, "This is unpleasant, I

want it to be different, how can I escape it, how can I fix it?" or "This is pleasant, I like it, how can I hang on to it, have more of it, hoard it?"

This link in the unfolding chain of experience, evaluation, and elaboration is where the inclination to meet life conceptually, rather than experientially, can be problematic. We overthink, ruminate about the past, worry
about the future, and compare our experience with other people's experiences,
using both upward and downward comparisons (better than, worse than). We
altogether lose contact with the experience itself.

Why does this process of labeling and evaluation create suffering? To
understand the process we need to look deeper to (1) what drives evaluation
and (2) the ways in which context powerfully shapes our experience.

Craving and Discrepancy Monitoring

There are three primary interrelated types of craving—all of them lead us to
abandon the moment and start to elaborate our experience. They each work
from a place of discrepancy between how things are and how we believe they
should be. Craving hinders us from living our lives fully in direct experience
and responsiveness. Unlike real appetites, which can be sated, cravings are
rarely satisfied.

• *The first type of craving is a craving for sensual pleasure.* The hunger for
sensual pleasure involves our desire to feel good and experience pleasure. It
accounts for much of the endless activity we engage in to protect ourselves
from the unpleasant and difficult in life. It is rooted in our sense that we are
not capable of tolerating discomfort and threat. Instead, we look outside ourselves for something that will make us happy, to deliver a sense of well-being
we feel unable to offer to ourselves. Sensual craving is not to be confused with
genuine happiness where we truly appreciate and delight in all that is lovely
in life.

On one level, the hunger for sensual pleasure sounds reasonably benign.
It is understandably human to want to feel good. However, this hunger can
lead us to live lives of agitated activity as we endlessly seek to find ways to
avoid discomfort. We do not always see how our preoccupation with *fixing* the
unpleasant continually reinforces a belief that we do not have the capacity
to be at ease with experiences that are uncomfortable. When we habitually
turn away from discomfort, we create the conditions for an anxious life as
we engage in the impossible task of defending ourselves against the inevitable discomfort that life brings. For Sam, these strategies included visiting
his favorite websites and then spending hours aimlessly looking at the website
links. It is not that these activities are themselves problematic; they can all be

intrinsically pleasurable. The problem was that Sam turned to these as strategies to numb discomfort.

- *The second type of craving is to become the kind of person who we believe we ought to be.* The continual drive to be someone other than who we are sabotages our well-being, our health, and our capacity to live wakeful, meaningful lives. Instead of lessening our discontent and distress, this craving disconnects us from meeting ourselves and the moment fully. Most of us want to be the kind of person who is admired, loved, successful, and praised. The kind of person who only has pleasant experiences, who doesn't become ill or age, whose children succeed, whose vacations are always perfect, whose life is under control. We find our minds leaning forward into the future, with hope and longing and planning. Our present moment is dismissed as *not being good enough* and becomes simply the waiting room of a perfect future. Equally, we see ourselves as not good enough, a failure, or unworthy. This describes Sophia's inner critic well; it is this sense of *not being good enough* that undermined any sense of pleasure or accomplishment in teaching. Rather than being happy about the positive course evaluations, one negative comment triggered her inner critic and threatened her idealized image of being the perfect teacher, setting off a volley of self-criticism (or second arrows). Understandably, the perfect, idealized person we yearn to become remains elusive.

- *The third type of craving is to avoid, block out, and even annihilate our experience.* We don't want to be the kind of person who fails, who is continually striving for the unattainable, who is lonely, who feels invisible. We don't want to be the kind of person who is ill, in pain, who has unwelcome thoughts and emotions. We don't want to live lives where our children are troubled, our ambitions disappointed, our plans unfulfilled. As we busily try to fix ourselves and our lives, we try to annihilate what we cannot accept, judging and blaming ourselves or sinking into despair or numbness. In Sophia's case, she desperately wanted to avoid the dreaded image of a frozen teacher in front of a class of disruptive students; it was what drove her impulse to "pack it all in." In her 20s, when her anxiety morphed into depression and a period of time off work at home, Sophia closed down emotionally and mentally.

The extreme form of annihilating experience is suicide.

Mohammed's struggle with pain started in college during a football game that shattered several vertebrae in his back. In the aftermath, every moment of pain would be followed by a flood of rumination: "If only I had not gone into that tackle so clumsily, not been such an aggressive player in general, been warned off being so physical by earlier injuries." He blamed himself, the player he'd clashed with, and the unfairness of life. Mohammed saw only a future of unbearable pain—he hated the pain and wanted it all to end. In fact, when he imagined a future life living with his pain, he wondered whether he might not rather be dead. He said it took a long time to come to a place where he no longer "hated the pain." The movement toward health began in the place where blame began to end.

Context

The context for any moment powerfully shapes our experience (see Chapter 3). This includes other demands on our attention, what happened just before, our lifelong learning history, our disposition, our current mental and emotional state, the broader social and cultural context, and our evolutionary learning history. All will shape both the what and the how of the mind (Sapolsky, 2017).[3] For Sam, early in active addiction the trigger of passing his dealer's house would have led to a fix as surely as night follows day. However, in recovery, especially if he was looking after himself emotionally and physically, this same trigger would elicit a different response because the context of his mental state had changed. He was able to meet the trigger in a different frame of mind, at a different stage in his life. Ling described how "tiredness, and certain times of the year are things to be wary of because then anything can set me off." For Sophia, the context of the comment on her course evaluation is also key. "I knew it all before" can mean different things depending on who is saying it, and his or her intentions. If Sophia is feeling happy and secure, she is more likely to take the comment in her stride than if she is feeling tired and fed up. Also, whether a negative evaluation is placed first or last in the pile can also change how it is experienced. If it is placed last, it is experienced in the context of all the positive course evaluations that came before.

Concepts and language powerfully frame our experience. The moment we describe an experience with language, we shaped it. Concepts and language are powerful. Our mind is inclined to meaning and wholeness, and wants to package experiences neatly. For Mohammed, the words *chronic pain* were a cauldron of suffering—they encapsulated his injury and all the years of disability, struggle, and suffering. They were tied up with identity: "My chronic pain is 'me,' it defines who I am, what I can't do." Each person used as an example in this book has similar defining structures underpinning his or her suffering—*unlovability* for Ling, an *inner critic* for Sophia, a sense of *emptiness and disconnection* for Sam. But these are concepts, when examined carefully are artifices, something we return to when we consider the route map out from suffering to flourishing.

Finally, any moment unfolds in a social and cultural context. Consider the pain and suffering of someone living 2,500 years ago at about the time the Buddha was alive. Life expectancy was half of what might be expected in today's developed nations. For most people, the basic needs of shelter, food, and safety were priorities. Today, even though we are seeing trends toward greater security and well-being around the world (Pinker, 2011), many people still live in challenging circumstances where survival, safety, injustice, and discrimination are dominant themes in their lives. These basic preoccupations shaped by our life context will inevitably shape our minds and priorities. The human mind has not evolved much in the last few thousand years. There are many more commonalities than differences in the structure and function of the mind across social and cultural groups. But someone whose safety is constantly in question—or who is struggling to meet the basic needs of water, food, and shelter—will most likely, and understandably, be preoccupied with these themes. If we smell smoke and believe there to be fire, it is sensible to immediately seek safety. A person's context and learning history are imperative considerations for any mindfulness teacher.

> *The key insight is that we automatically label all of our experiences as pleasant, unpleasant, or neutral. This labeling of an experience as pleasant–unpleasant is the template from which we react to and elaborate experiences. We are prone to see discrepancies between how things are and how we think they should be. The driver for evaluative elaboration is craving—for pleasure, to be the person we think we should be, or sometimes to zone out.*

The Vicious Flower

A helpful analogy that summarizes how psychological distress and suffering are created and maintained is the "vicious flower" (Salkovskis, Warwick, & Deale, 2003). The analogy is especially helpful for explaining the sorts of issues that come up for us again and again over time and in different situations. It describes how our attempts to fix our unpleasant experience can loop back, like petals of a flower, into patterns of reactivity that inadvertently maintain and perpetuate our difficulties (see Figures 5.5 and 5.6). We outline the vicious flower analogy through its stages of development.

1. *The center of the vicious flower is an experience coming into awareness.* Typically, it starts with an experience coalescing into a familiar pattern, made up of recognizable parts. This is the *what* of sensations, emotions, thoughts, and impulses/behaviors, with associative links that have formed through previous learning. As we've already seen for Sophia, the trigger of an actual

or perceived criticism quickly coalesces into the first level of the artifice of her inner critic—namely, a particular constellation of sensations, emotions, thoughts, and impulses.

2. *A discrepancy monitor continually evaluates our experience against how it should or ought to be.* Very early in the process of an experience coming into awareness, the mind appraises it as pleasant, unpleasant, or neutral. When an experience is judged as unpleasant, this triggers the discrepancy monitor— what we in Chapter 2 called the "judging mind." Our discrepancy monitor is finely tuned for evaluating the gap between how things are and how we feel they should or ought to be. It is driven by craving. Unpleasant sensations, emotions, and thoughts are hard to bear, and we understandably want them not to be there—we want to feel good, we want to be the person we think we should be. In Sophia's case, the thought "My teaching is not good enough" and a vivid memory of a class she could not control 30 years ago were hard to bear and associated with a set of unpleasant emotions and sensations. She had an idealized view of the sort of teacher she should be, and the gap between how she thinks she is, in this moment, and how she should be, drives the next stage of the vicious flower's development.

3. *Strategizing to fix and/or avoid the problem.* To bridge the gap between how things are and how we think they should be, we start a process of strategizing to fix and/or avoid. We use these strategies for a good reason—because they are often effective in providing some relief from distress, at least in the short term. These strategies can be broadly categorized into elaboration (e.g., rumination, worry, preoccupation, debating with ourselves, getting stuck in attempted problem solving) and avoidance (e.g., blaming others, distraction, safety behaviors, reassurance seeking, and numbing with food, drink, TV, or computer use). Sometimes these strategies may be skillful, even the reactive and avoidant ones. They can be part of protective mindfulness—that is, the mind recognizes destructive thoughts and impulses and acts to protect itself. The strategies are understandable ways of managing psychological, physical, and life challenges. Sophia's range of strategies are shown in Figure 5.6 and include extensive rumination, a tendency to try to do things perfectly next time by overpreparing, and if all that fails, zoning out by surfing the Internet, comfort eating, or sleeping excessively.

4. *These strategies can inadvertently loop back to exacerbate and perpetuate the problem.* The irony is that the reactive strategies that are intended to fix our problems and protect us can inadvertently exacerbate our problems and even maintain them in the longer term. This is because they do not address the root causes and the short-term relief reinforces the behaviors—that is, we

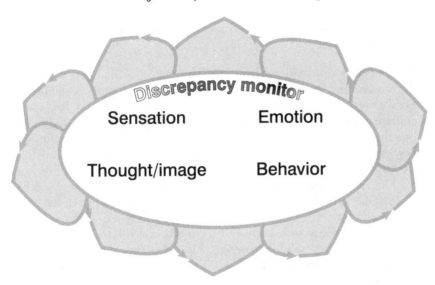

FIGURE 5.5. The vicious flower: How distress and suffering are maintained and perpetuated.

learn that the strategy works in the short term and that's why we do it again and again. The strategies entangle us in cycles of reactivity. In Sophia's case, overpreparation for teaching was in part what made her such a good teacher, but it reinforces the inner critic because it is premised on a dysfunctional conditional assumption: "If I prepare really well, the fact that I am not a good teacher will not be exposed." Underneath the conditional assumption lies a core belief around inadequacy and unworthiness that cannot be challenged or rebuilt. Avoidance, sleeping, and comfort eating provide short-term relief, but our problems are still there waiting in the crevices of our minds. It is called a "vicious flower" because the strategies loop back to the problem forming petals around it.

The vicious flower metaphor was first developed in cognitive therapy to explain how health anxiety is maintained (Salkovskis et al., 2003). Clinical psychologist Melanie Fennell went on to use it in mindfulness programs with people prone to suicidal thinking and behavior (Williams, Crane, et al., 2014). However, it can equally well be used to explain any recurrent problems that entangle us from spending excessive amounts of time on our phones, from surfing to changing jobs as soon as the going gets tough, feeling trapped in relationship patterns, such as criticizing or blaming a partner or child, letting procrastination repeatedly sabotage us, to unhealthy lifestyle habits such as yo-yo dieting. In short, the vicious flower can be used to explain many problems that tend to recur.

> We summarize again with Sophia's case. The immediate imprint of criticism is the center of the flower, which would very quickly coalesce into familiar sensations, emotions, thoughts, and impulses (see center of Figure 5.6). For Sophia, criticism triggered a major discrepancy between her perceived and ideal self, how she felt herself to be (inadequate and unworthy), and an idealized image of how she thought she ought to be. When Sophia's inner critic was activated, her fix-it mind would respond with ruminative thinking (e.g., "I'm going to give up teaching, it is too much trouble, and I am no good at it. Anyone can teach better than me. Why am I so hopeless?"), she would try to make herself feel better (e.g., spend time surfing the Internet), and eventually she would resolve to prepare her course to such a standard of perfection that no one could possibly criticize it (see the petals in Figure 5.6). All of these would provide temporary relief but would not do much to address the root of the inner critic: an underlying sense of inadequacy and worthlessness. In fact, the negative self-talk and overpreparation only served to strengthen her beliefs about her worth being contingent on always doing well.

The vicious flower analogy can accommodate many of the psychological science and Buddhist psychology ideas we covered in Chapters 1–4.

1. The center of the flower is the stimulus; the petals are the reactions.

2. The center of the flower is where experience can be seen as it is, differentiated and described close to its lived experience.[4]

3. The center of the flower is the first arrow; the petals are the second arrows.

4. The coalescence of an experience in the center of the flower arises when an experience is labeled as pleasant or unpleasant—the first link in the chain of reactivity.

5. The constructive process of evaluative elaboration drives the generation of the petals.

6. Craving (denial, attachment, and aversion) underlies the discrepancy monitor's continual judging, as we seek to feel better and to escape distress.

7. The center of the flower can be both conceptual and experiential ways of being and knowing, but the conceptual mode is more likely to elicit the discrepancies and petals of the flower. If an experience is known experientially, it may well still be unpleasant, but it will be less likely that the chain of reactivity unfolds through attempts to fix the problem conceptually.

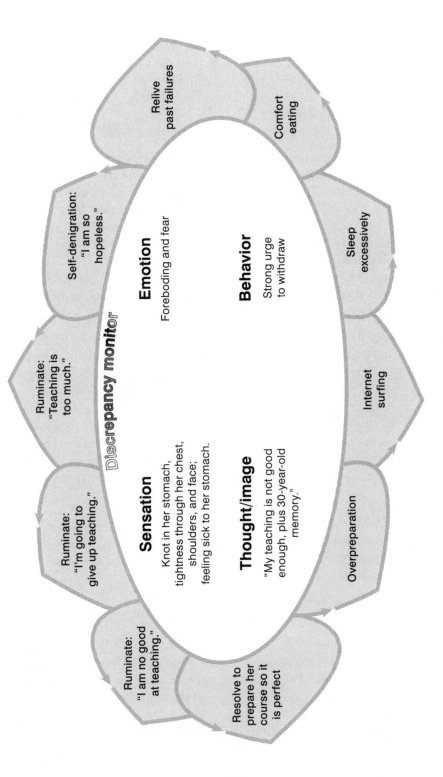

Discrepancy monitor

Emotion
Foreboding and fear

Behavior
Strong urge
to withdraw

Sensation
Knot in her stomach,
tightness through her chest,
shoulders, and face;
feeling sick to her stomach.

Thought/image
"My teaching is not good
enough, plus 30-year-old
memory."

Relive
past failures

Comfort
eating

Self-denigration:
"I am so
hopeless."

Sleep
excessively

Ruminate:
"Teaching is
too much."

Internet
surfing

Ruminate:
"I'm going to
give up teaching."

Overpreparation

Ruminate:
"I am no good
at teaching."

Resolve to
prepare her
course so it
is perfect

FIGURE 5.6. The vicious flower: Sophia's inner critic.

113

8. The vicious flower can be seen through the lens of some of the definitions of mindfulness. Simple knowing would be standing back to see the content and process of the vicious flower and would likely do much to break it up. Elements of the flower involve protective awareness, as the mind seeks to protect itself from mental and physical pain, albeit gone astray.

9. The analogy can be extended to include the context in which any experience arises and forms into a vicious flower. This can be proximal—the prevailing mood state (happy, sad, irritable) shapes how a moment is experienced and appraised. These are like the weather conditions determining whether the plant flowers or not. It can also be distal, our life's learning history, our genetic predisposition, and the evolutionary story of our species as a whole. For example, our long-standing beliefs and habits will create the tendency toward certain repeated patterns of reactivity. The underlying core beliefs, conditional assumptions, and ways we have learned to react within the analogy can be the roots and stem of the vicious flower.

10. Finally, the analogy can be used to frame change in several ways. First, it can be interrupted at each stage of its development. Like the links in a chain, any link can be broken. Second, like a flower, it requires a range of conditions: sun, soil, and water—if these conditions are not present, it will not flower. In the same way, by denying some of the supportive conditions (e.g., judging our experience, strategizing to fix unpleasant emotions), we can prevent the vicious flower from flowering. Finally, the analogy can equally well be used for the cultivation of compassion, joy, and wholesome mind states and behaviors. These themes of transformation and flourishing are the subject of the rest of the book.

The key insight from the vicious flower analogy is that we all use reactive ways of coping that at one level are completely understandable, even protective. But when examined, we see that these coping strategies can often inadvertently maintain the problem and sometimes even make it worse.

SYNOPSIS

This chapter returned to the questions we asked at the start of the book: What creates distress and maintains distress and suffering? How can we use theory to map the mind? We have developed hypotheses from psychological science and Buddhist psychology and provided a sketch of the landscape of the mind caught in distress and suffering. This linchpin chapter converged on several key ideas.

1. First, the mind can be described and understood, at least in part, to a degree that helps us.

2. Much of the time we process the many stimuli that make up the landscape of our lives quite automatically and rapidly. We are often not even aware of our reactions. Awareness and understanding opens up a space between stimulus and reactivity, and in that space, we start to have a choice to respond more flexibly, creatively, and skillfully.

3. The direct path from stimulus to reaction is like a single direct arrow, where we experience the stimulus as a bodily sensation or mental state, which in turn triggers an immediate reaction. We react to these concerns in understandable ways—in ways that serve us and can provide short-term relief from pain and distress. But some of these reactions add to our suffering. These can be described as the second arrow(s) of suffering.

4. The ways distress and suffering are maintained and exacerbated can be divided into the "what" and the "how." The what refers to deconstructing our experience into sensations, emotions, thoughts, and behaviors. The how refers to the labeling (pleasant, unpleasant, or neutral) and subsequent elaborative evaluation of our experience influenced by context. This is driven by craving for pleasure, an ideal of ourselves and our lives, and sometimes a wish for oblivion. Reactivity stems from a difficulty recognizing and allowing experience to be as it is—an inability to meet challenging experiences in any moment.

5. The vicious flower analogy is a deceptively simple way of describing and explaining how distress and suffering are maintained. We all use reactive ways of coping that at one level are completely understandable, but which can inadvertently exacerbate and maintain our problems.

6. Health and mental health are borne of understanding how distress is created and re-created in our minds, so these processes can be seen and transformed; it then becomes possible to respond in new ways.

In the next three chapters, we build on this map to create a route map that helps us navigate toward greater health, well-being, and flourishing (Chapter 6). New ways of being, knowing, and responding provide the ground for well-being and flourishing (Chapters 7 and 8).

CHAPTER 6

Transformation

A ROUTE MAP THROUGH MINDFULNESS TRAINING

> Through constant familiarity, we can definitely establish
> new behaviour patterns, using our tendency to form
> habits to our advantage. If we make a steady effort, I
> think we can overcome any form of negative conditioning
> and make positive changes in our lives. But we need to
> remember that genuine change doesn't happen overnight.
> —DALAI LAMA (2011a)

At the start of Chapter 2 we pointed to research suggesting that without a map people tend to walk in circles (Souman et al., 2009). The last four chapters have articulated maps that can help us navigate the landscape of the mind; they are the tools we need to live meaningful lives characterized by contentment, joy, ease, and meaning.

In this chapter, we set out a route map for change and transformation. These maps enable the richness of Buddhist psychology and contemporary science to inform mindfulness-based programs, so that mindfulness training can be used with precision and skill to effect positive change. Every situation, every person, every moment is different. The maps enable us to know what is needed in a particular situation, for a particular person, at a particular moment. They point to different routes and even methods of change. The path out of distress is not the same for everyone. The route to cultivating mindfulness and compassion is also likely to be different for different people at different points in their lives. Maps also enable obstacles to be anticipated and worked with. Agitation, striving, skepticism, fatigue, self-doubt, and intellectualism—all are obstacles in this work, and maps provide routes through these obstacles. Without a map, mindfulness is just a set of techniques that may, or just as likely may not, be helpful. With a map we have a route out of distress and suffering, a route to joy, well-being, and realizing our potential.

Consider Sophia, the person whose journey with mindfulness we have been tracking from when she first suffered a serious episode of mixed anxiety and depression in her 20s to her work now in her 60s as a mindfulness teacher.

Through many years, Sophia had learned first to recognize and then befriend her punitive inner critic. When her inner critic appeared, she could stay steady with the feelings, sensations, and thoughts it elicited and allow them to be there. She could affectionately say to herself, "Hello there, dear friend, have you come to give me a hard time? I know you well, dear friend, and I see what you are trying to do." She could see the potential for the reemergence of her inner critic and the vicious flower it could easily regenerate (see Chapter 5, Figure 5.6).

In a process that took many years, Sophia was able to drop beneath the inner critic's sabotaging and undermining qualities to a more wholesome intention. When she did this, she could see the inner critic as a well-intentioned friend who had trouble expressing herself well. She could see that at the root of the critic was a wholesome intention to be a good teacher, to do the best by her students, to enjoy her teaching for teaching's sake, to be a good mother, grandmother, wife, and friend. To not be motivated by fear or a sense of lack. When Sophia connected with this intention, the harshness went out of the inner critic. She described a moment when she said to herself, "Aw, bless, you're doing the best you can." She connected with an intention to serve, to see others flourish, to take pleasure in her work and life. Her work and her life became infused with meaning and joy.

The mind can be our greatest friend and our worst enemy. It holds an equal capacity for suffering and for joy. We can be tormented by rumination, denigrate ourselves, act on impulses, be flooded by negative feelings borne of reactivity, and create *vicious flowers* that lock us into suffering. As well as great joy, the mind also has an equal capacity for clarity, creativity, and responsiveness. It has the potential to be a true friend. However, if we drive today using yesterday's route map, we will not get to where we're trying to go. What is the route map from suffering to well-being? What route map leads to joy and flourishing?

After introducing mindfulness (Chapter 1), we drew on psychological science (Chapters 2 and 3) and Buddhist psychology (Chapter 4), and then set out a map of the mind (Chapter 5). Just as a careful cartographer precisely and accurately describes the landscape using images and colors, so skilled map readers are able to navigate their way through the terrain to reach various places. In this chapter, we use the map to set out the key waypoints for someone undertaking mindfulness training, including:

- Stabilizing attention;
- New ways of knowing and being;
- Responding skillfully;
- Reappraisal, insight, and wisdom; and
- Embodiment.

The map alone isn't enough—skill and knowledge are needed to interpret and guide ourselves safely through the landscape. We conclude the chapter with how mindfulness-based programs support this transformative journey.

Stabilizing Attention

Mindfulness training enables us to learn how to choose more intentionally *what we pay attention to* and *how we pay attention to it.* We can shine the beam of attention on whatever object we want to illuminate. The stimuli in the center of the flashlight beam become brightest; those on the edges are less bright, and those outside the beam are not visible. We can choose different lenses for the flashlight (e.g., the different senses of seeing, hearing, touching, etc.) and even change the flashlight's lens filters (e.g., with attitudes of curiosity, care, equanimity, etc.). These are the attitudes of mind we cultivate in mindfulness practice.

We highlight several facets of attention that are key to mindfulness and mindfulness practice. These include that attention:

- Is the gateway to experience;
- Is rooted in protective awareness and intentionality; and
- Can be trained, but is also, in part, automatic.

Attention Is the Gateway to Experience

The nature of our experience is determined by which stimuli we attend to, which we only peripherally attend to, and which are ignored (see Chapter 2). What we pay attention to, and how, are trained throughout mindfulness programs.

As we discussed, our attention tends to be drawn to the difficult and unpleasant, and we gloss over the lovely and the pleasant. Clinical psychiatrist Rick Hanson has described it as the Velcro and Teflon mind (Hanson & Mendius, 2009). Like Velcro, the mind can clasp on to the unpleasant. Like Teflon, the mind can move over pleasant experiences without making direct contact. Mindfulness practices show us how attention orients to and becomes preoccupied with difficult body and mind states (agitation, sleepiness, aches, and pains)—like Velcro. We can also see how it glosses over all that is lovely and right with the mind and body—as though it were covered in smooth Teflon.

With mindfulness, we are *taking back possession of the mind* to begin to intentionally bring attention to our experience. Attentional training reveals the automaticity of our tendency to either the Velcro or Teflon mind, but when we have sufficiently stabilized our attention, the richness of our experience becomes more apparent.

Mindfulness practice builds our capacity to stabilize attention. We learn to focus and see not only the contents of the mind (sensations, feelings, thoughts, and impulses) but also the dynamic processes of the mind. We can see the gap between stimulus and response, which allows us to take time to consider the best response before speaking or acting. We can play with ideas and be creative. When faced with novel challenges, we can see them more clearly. With inevitable temptations and urges, we can resist them, if we choose to, or we can choose to indulge our impulses with awareness. When attention is imbued with curiosity, friendliness, and care, we can bring a *beginner's mind* (i.e., the capacity to meet the present anew) to our experience. This develops our capacity to meet experience, whether pleasant or unpleasant, without being carried away by reactivity. Such control of our attention (also known as executive control) can enrich any experience (like eating mindfully, a body scan practice, smelling coffee, being with a loved one), with depths and details that were until now glossed over.

Stable Attention Is Rooted in Protective Awareness and Intentionality

Bringing intention to our attention is the first pivotal step in the journey toward thriving rather than surviving, the shift from habitual reactivity to responsiveness. This protective dimension of mindfulness allows us to step back from our reactive patterns and, instead, approach situations with a more effective responsiveness. Rather than our actions, thoughts, and emotions being habitually driven by our craving and discrepancy monitoring, we can pause to ask ourselves, "What does this moment need?" Is it greater compassion, investigation, calm—qualities we can intentionally cultivate? Is it a different response or indeed no response at all? Mindfulness practice teaches us that even in the face of habitual and unhelpful patterns, it is possible to bring attention, intentionally, to what is happening and choose to anchor ourselves. Having anchored ourselves, protective awareness enables us, like a gatekeeper or security guard, to allow access to what will help us and deny access to what will create suffering. For example, in the face of a stressor, we can focus our attention on present-moment bodily sensations rather than being overwhelmed by habits of mind and body that feed stress and suffering. Here attention is deployed protectively, by choosing skillfully what to bring into awareness and what to deny access.[1]

George Eliot (1860) wrote, "It seems to me we can never give up longing and wishing while we are thoroughly alive. There are certain things we feel to be beautiful and good, and we must hunger after them." When people attend mindfulness programs and when students search out pathways of traditional contemplative development, they share the same longing for happiness, fulfillment, and wakefulness. They also share the same cravings, such as to feel good, not bad, and to be the person they imagine they should be. Mindfulness is not about living in some mythical, eternal ideal now, since that would add a new suffering. Instead, it is about developing an intentional capacity to meet the present with courage and awareness. In so doing, we begin a process of transforming the mind. As we learn to attend carefully and intentionally to our present-moment world of experience, we can step out of the grip of the impulsivity and reactivity that binds us to distress.

Attention Can Be Trained, but Is Also, in Part, Automatic

Attention's automaticity is necessary, freeing us from having to pay deliberate attention to everything, which would be impossible. As outlined in detail in Chapter 2, attention alerts us quickly and automatically to any stimuli that need urgent attention (threat and pain are two obvious examples). More than this, much of what we do routinely day-to-day is done automatically, in the background beyond awareness (registering temperature and maintaining balance are two obvious examples). This automaticity enables us to process a great deal of complex information throughout the day without being overwhelmed. Although this automaticity is a great asset, it is potentially also a liability. For example, the attention of someone who is prone to anxiety will be drawn to threat and a sense of vulnerability; his or her awareness can unknowingly become clouded by biases, allowing reactivity to blossom. This is true for all of us to a greater or lesser degree; our attentional biases, unknown and unchecked, color our experience.

When we stabilize our attention, our unfolding moment-by-moment experience slows down. We can see the content and processes of the mind more clearly. It provides the possibility of responding with freshness, insight, and discernment. Mindfulness training encourages greater familiarity with the mind, enabling us to see that attention structures and is structured by our world. By shining light on both the *what* and the *how* of the mind (Chapter 5), we see stimuli more clearly as they enter our awareness because we are more attuned to our bodily sensations, emotions, thoughts and images, and behavioral impulses. We can start to see the moments when we label experiences as pleasant, unpleasant, or neutral. We can see our discrepancy monitoring and evaluation kick in. These are the moments when the second arrows of suffering are fired (Chapters 4 and 5). We see how distress and suffering are created and perpetuated (the vicious flower; Chapter 5).

The formal exercises in mindfulness programs are intended to train attention, first by stabilizing it, and then by providing the space for these insights to emerge. For example, the body scan involves moving the beam of attention through the body—with qualities of curiosity, care, and patience, as well as a disciplined steadiness—noting each time our mind wanders and then firmly, but kindly, escorting our mind back to the body. This practice involves holding the flashlight beam steady, focusing the lens with the attitudes of curiosity, friendliness, and care, so that we can really see what is there. Over time, this kind of practice builds our capacity to choose where and how to deploy our attention. It also reshapes our mind so the attitudinal dimensions of curiosity, care, and patience become second nature.

Like stepwise improvements in telescopes over centuries, mindfulness training over weeks and months can stabilize our attention so we see ever-greater detail in our experience. This is true both in a static sense, where in any given moment we can discern greater granularity in our experience, and also in terms of the dynamic shifts in the landscape of our minds over time.

When Sophia's inner critic is triggered, she has learned, in that moment, to discern and parse present-moment bodily sensations, emotions, mental events, and impulses. At these times, rather than being triggered into reactivity, she is able to see the unfolding process, the moments when the experience is powerfully labeled as unpleasant, and the moment when different types of craving set in (e.g., to feel OK, to be the perfect teacher, mother, grandmother, wife). These are the moments just before the volley of second arrows are about to be fired. Each of these steps in the process, once seen, can potentially be prevented.

When attentional control is strengthened, we begin to have choices. In the gap between stimulus and reaction, we can choose to pause and consider the response that is most likely to be helpful. The more we are able to pause, the more we are inclined to bring (and feel confident bringing) intentional attention to our experience, giving ourselves the chance to exercise choice and act skillfully. We invoked William James (1890), one of the first psychologists, in Chapter 2, and come back to him again here since it is as good a description of the importance of attention in transformation as we can find.

"The faculty of voluntarily bringing back our wandering attention, over and over again, is the very root of judgment, character, and will. No one is compus sui if he have it not."

Mindfulness programs train this faculty precisely to support people to better understand, manage, and transform their minds. It is the first waypoint on the route map in a mindfulness training.

Ways of Knowing and Being

The beauty and mystery of this world only emerges through affection, attention, interest and compassion . . . open your eyes wide and actually see this world by attending to its colors, details and irony.
—ORHAN PAMUK (2002)

We can experience the world in different ways by engaging different modes of mind (McGilchrist, 2009; Teasdale, 1999; Teasdale & Barnard, 1993; Teasdale & Chaskalson, 2011a, 2011b). As we outlined in Chapter 3, we know the world experientially and conceptually. Experiential mode involves present-moment direct experience, continually unfolding moment to moment, with our experience forming and reforming, in all its embodied particularity. Conceptual mode, on the other hand, represents our world as abstract ideas, concepts, stories and narratives, and working models, allowing us to remember the narratives of our past and to plan for our future. It is often heavily language based and has a level of evaluation and analysis. McGilchrist (2009) uses the word *represent* to capture this sense of the mind-taking experience and *presenting it again* but conceptually. It is important to note that concepts can also be experienced in experiential mode, but here thoughts and images are like bubbles forming as a pot begins to boil, experienced in the moment as mental events, as passing phenomena.

Experiential and conceptual modes lead to profoundly different ways of knowing and being in the world. Each mode is supported by a different mental architecture and activates different brain structures and functions (McGilchrist, 2009). Like an orchestra, each mode uses a different combination of instruments, perhaps played in a different key. Rather like the conductor of an orchestra, we can intentionally choose to switch modes and create different sounds and mood—or in the case of the mind's climate, create different ways of knowing and being (Barnard & Teasdale, 1991). Different music creates different states of being—so, too, different modes of mind create different ways of being. Try the exercise in Box 6.1 to get a clearer sense of what we mean by the mind's climate.

BOX 6.1. Mindfulness Exercise: Noting the Mind's Climate

Pause just now, and turn your attention inward. Sense the climate of your mind right now. Does your mind feel agitated or calm, contracted or spacious? How aware have you been today of how the psychological climate has changed throughout the day, affected by a range of conditions you neither chose nor controlled? Sense how the climate of your mind is shaping the kind of thoughts that are present. Turn your attention to your body so that you can begin to sense how the mind's climate is imprinting itself on your body. You may begin to have a felt sense of how your body is impacted by agitation, and how it is impacted by calm.

Learning mindfulness involves first learning to see and recognize the climate of our minds. Are we in automatic pilot, running off habitual ways of thinking and behaving? Are we in a more receptive, present-moment aware-ness that can *be* with what is? Are we conceptual, ruminative, or overthink-ing things? Are we conceptual, but in a creative free-flowing mode of mind? Stabilizing and training our attention enables us to better see the current climate of our minds, including seeing:

- The mind switching in and out of modes;
- The space between stimulus and reactivity;
- The point at which stimuli are assigned a feeling tone (pleasant, unpleasant, or neutral);
- The beginnings of evaluative elaboration;
- The points at which the volley of second arrows of reactivity are fired; and
- The effects of this volley of second arrows.

Mindfulness training supports the development of this capacity to rec-ognize and begin to understand the *what and the how of the mind* (Chapter 5). But this understanding is not a form of introspective navel gazing; it is pragmatic—that is, it is developed to help us move toward well-being and flourishing, and out of suffering.

A good example is how we know and understand pain. Someone who suffers back pain may say, "My chronic back pain is excruciating," or "This pain will never go away." Whatever is directly sensed in the body is translated into the concept of *pain*, given an intensity rating of "excruciating" and a duration as "will never go away." It may even be associated with a personal identity: "I am a chronic pain patient." Although the direct experience is likely unpleasant, even agonizing, it is most likely more nuanced and dynamic than the concepts "back pain," "excruciating," and "chronic" convey, especially when placed together into the narrative of "I have excruciating and chronic back pain," or "I am a chronic back pain patient."

Mohammed used the core mindfulness practices to explore his mind and body. This enabled him to know his experience in a different way. What he noticed was that pain was stabbing, and pulsed, but was also fairly consistently in a particular part of his body. The sensations were no less unpleasant, but he discovered that in each moment it had a particularity and it changed from moment to moment. When Mohammed examined his pain experientially, he could observe more directly his bodily sensations, the thoughts that were like bubbles in a boiling pot of water ("This is unbearable"), and his understandable desire to fix or escape the sensations. When doing the body scan, he had an extraordinary insight: "In most moments there is more right with my body than wrong."

Mastering Both Modes of Mind

Mindfulness training involves knowing the landscape of our inner world by developing a deep familiarity with both the experiential mode of mind and the conceptual, verbal mode of mind. Over time, we can learn when they serve us well and when they become problematic. We can then use this understanding to navigate out of dis-ease and distress into greater well-being. This involves being able to intentionally orient our attention and switch modes.

While much of this shifting happens quite automatically, we can, to some degree, learn to bring these shifts under our intentional and voluntary control (Norman & Shallice, 1986). We are more likely to shift into an intentional, deliberate, controlled mode of processing when we are learning something for the first time (e.g., a skill like riding a bicycle) or when we want to analyze a situation quite deliberately (e.g., a decision we have to make or problem we have to solve). However, much of the time there is a large degree of automaticity (Bargh et al., 1996; Kahneman, 2011). Mindfulness practice enables us first to see these processes, and then train our attention so we can exercise choice when possible.

Mastering both modes of mind supports investigative awareness (Chapter 1). It enables an inquiry that is both conceptual and experiential, where ideas and their resonance in our feelings and body are given equal weight. With humility, we open to listening and learning from our experience. This is the work of investigative awareness both in our everyday life and in our mindfulness practice—namely, to stabilize attention and open up to conceptual and experiential ways of knowing and being, so that we can unlock the extraordinary potential of the mind to see, to understand, and to learn.

These inner shifts are not easy. The practicalities of mindfulness practice and the integration of new learning can be challenging. But even in the time frame of an 8-week mindfulness-based program, participants can find themselves experiencing profound changes in how they attend to experience. To learn that our well-being is something we can cultivate through mindfulness training is new for many of us. It offers us new choices in the face of difficult experiences, such as depression, pain, and long-term physical ill health, so that we are increasingly empowered to think and act differently.

For most years since her mid 20s, Sophia had gone on a silent mindfulness retreat as a way of stepping back from life, developing her mindfulness practice, and enjoying silence in a supportive community of other practitioners. These retreats supported her learning in numerous ways.

In the last few years, Sophia's retreats enabled her to see how her Parkinson's diagnosis was a vortex for anxiety and many of its symptoms acted as potent triggers for anxiety. A rush of thoughts was never far away: "How will this play out?"; "What do these symptoms mean?"; "I will miss my grandchildren growing up"; "I have so much I still want to do"; "I'm not brave enough to face the decline in my mind and body"; "People will see me as weak and needy."

On a mindfulness retreat, the silence, spaciousness, and teachers enabled Sophia over and over again to anchor her attention in her breath and body, to return to her direct moment-by-moment experience. Over the course of a retreat, the crushing grip of anxiety usually weakened, and she could relate directly to her mind and body. Yes, she had fatigue, tremors, and some loss of initiative, but there was also the richness of seeing and tasting. There was more right with her than wrong. This expansion of awareness opened a great sense of love for her husband, children, grandchildren, friends, and of life itself.

As well as being a teacher, Sophia was also a writer and had published a few short stories and some poetry. She loved learning, ideas, words, and language but always felt she sabotaged herself. One of the main things she learned through mindfulness retreats was how the pervasiveness of her harsh inner critic crippled her creativity, spontaneity, and productivity. As she moved between experiential and conceptual ways of knowing during the course of a retreat, she had a flow of creative ideas for short stories, books, and things to do with family and friends, a bucket list of things she wanted to do before her illness disabled her further. These were ideas she could hold in awareness and let go with a note to herself to perhaps journal them later that evening. Each time she was gripped by anxiety, she named it, using the anchor of her breath and body to avoid being overwhelmed. This was not always easy. Sometimes she was sucked right down into the vortex of anxiety before being able to steady herself. A sense of steadiness and ease emerged and began to stabilize, which she was able to carry into her life at the end of the retreat.

Knowing the experiential and conceptual modes of mind and being able to switch between them is empowering. It is quite liberating to be able to relate to difficult thoughts as just thoughts that arise, and then fade. Although thoughts can powerfully grip the mind, we can come to know that these same thoughts can be experienced as mental events in this moment. People learn that thoughts are not facts and that they do not have to have power over us.

The Three-Step Breathing Space

One of the key mindfulness practices learned in mindfulness-based cognitive therapy (MBCT) is the three-step breathing space (Figure 6.1; Segal et al., 2013). Try it and see for yourself by following the steps in Box 6.2.

The three-step breathing space has a number of functions and each step is important. Each time we take a three-step breathing space, we become aware of the particularity of our mind and body in any given moment—preoccupied, at ease, angry, interested, slothful, and so on. In his teaching, Chris Cullen describes this as "the many faces of the Breathing Space." As Heraclitis put it, we can never step into the same river twice, the river has changed and so have we. While the three-step breathing space's function is the same—to pause and come to our senses—our experience each time will be different and particular. Participants learn that it's a doorway to greater steadiness and also greater understanding. Like a series of doorways, it opens us up to a series of different rooms.

The key insight is that we can be in and know the world both experientially and conceptually. This capacity can enrich our lives.

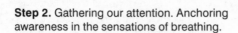
Step 1. Aware of our body sensations, moods/feelings, and thoughts.

Step 2. Gathering our attention. Anchoring awareness in the sensations of breathing.

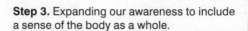
Step 3. Expanding our awareness to include a sense of the body as a whole.

FIGURE 6.1. The three-step breathing space.

BOX 6.2. Mindfulness Exercise: Three-Step Breathing Space

Step 1. Becoming Aware

Become more aware of how things are in this moment by deliberately adopting an erect and dignified posture, whether sitting or standing and, if possible, closing your eyes. Then bringing your awareness to your inner experience and acknowledging it, asking yourself:

- What **body sensations** are here right now?
- What **moods and feelings** are here?
- What **thoughts** are going through the mind?

Step 2. Gathering

Then redirecting your attention to focus on physical sensations associated with breathing. Bringing the mind to settle on the breath, wherever you feel it most vividly. Tuning into these sensations for the full duration of the in-breath and the full duration of the out-breath.

Step 3. Expanding

Then expanding the field of awareness around the breath, so that it includes a sense of the body as a whole, your posture, and facial expression.

As best you can, bring this wider awareness to the next moments of your day.

Note. Adapted from Teasdale, Williams, and Segal (2014, p. 183).

Responding Skillfully

A mindfulness teacher was asked, "What is the purpose of a lifetime of mindfulness practice?" She answered, "An appropriate response." Between stimulus and reactivity there is a gap. We have seen how when we live without awareness, reactivity can feed dis-ease and mental health problems. We get locked into trying to fix our dis-ease with well-intentioned, but ultimately unhelpful strategies, the petals of the vicious flower.

The three-step breathing space can in time support responsiveness. Stabilizing and anchoring attention, and opening more fully to the mind and body can be followed with questions like:

- "What does this moment need?"
- "How might you bring a wise and compassionate response to yourself and to your situation?"
- "What would support your well-being and the well-being of others?"

In the breathing space, these questions can yield a broader, more creative, wiser array of responses. These might include bringing the attention to the body, using the body as a way of turning toward difficulty rather than using the analyzing, conceptual mind. Although we are processing the same raw material, it is held within a different mode of mind, letting the deepest, wisest part of the mind–body do its own work.

Freedom from unhelpful negative thinking comes directly out of the three-step breathing space. During the three-step breathing space, we can decenter from our thinking by watching thoughts come and go, labeling thoughts (e.g., judging, planning, worrying, catastrophizing, perfectionism, all-or-nothing thinking, mind reading) and taking a more intentional, balanced perspective (e.g., "What would my wisest mind have to say about these thoughts?"). Finally, this space enables us to bring responsiveness to moments of happiness, humor, beauty, and love. We are better able to recognize and turn toward these experiences. "Ah, here is gladness . . . it's like this." Savoring and appreciating these experiences more fully, especially when felt in the body, can nourish us and support our well-being. We can then cultivate the habit of opening our eyes to all that is good in our lives, including the many blessings that we tend to overlook.

Stable attention shines light on the unfolding processes of the mind. It makes it possible for us to directly experience bodily sensations, thoughts, and feelings, and to see behavioral impulses as just that—impulses. We can then experience pain as pain and joy as joy. These stimuli can be experienced directly, moment by moment. This is the center of the vicious flower (see Chapter 5, Figure 5.6).

Turning toward and allowing the experience to be as it is, with patience, kindness, and care, is the beginning of a different kind of response. It can deactivate our discrepancy thinking and provide the space for craving to abate. It opens the possibility of a more embodied response, a response that draws on experiential knowing. It reveals our intentions and allows our response to be based in intentionality. Experiential mode of mind helps us slow down the dynamic mind, revealing the unfolding cascade of sensations, feelings, and thoughts. It creates the gap for us to respond in a way that is rooted in intentionality and imbued with friendliness and care.

Stable attention, interwoven with friendliness and care, alters our psychological landscape. It is what sets us on a path of responsiveness. We cease to divide the world, inwardly and outwardly, into friends and enemies, experiences to be pursued or avoided. Pain, dis-ease, discrepancy thinking, self-criticism, resentment, and conflict—all the habits of thinking and behavior that drive reactivity—are seen as just that, understandable but unhelpful habits. This cuts off at its source the patterns that trigger and maintain reactivity.

We discover that our capacity to establish caring and compassionate relationships in the world is deeply rooted in our capacity to establish a caring and compassionate relationship with ourselves. Over time, our capacity for skillful responding and our confidence grow.

Being more responsive does not just help us deal more effectively with the first arrows of pain and dis-ease. It also opens us up to the moments and experiences that uplift our heart and mind, such as the lovely, moments of joy, beauty, accomplishment, and love. These moments are recognized, allowed, and savored. It is not rocket science. Like gardening, whatever we cultivate will flourish. If we cultivate the plants to produce vicious flowers, they will flower. But joy, connection, and beauty can equally be cultivated through providing the right conditions—stable attention, attitudes of curiosity, patience and care, and savoring—an alternative to both the Velcro and the Teflon mind. Like water, light, and nutrients for a garden, mindfulness deployed skillfully enables the mind and body to flourish.

The more we cultivate the conditions for responsiveness, the more likely it is to happen. What the mind attends to, and is inclined toward, is what shapes the mind. Importantly, responsiveness is an antidote for fear, anxiety, and disabling reactivity.

The key insight is that mindfulness training creates a space in which we can choose to respond more skillfully.

Reappraisal, Insight, and Wisdom

The introduction of mindfulness into our psychological landscape reveals that the story and narrative that had previously seemed like fixed *reality* is a process that is unfolding and dynamic, open to change and possibility. This is a radical insight because it redefines our beliefs and views them as *processes* instead of fixed entities.

Reframing perception and views was the fourth function of mindfulness we set out in Chapter 1. Habitual reactivity freezes us into self-descriptions, views of the world, and identities within that world that are broken, tangled, and imperfect.[2] The first transformative step of mindfulness is to loosen the grip of identification and identity formation by attending to the moment free of bias and preference. Reframing our perceptions and views, which we refer to as decentering,[3] is a movement toward health.

Ling's work in the court system, a cauldron of suffering, was stressful. Given her history and sensitivities, exposure to this suffering day after day was

particularly trying for her. There was a path not far from the courts that took
Ling up into some hills around the city. Often during her lunch break, she
would take a brisk walk up into the hills where she would sit on a bench and
eat her lunch. From this vantage point, she could look down at the town and
see the city's courts, town square, shopping district, and suburbs. Looking down
on the courts in this way enabled Ling to put into perspective the stresses and
challenges of her day. It helped her to decenter from the stress and suffering of
the many upsetting cases she listened to throughout her working day. It took a
few years, but Ling eventually came to see that she needed to find a new job—a
job that nourished her and provided her with the space to be there for her teenage children in a way no one was there for her as a teenager.

Mindfulness training enables us to decenter, to see our experiences from
a different perspective, from a new vantage point. This can be as we saw
with Ling at the level of life choices, but also at the level of any momentary
experience. We are able to see our experience like Ling did while sitting on a
bench looking down on her hometown. This allows greater clarity and understanding, and in time can enable greater equanimity and responsiveness. Normally, our experience is foregrounded and awareness itself is backgrounded.
With decentering, this is reversed. By bringing awareness into the foreground,
our experiences can be held in a wider field of perception. Instead of being
stressed, sad, in pain, driven, or carried away by addictive impulses and/or suffering, we can recognize and hold these states in our field of awareness—"Ah,
here is stress, sadness, suffering. . . ."

We do not have to be the person we believe ourselves to be. Nor are we
obliged to strive to be the person we feel we should or ought to be. With mindfulness, we discover that just as our mind is a process, our sense of our *self* is
also a process, impossible to adequately pin down by any one definition. Over
time, we learn new ways of knowing, using both experiential and conceptual
ways of knowing, and we develop wisdom as we come to see first that experiences, including the experience of a fixed self-identity, are impermanent.

A healthy mind is malleable and flexible, not gripped by reactions but
able to investigate and question present-moment experience. Like the hands
of a skillful artisan shaping a piece of clay on a potter's wheel, we too can
shape our minds. As we discussed, mindfulness develops our capacity to discern and investigate the state of our mind in the present moment. It helps
us recognize unhelpful patterns of anxiety, agitation, and aversion, as well as
patterns that we have engaged with for years, or ones that are generational.
Yet just because something has a long history does not mean it has an equally
long future. Learning to see a thought as a thought, a feeling as a feeling, and
a sensation as a sensation helps us develop a capacity for flexibility rather than
rigidity, for responsiveness rather than reactivity. Whereas reactivity is rooted

in past experience and imagined future experiences, responsiveness is rooted in our capacity to engage with the present moment, just as it is, free from the burden of association.

A healthy mind is a mind that is a friend that we need not fear. It is characterized by a sense of well-being, ease, and the capacity to embrace difficult emotions and mental states without being overwhelmed. A healthy mind is a resilient mind that can be deeply touched by affliction, yet able to meet it with balance and compassion. Mindfulness is not indifference. Although we may be touched and saddened by loss, disappointment, illness, and separation from those we love, we come to learn that moments of pain and sorrow are never the end of the story. We can continue to breathe, to move through life and to love, without being broken.

When we analyze problems in overly conceptual ways, we produce a lot of hot air, but not much nourishment or insight. Having stable attention and bringing care to our inner and outer worlds help us see things more clearly, so we are better able to find answers to the question "What does this moment need?"

Stabilizing and then accessing a more expansive experiential mode can clarify what this moment needs. It is common for people to say, "Ah, it is much clearer now. I can't believe how much I was overthinking this." As we learn to address problems in this new, helpful way, the more likely we are to discover new beliefs and try new approaches. For example, new beliefs develop, such as "This, too, shall pass" and "I have faith that it will turn out OK."

Through formal mindfulness practice and also by applying the learning in everyday life, we come to see that what feels intractable and worrisome is, in fact, something that is temporary and/or something that we have to accept that we have no control over. This is illustrated by one of the cognitive therapy strategies for people who suffer generalized anxiety disorder (repetitive, uncontrollable worry about almost everything, small and large; Beck, Emery, & Greenberg, 1985). People with this disorder are asked to write their worries down, put them in a jar, and then return to them later, perhaps a week later. They come to see that what dominates their mind today can seem trivial a week later. The issue that had preoccupied them has usually passed and is no longer so relevant or important; today something different may be dominating their mind. The key learning—for people with generalized anxiety disorder—is that their distress did not stem from the *content* of the worry, but rather the *process* of their mind latching on to something like Velcro and then repetitively, uncontrollably, trying to solve it conceptually. In some ways, generalized anxiety disorder is a caricature of all our mind's tendencies. The insight is that this is optional; we can decenter from worry and cultivate different, more helpful ways of knowing and responding.

As I (CF) approached the counter in the post office, I was aware of a young woman approaching from the opposite direction. I invited her to go first and a startled look came over her face as she said, "That's amazing." I asked what was so amazing and she replied, "I am the kind of person people never see and they always jump ahead of me in line."

Identities can have a long history, rooted in distress. Self-identity is also shaped in the moment through identifying with prevailing thoughts and emotions that are endowed with authority. To see reactivity and not feed it and instead sow and cultivate responsiveness are moments that have within them the seeds of change. In the case of the woman in the post office, she can *lift her gaze* to more fully see and be seen by others.

The key insight is that mindfulness training can create important shifts in perspective about ourselves, others, and the world.

Embodiment

The route map to well-being leads to embodiment. Embodiment occurs when there is an alignment among our intentions, thoughts, physical bodily expression, and actions. Stephen Pinker (1997), a cognitive neuroscientist, describes this as a "society of mind," applying the analogy of functional societies that have shared understandings, systems, and collective action. So, too, the mind can function as a healthy society. When this happens, we can be present with a certain ease of being, living with intentionality, presence, and care. Embodiment is fundamental to mindfulness training and we dedicate a whole chapter to it (Chapter 8).

The key insight is that mindfulness in its deepest sense is about more than attention and attitudes of mind. It is also a way of being in the world with clarity, care, and ease—a state of being that can be characterized as calm abiding.

How Mindfulness Programs Support This Transformative Journey

The waypoints on our route map to transformation are stabilizing attention, new ways of knowing and being, responding skillfully, reappraisal, insight, and wisdom, and embodiment. How do the structure and core components of a mindfulness program support people in moving through each of these way-points? Mindfulness programs are structured to enable participants to learn each of the key building blocks in turn. Mindfulness programs typically start by examining everyday activities (e.g., eating) to illustrate how much of our experience is beyond awareness and how much of our lives are lived on automatic pilot. Early mindfulness practices begin to stabilize our attention and teach skills to help us recognize and understand how our mind and body can create distress and perpetuate suffering. Both the mindfulness practice and teacher's embodiment help us to develop an ability to turn toward experience with friendliness and care.

Later sessions map out how suffering is created and maintained, and participants begin to apply their learning to stepping out of habits of thinking and behaving that perpetuate suffering. Capacity and confidence grow alongside more stable attention and a shift in perspective. These later sessions support participants to consider what sustains and nourishes them so we are better able to apply all we have learned in our lives beyond the end of the mindfulness program.

In Chapter 1, we said that learning mindfulness is like a kayaker learning to navigate a turbulent river. The structure of mindfulness training is like providing training in kayaking as well as a route map for the river. The practices and exercises teach the kayaking skills, applying them in ever more challenging situations. Over time, this enables the kayaker to have the understanding and skills to navigate the river, anticipate problems, and safely find a way through turbulence and danger. The aim is that by the end of the program, participants have developed the understanding and competencies to navigate in the mainstream of their lives.

Mindfulness programs have essential ingredients that define their intentionality, underlying theoretical premise, content, and pedagogy, alongside ingredients that can be tailored for particular contexts and populations (Crane et al., 2017; see Table 6.1).

Mindfulness programs are structured intentionally so that across the sessions there is a program of sequenced and incremental learning. We set out some of the prototypical learning and session content in a mindfulness program in Table 6.2.

Challenges and Hindrances

There are predictable challenges in learning mindfulness. They are not problems that block the route, but are part of the path we walk when learning mindfulness. The challenges include impatience, boredom, agitation,

TABLE 6.1. The Essential and Flexible Ingredients of Mindfulness-Based Programs

Essential	Flexible
• Is informed by theories and practices that draw from a confluence of contemplative traditions, science, and the major disciplines of medicine, psychology, and education. • Is underpinned by a model of human experience that addresses the causes of human distress and the pathways to relieving it. • Develops a new relationship with experience characterized by present-moment focus, decentering, and an approach orientation. • Supports the development of greater attentional, emotional, and behavioral self-regulation, as well as positive qualities, such as compassion, wisdom, and equanimity. • Engages the participant in a sustained intensive training in mindfulness meditation practice, in an experiential inquiry-based learning process, and in exercises to develop insight and understanding.	• The core essential curriculum elements are integrated with adapted curriculum elements and tailored to specific contexts and populations. • Variations in program structure, length, and delivery are formatted to fit the population and context.

Note. From Crane et al. (2017, p. 993).

sleepiness, craving a more pleasant experience, worry, and doubt. When we recognize and work with these challenges, we can stabilize our attention and deepen our understanding. We outline the most typical challenges in Table 6.3, alongside suggestions of ways to respond and work with each challenge.

All of these typical challenges benefit from being recognized for what they are, understood in terms of the *what* and the *how* we outlined in Chapter 5, and met with stable, friendly, and caring attention. Challenges can teach us about the mind and how distress is created and perpetuated. Working with them also teaches us how distress can be ameliorated and how obstacles can be met and overcome.

Much of the force of these challenges comes from their habitual nature. The vicious flower analogy can be used to really see these challenges clearly. Although seeing and interrupting habits is not easy, doing so robs challenges of much of their power and creates a space in which alternatives can emerge. We can see that beneath and around the challenging state lies a realm of possibilities. Rather like shining a flashlight in the forest, we shine the flashlight beam of our attention first on the challenging situation—perhaps ensuring a lens of friendly curiosity is in place on the flashlight beam—and then we can choose to expand the awareness or shift it elsewhere. Like any well-ingrained habit we have to be persistent and patient, because it takes time to change.

TABLE 6.2. Outline of a Prototypical Mindfulness Program, with Indicative Session Topics, Key Learning, and Core Mindfulness Practices

Session topic	Key learning	Key session and home practice content
1. Waking up from automatic pilot	• Automatic pilot • Stabilizing attention • Attitudinal dimensions of mindfulness	• Welcome, introductions, and orientation • Raisin exercise • Body scan • Home practice: body scan, routine activity
2. Another way of being: keeping the body in mind	• Stabilizing attention • Attitudinal dimensions of mindfulness • A new way of knowing and being, experientially • How the mind creates meaning	• Body scan • "Thoughts and feelings" exercise • Home practice: body scan, experiences calendar
3. Gathering the scattered mind	• Stabilizing attention • Attitudinal dimensions of mindfulness • A new way of knowing and being, experientially • Coming home to our senses through mindfulness practice • Bringing mindfulness into everyday life	• Seeing/hearing exercise • Sitting practice and mindful movement • Breathing space • Mindful stretching • Home practice: mindful movement and sitting practices, breathing spaces, experiences calendar
4. Recognizing reactivity	• Stabilizing attention • Attitudinal dimensions of mindfulness • A new way of knowing and being, experientially • Recognizing and allowing reactivity • Learning experientially how cycles of reactivity play out to maintain and perpetuate distress and suffering	• Seeing/hearing exercise • Sitting practice • Breathing space • Mindful walking • Home practice: sitting practice and/or mindful movement, breathing spaces, experiences calendar, walking practice
5. Allowing and letting be	• Stabilizing attention • Attitudinal dimensions of mindfulness • A new way of knowing and being, experientially • Developing stability and spaciousness • Disempowering reactivity with allowing and befriending	• Sitting practice • Sitting and movement practices, explicitly including difficulties • Befriending practice • Poem: "The Guest House" (Barks & Moyne, 1997) • Home practice: sitting practice, working with difficulty, breathing spaces

(continued)

TABLE 6.2. *(continued)*

Session topic	Key learning	Key session and home practice content
6. Responding skilfully	• Stabilizing attention • Attitudinal dimensions of mindfulness • A new way of knowing and being, experientially • Responding with discernment and skillfulness • Reappraisal, insight, and wisdom: learning that thoughts are not facts	• Sitting practice • Psychoeducational exercises • Breathing space • Home practice: selection of guided practices, breathing spaces
7. How can I best take care of myself?	• Stabilizing attention • Attitudinal dimensions of mindfulness • A new way of knowing and being, experientially • Taking skillful action in the face of challenges • Learning to nourish ourselves • Cultivating compassion, joy, and equanimity • Reappraisal, insight, and wisdom	• Sitting and/or movement practice • Nourishing/depleting review and rebalancing • Breathing space • Mindful walking • Home practice: establish ongoing formal and informal mindfulness home practice pattern
8. Mindfulness for life	• Review of the course and key learning • Stabilizing attention • Attitudinal dimensions of mindfulness • A new way of knowing and being, experientially • Reappraisal, insight, and wisdom • Embodiment planning for ongoing learning and practice	• Body scan • Course review • Personal reflections questionnaire • Resources for maintaining and sustaining practice • Concluding mindfulness practice
9. Beyond the 8-week course	• Maintaining and sustaining practice • Revisiting the program but with greater depth and building • Appreciation/gratitude, befriending, compassion, and mindfulness in everyday life • Fuller application and integration into life: embodying what has been learned	

Note. Many mindfulness programs include a full day of mindfulness practice around Sessions 6 and 7 to enable people to drop into an extended period of practice, experiencing directly the nourishing effects of extended mindfulness practice and consolidating their learning.

TABLE 6.3. Challenges Present in Mindfulness Practice and Ways of Working with Them

Challenge	Response
Craving for pleasant experiences and stimulation	Cultivating interest in present-moment experience in the body and mind; seeing clearly the experience of craving, desire, and wanting. When is it present? When is it absent? What happens just before it arises? What happens as it passes by? What are the links in the chain of our experience? If we follow the links of the chain, where does it take us? What links can be broken? What happens when we break them? Beginning to find a greater sense of ease and well-being in the body and mind, as it is. Exercising letting go and restraint.
Aversion, wanting things to be other than how they are, anger, criticism of ourselves and others, and continual harsh judging	Befriending the difficult and turning toward it, allowing the experience to be there exactly as it is, but cultivating curiosity, patience, and equanimity. Bringing compassion to our experience. The same questions can be posed as with craving for pleasant experiences. When is aversion present? When is it absent? What happens just before it arises? What happens as it passes by? What are the links in the chain? If we follow the links of the chain, where does it take us? What links can be broken? What happens when we break them? Consider shifting attention to another object that elicits appreciation, gratitude, or joy.
Restlessness and worry	Learning to sustain attention in body and mind; steadying, stabilizing, and anchoring attention with qualities of patience, discipline, and care (this hindrance often has deep roots). There is a need here to bring concentration and energy into balance, so there is enough concentration and stabilized energy to respond to restlessness. It can help to have quite precise concentration by choosing a very particular object for attention and really drawing attention to this object with steadiness. Knowing that we can hold restlessness in awareness, perhaps with some care or humor, can be helpful too: "Ah, here you are, restless mind, I see you." As with aversion, really looking into the body and mind.
Numbness, boredom, and sleepiness	Moving attention to the body. Invigorating the mind and body either with mindfulness practices such as intentional and active practices that cultivate attention (e.g., opening the eyes if they are closed, or really closely sensing the breath) or getting some fresh air or movement of the body. Choosing an object of attention that supports alertness and staying steadily with this object. Knowing that this hindrance is about withdrawal is helpful, enabling us to see that the mind is trying to protect itself like a rabbit backing into its warren. If we are very tired, rest!

(continued)

TABLE 6.3. *(continued)*

Challenge	Response
Doubt	Not buying into doubt but instead looking deeply into the bodily sensations, feelings, and thoughts that comprise and are precursors to doubt. Experientially learning the capacity to respond with mindfulness to doubt, rather than habitually. Learning to step out of the narrative of doubt through sustaining attention within the body. Crucially, first recognizing and then seeing doubt for what it is: *a layer of thinking that obscures our direct experience.*

Some challenges undermine and sabotage our intentions and aspiration. In developing a mindfulness practice, many practitioners report a sense of relief in learning about them, understanding they are not just personal challenges but universal patterns that are part of anyone's experience when they stop and begin to look at their minds. We develop a simple knowing when craving, ill-will, dullness, doubt, and agitation are present, and also when they are absent. We know with mindfulness that these are not static states, nor do they define us (e.g., "I am not a lazy person"), but like everything else they are states that arise and pass (e.g., "Laziness and apathy come and go"). We begin to develop the capacity to meet these changing patterns with mindfulness and care, rather than being overwhelmed by them or identifying with them. When met with friendly curiosity, these patterns can be investigated and we can learn a lot through the investigation itself.

These hindrances and challenges help us develop attentional control, attitudinal dimensions of mindfulness, and understanding. Repeated practice in the face of challenges (e.g., agitation and doubt) develops our capacity for sustaining attention. Understanding comes from seeing how the body and mind states arise and pass away. This work, though, is nuanced and subtle. Dullness and fatigue may be the result of being overextended in our lives. The *solution* to dullness and fatigue, however, is not always to slow down or withdraw, but can also be to question how we live our lives. Doubt can also support us in asking key questions in our life and our practice. We may find it is rooted in a deep sense of doubting ourselves or others, disabling our capacity to trust, commit, and develop a sense of capacity for connection and love.

Mindfulness teaches us to develop our capacity for sensitivity and appreciation, qualities quite distinct from the sensual craving employed to solve discontent. Although we may be appropriately disturbed in the face of suffering, this can lead to skillful responses, rather than automatic aversion.

The key insight is that when we become aware of our minds and bodies and start the work of stabilizing and transforming the mind, we inevitably meet certain challenges—meeting these with aware-ness, friendliness, and care is an important part of mindfulness.

In this chapter, we outlined the transformation and route map through a mindfulness training program. We now conclude with some illustrative exam-ples of what this journey might look like, highlighting the waypoints.

In this first example, one of us (WK) was teaching Session 6 of a mindfulness program for a group of people with a history of recurrent depression. I was sup-porting participants *to stabilize their awareness* on the breath in the body "as best you can, attending to your breathing, as it is experienced in your body, just now, nowhere to be, nothing to achieve, simply being with, attending to moment by moment this breath . . . breathing in, breathing out." This practice was intended to develop the intentional choice of awareness, choosing to focus on the breath, steadying attention.

While we were practicing, a bee flew into the room and started to fly around, the sounds of its flight moving around the room, and I looked up. It was not agitated, simply flying around, and while I was sure most would be aware of the bee, no one in the group looked visibly panicked. Aware that this bee had probably hijacked many people's attention, I decided to use it as a teaching moment. "Noticing where the mind is just now, if it is taken by hear-ing and noticing the sounds, their tone, volume, where they are in the room, where they begin, end . . . the breath all the while as an anchor." I wanted to encourage people to *recognize reactivity and be with their experience, to create a space between stimulus and reaction, and know it experientially.*

The bee was flying around and then settling, so the sound was coming and going and moving around the room. When it flew past my head, I myself had a sense of fear rising and then easing as it flew past and settled. This hap-pened three or four times. "As you bring awareness to listening, noticing what happens in the mind and body, in this moment . . . and this moment . . . As best you can, attending to the sounds, as sounds with volume, pitch, experienc-ing them in space, near, far, left, right . . . Noticing where the mind is just now, how it is with your experience, *bringing patience and affectionate curiosity to your experience. . . .*"

In the inquiry following the practice, one person described his experience: "When the bee came in, I had a strong impulse to get something to swat and kill it. [Reactivity] But I followed your invitation and noticed how the sound had just taken me into a place of fear and annoyance. I thought to myself, 'Is this bee going to sting one of us?'; 'Why can't they shut the windows so our mindfulness practice isn't interrupted?' [Conceptual understanding and judg-ing] But as I stayed with it, I could see how these thoughts and feelings were spiraling, quite powerfully, and I was gripped by a fix-it mode that was compelling. [Unpleasant tone, craving, and impulse to fix]

But when I slowed down, the sounds became a rich tapestry of experience, so pressing and insistent, and then each time the bee settled somewhere, my thoughts and feelings slowly settled down, too. [Experiential knowing] I noticed how automatically my mind stepped up and settled down as the bee flew and settled. My body followed, agitated and gripped, and then easing. You know, as the practice went on, after about 5 minutes or so, I could actually begin to have experiences alongside the bee, of my breath as an anchor. I looked up to see others sitting here looking so steady, which supported me to be steady. With this cool sense of steadiness I could see it all playing out. [Reappraisal and insight] It was extraordinary to just step out of what every fiber in my body wanted to do, swat the bee." [Different response; choosing to do nothing is a response]

With mindfulness we begin to discern the distinction between the *story* of what is being experienced and the *actuality* of the moment. The example above shows how mindfulness practice, even during a seemingly trivial experience, enables this transformation. The sound of a bee is experienced as a sound that changes and moves, and that over time, the sound can be experienced alongside other experiences. Thoughts such as "Why can't they shut the windows?" and strong impulses to swat or escape the bee are seen as thoughts and impulses, arising and inevitably, with time and steadiness, falling away.

In the same way, Ling's plummeting mood, Sam's craving, Mohammed's stabbing back sensations, and Sophia's inner critic can all be seen as a matrix of experience that is constantly changing rather than a solid entity that defines us. Mindfulness enables a new way of knowing, supporting decentering from our states and experiences. We learn that we are not our bodily sensations, thoughts, impulses, emotions, or moods. They can be seen and held in the light of awareness. Thoughts arrive uninvited—impulses and bodily sensations appear and fade, often beyond the realms of our control. The agitated thinking that creates and re-creates distress begins to calm as we increasingly learn to cultivate a sustained, present-moment experience. As the mind calms, so, too, does the body begin to calm. Mindfulness brings an experiential awareness of change, softening the tendency to react to what is often reified through identification.

This new way of knowing, paired with affectionate curiosity, allows a more friendly and caring relationship to mind and body to emerge. We can begin to see that our patterns of judgment and self-blame are habits that create further distress, and that we merit compassion rather than self-criticism. Awareness of the coexistence of different experiences at any given time challenges the belief that the difficult has to disappear for wellness to appear. They coexist and we can choose where we place our attention. We can begin to embody the whole of our experience.

When Sophia had her "breakdown" in her 20s, the first step in her recovery involved seeing her family doctor and starting on a course of antidepressant medication. Over several weeks, the vice of anxiety and depression that had gripped her mind loosened. Even though she started doing a bit better, she barely comprehended what had happened. At the suggestion of her family doctor she started cognitive-behavioral therapy. She learned how powerful imagery drove her anxiety, how pervasive her inner critic could be when she was low. Her therapist taught her a range of strategies for challenging her negative thinking. She gradually returned to her teaching job with the support of her school principal and colleagues.

In her late 40s, when her family had grown up, Sophia decided to train as a mindfulness teacher. Training as a mindfulness teacher starts with going through an 8-week mindfulness program as a participant, learning mindfulness from the inside out. In these 8 weeks, Sophia learned a lot more about her inner critic and how powerfully it had shaped her life. She learned how her mind could create and exacerbate mind states that fueled anxiety and depression. She developed a familiarity with her inner critic that had always been just below the surface, ready to pounce on any thought or action, stifling her creativity and spontaneity. She learned to befriend her inner critic and to respond with compassion to herself.

Sophia used what she learned in her life more generally: to live with greater meaning, compassion, and dignity. She came to see that the understanding and strategies that she first learned to help her with anxiety and depression in her late 20s could be combined with what she learned in the mindfulness program to help her in her life more generally, in her work as a teacher, in her relationships with friends and family, and in managing the inevitable challenges of life, ill health, and aging.

After training as a mindfulness teacher, Sophia worked part-time teaching mindfulness classes to people in the community, and established weekly evening mindfulness practice groups for all the graduates of her mindfulness classes. These became quite an event; sometimes the room would be packed to capacity with graduates returning to deepen their learning and join in the sense of community.

In her 60s, Sophia was diagnosed with Parkinson's disease. She said to her family doctor: "Even though I know the Parkinson's disease is going to wreak havoc on my life and take me to some dark places, I can't imagine ever going down into depression again." Her doctor, surprised, asked her how she could know that and she replied, "My mindfulness practice has given me a deep faith in my capacity to manage even the most frightening and darkest thoughts and feelings. I know deep down they will pass—my life has much more meaning than that."

Sophia told a story about how her Parkinson's tremor meant she knocked over a cup of tea in her living room.

"I was in my living room this week with my grandson, Noah, and Rufus, my dog. Noah was playing with his trucks and Rufus was asleep in his bed. I had put the mug on the arm of the chair where I was sitting because my tremors were quite bad, but it crashed to the floor. The tea spilled and the mug's handle broke. Rufus looked up from his bed, came over to see what had happened, sniffed the liquid to see if it was worth drinking, decided no and then went back to his bed. Noah looked on with delight at the whole scene, the noise, the cup breaking, the spill, and the dog's reaction. He came over as well to explore the situation in much the same way, although he used his hands to explore the liquid, mug, and broken handle. I watched this really interested as Rufus and Noah did not react the way I instinctively had.

"When I knocked the mug over I had an automatic reaction of horror and anger, and before I knew it, the words formed in my head: 'You stupid idiot.' When I was a girl, there were such high standards in my home. My parents wouldn't tolerate mistakes and I would feel so ashamed when I did something wrong. If I did something wrong, I would be chastised. Over time I learned to chastise myself. If I did something 'wrong,' it always produced a powerful reaction of 'Uh oh, I am going to get into serious trouble. Why am I such a stupid idiot?', with a palpable sense of horror.

"But this time, I saw the mug fall, and did not react. In that short space, I had a chance to respond differently. I was also interested to see how Rufus reacted and how Noah reacted. Noah's parents, my son and daughter-in-law, are balanced and caring; he hasn't internalized the same self-critic I have. He was just curious, even joyful in this interesting experience. All three of us in this little scene—me, Noah, and Rufus—had an initial experience as our attention was drawn to the spill and broken mug (the first arrow). My mind was ready to fire a second arrow stemming from what I had learned growing up: 'I should behave perfectly, making mistakes is evidence of stupidity.'

"Instead of chastising myself or getting upset, I chose to get down on the ground with Noah and we laughed together. It was a wood floor, so no harm had been done. I want Noah to have good memories of me and, more than that, I want him to be happy, without being crippled by the inner critic that has been part of me for so long. Moments like this suggest he will have this gift, which gives me great joy. I mostly did OK with my son, but Noah seems so together, so happy—that gives me great joy."

Each of these examples illustrates the transformative journey and the waypoints along the journey. A participant in one of our classes said, "It changed me in just about every way possible" (Allen et al., 2009). Our life experiences will, of course, be unique to each of us, but there are many commonalities in how our minds create distress and suffering and also joy and a journey to flourishing and well-being.

SYNOPSIS

Our key premise is that mental health and well-being are supported when we learn to stabilize and harness our attention, intentionally and effectively. We access new ways of knowing and being, both experiential and conceptual, and master when and how to shift between them. Mindfulness training enables us to intentionally and effectively deploy our attention, and opens up a space that enables greater discernment, wisdom, and responsiveness (see Figure 6.2).

Many of the philosophical, contemplative, and religious traditions have a version of this imploration:

> Grant me the serenity to accept the things I cannot change,
> the courage to change the things I can, and
> the wisdom to know the difference.

The transformation that takes places through mindfulness training is intended to support this understanding, acceptance, courage, and discernment. It supports new ways of knowing and being. Finally, it cultivates the conditions for living our lives with greater friendliness, compassion, joy, and equanimity, which we explore next in Chapter 7.

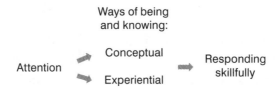

FIGURE 6.2. The transformational journey of change in mindfulness-based programs.

CHAPTER 7

The Heart of the Practice

BEFRIENDING, COMPASSION, JOY, AND EQUANIMITY

> Out of the soil of friendliness grows the beautiful bloom
> of compassion, watered by the tears of joy and sheltered
> beneath the cool shade of the tree of equanimity.
> —LONGCHENPA (1976)

In Buddhist psychology, befriending, compassion, joy, and equanimity are pivotal to the transformation and liberation of the mind. These qualities are seen as the foundations of all our development as we embark on a path of mindfulness practice. They are seen as being potentialities and capacities of every human mind that can be cultivated, trained, and naturalized in the same way that attention can be trained and developed. In the face of great distress, though, befriending, compassion, joy, and equanimity can disappear just when they are most needed. In Buddhist teachings, these qualities are developed more explicitly so that they are available and effective when we need them the most. Regardless of how they are taught or learned, it is important they are learned for transformational change to occur.

When Mohammed's mind became contracted by his 24/7 pain, he could bring some steadiness to his experience and also care and friendliness.

In the midst of a flurry of negative thinking, Ling could anchor her attention in her body, a place that was now available to her as a refuge.

Sophia could draw on a lifetime of mindfulness practice to hold the tremors of Parkinson's with some equanimity.

Sam could recognize the triggers for addictive cravings. He could know, at an experiential level, that he did not want to revisit that rock bottom in his life where addiction had taken him—he had committed to living a better life.

144

In Chapter 5, we set out a map of how distress and suffering are created and maintained. In this chapter, we build on the route map of mindfulness training (Chapter 6) by exploring the four attitudes of mindfulness. These four attitudes, which are fundamental to mindfulness training, are:

1. Befriending: an intrinsic orientation of mind or underlying tendency toward experience that is curious, friendly, and kind;
2. Compassion: an orientation of mind that recognizes pain and the universality of pain in the human experience, and our capacity to meet that pain with kindness, empathy, equanimity, and patience;
3. Joy: an intrinsic attitude of mind that includes gladness of the heart, softheartedness, and tenderness. It supports a capacity for appreciation, contentment, and gratitude; and
4. Equanimity: a quality of inner balance imbued with awareness, care, and compassion that is fully engaged with the events of every moment, both inwardly and outwardly.

We conclude this chapter with a short overview of relevant psychological science.

Mindfulness Training and the Cultivation of the Four Attitudes of Mind

These four attitudes allow us to turn toward our reactivity and work with it. They help us create the conditions for flourishing. They are interwoven, as Longchenpa (1976) noted in the text that opens this chapter. They are in a chain reaction with intention, views, and ethics, and are the foundation on which we can walk the path of a mindful life.

Mindfulness training uses the fact that we have already experienced these qualities of mind, even if only momentarily in our lives. These are not abstract, remote, esoteric, or metaphysical concepts. Mindfulness makes understanding and wisdom *everyday*, something each of us can access in our own experience. We are always practicing something, and whatever we practice tends to grow stronger. So we may as well practice qualities of mind that support our well-being and the well-being of those around us.

Even in the midst of the most difficult and challenging times, there will have been moments when we have been touched by the kindness, the befriending of another, or we have been able to extend the hand of friendship to another. Compassion is no stranger to any of us. There are moments when we encounter distress and pain and sense an unhesitating compassion arise inwardly—moments when we have been touched by the care of another. Joy and appreciation are not unknown to us—they are qualities that gladden the mind, enabling us to delight in the loveliness we encounter, that lighten our hearts. In moments of difficulty, we have perhaps glimpsed the possibility of standing in the midst of all things with poise and balance, able to find an inner stillness. These moments of warmth, happiness, compassion, and poise cannot be contrived, yet they can be cultivated. We can learn and develop the inner capacity and intentionality that incline the mind toward the lovely, healing, and liberating qualities within us all. These qualities, like mindfulness itself, are always present-moment experiences; we do not experience yesterday's compassion or tomorrow's joy. They are a present-moment awareness, an immediacy of connection with our inner worlds and the life we live together with others.

These moments may be fewer and more fleeting than we would like and too often we find ourselves again immersed in habits of despair and struggle. Yet they are memorable, offering a glimpse of a way of being present in our life that is alive, receptive, and engaged.

These qualities of kindness, compassion, joy, and equanimity are the attitudinal foundations and qualitative tone of mindfulness. Without the conscious cultivation of these qualities, developed experientially, it is not mindfulness training. Cultivating these qualities plays a central role in freeing the mind from patterns that create and re-create distress.

The cultivation of these qualities takes mindfulness out of the classroom and into our lives. Because our lives are essentially relational, mindfulness concerns itself not only with inner development but also with a deepening awareness of how we engage with and participate in the world around us, with the people we care for, those we struggle with, and the many we do not know.

As Ling learned to respond to the reactivity of her mind and body, she could see the applications not only to her own well-being but her capacity to parent her children.

Sophia's mindfulness practice helped her to be more embodied as a school teacher and later as a mindfulness teacher.

Once Sam had stepped out of the reactivity of craving and addiction, he was able to see the people around him with new eyes, and start over with the relationships in his life.

Mohammed started by bringing kindness and care to his "pain." Over time, these qualities extended to his body as a whole, to all that was right with it, and to the moments of joy in his marriage, his parenting, his caring for his elderly mother, and his work. He put it this way: "I am . . . umm . . . aware more of what bits of my body are good and which aren't good, and it changes every time I do a body scan, if you know what I mean."

Mindfulness, resting on the foundations of kindness, compassion, joy, and equanimity, enables us to contribute those much-needed qualities to a world so deeply scarred by mistrust, alienation, and anxiety. The kind of relationship we have with ourselves, our own minds and bodies—whether imbued with anxiety, aversion, and agitation, or with care, compassion, appreciation, and balance—offers a microcosmic view of the relationships we form with others. Anxiety and aversion lead us to turn away from the world and withdraw from relationships. It is easy, for example, to understand how Mohammed's chronic and intense pain created an impulse to contract and withdraw. Care, compassion, joy, and equanimity have the opposite effect, inclining us to turn toward all moments of our experience with generosity, empathy, and intimacy, even in the midst of physical pain and psychological distress.

In the early texts, the word *meditation*[1] is translated as *cultivation*, or *to bring into being*. What is being cultivated through mindfulness practice is our capacity to be more awake and responsive, including our capacities for befriending, compassion, joy, resilience, and balance. These qualities are attitudinal commitments, intentions, cultivated inclinations, and practices that are developed and trained.

Remember: "That which we frequently dwell upon, to this does our mind incline." Mindfulness reveals to us where our minds most frequently dwell and the ways our attention inclines. Discernment reveals whether our habits of dwelling lead to distress or toward greater freedom and capacity. When we understand this, we cultivate the qualities of befriending, compassion, joy, and equanimity that are the foundations of easeful relationship, both inwardly and outwardly.

Ill equipped and underresourced, we find ourselves left feeling helpless and despairing in the face of vulnerability. We even learn individually and collectively to equate vulnerability with weakness and failure or self-blame. We learn to fear vulnerability. Heroically, we try to construct the *perfect* life that is invulnerable to change, uncertainty, and pain, but we often end up floundering because we can't control and protect ourselves from the awareness of our core vulnerability and from life itself. At other times we simply *escape* by engaging in personal and collective forgetfulness, filling our days with busyness and distractedness that distance us from the awareness that our lives could crumble in a moment.

Mindfulness training, however, can help us embrace vulnerability with understanding, kindness, compassion, joy, and equanimity. These are the keys to our freedom and to meeting life as it is, rather than how we wish it to be. Kindness, compassion, joy, and equanimity can be cultivated in the midst of the difficult, whether it be physical pain or chronic illness, the stress, anxiety, and depression that can beset us, the painful thoughts and emotions that we are prone to flee, and the conflicts with others that are an inevitable part of living and working with others. When Ling's teenage children are at their most challenging, for example, this is an opportunity for her to develop the capacity for responsiveness both to herself and in how she responds to her children. Kindness, compassion, joy, and equanimity can also be cultivated in the midst of moments of beauty, love, connection, and rapture, as well as the everyday. We are invited to explore the possibilities of standing in the midst of all of this with kindness and compassion, opening the door to the possibilities of ease and poise.

The key teaching is that mindfulness training cultivates four inter-woven qualities that are part of the attitudinal landscape of mind-fulness.

Befriending

Befriending involves being curious, friendly, and kind, and is a capacity that we can all develop toward ourselves and our experiences. It is available to all of us, and is "the home where our hearts and minds dwell" (Feldman, 2017, p. 12). Although befriending, compassion, joy, and equanimity are interwoven dimensions, befriending is the foundation for the other three—they only arise when we can establish a relationship of caring curiosity with all experience.

The root of the Pali/Sanskrit word *metta* helps us to understand the meaning of befriending; it can be translated as friendliness or *spreading out* with kindness. When translated as a verb, it means befriending all of our experience, whether it is pleasant, unpleasant, or neutral; befriending our relationship to ourselves and others; and befriending all events and circum-stances. It does not distinguish thinking, feeling, and action tendencies—rather, it is a friendly *heartfulness* that imbues our thinking and action tenden-cies. Befriending describes a way of being that is all-inclusive, of our minds and hearts as well as all that we encounter in the world, both the challenging and the lovely. Its affective tone is warmth and tenderness. Its underlying intentionality is uprooting ill-will and cultivating generosity, gratitude, and care. The *near enemy*[2] of befriending is conditional kindness, extended only to what we like and denied to what we don't like. The *far enemy* is ill-will, resentment, and hatred.

There is vulnerability in living in an unpredictable world of conditions that are endlessly shifting and that we cannot control. This feeds the craving to be an idealized person. If we look closely at the realities of pain, change, uncertainty, beliefs in insufficiency and unpredictability, and widen the field of our awareness to include all people, we see that there is no one who is exempt from these vulnerabilities.

The first psychological gesture of mindfulness is to turn toward present-moment experience so as to understand it—this is the first step in developing the willingness to meet vulnerability rather than to flee from it or fear it. The second gesture of mindfulness is to develop the capacity and willingness to stand near to present-moment experience with an attitude of *caring curiosity*, no matter how difficult the present experience.

Developing the capacity to befriend does not mean that we have to *like* the painful or the difficult. When we learn to stand near to it and befriend it without being overwhelmed, we become free to explore the landscape of the difficult. Befriending is the beginning of accepting our vulnerability. It is a fading of the familiar strategies and mechanisms of avoidance that are triggered by our fears of vulnerability and our concerns about worth, lovability, and abilities (the vicious flower we set out in Chapter 5).

Learning to befriend the moment with all of its challenges and to develop our capacity to meet vulnerability in a fearless way is an important step. This attitude of *caring curiosity* is taught through the language and guidance of skilled mindfulness teachers, encouraging a gentle, interested, and tender exploration of physical and psychological pain. Participants in mindfulness trainings discover that it is increasingly possible to approach their personal story of grief, pain, depression, and hopelessness with care and curiosity. During the group dialogue, they also discover that what they had thought was only their personal story of distress is actually a universal story of vulnerability. When Mohammed said in a mindfulness class, "I just don't know if I can live with this pain for the rest of my life," there was a ripple of recognition through the group of all those living with chronic illness—the ripple was as if to say, "We, too, know this territory." When Ling described negative thoughts (e.g., "I am a terrible parent and I am going to mess up my kids") as "wrecking ball thoughts," there was palpable relief as the others with a history of depression were able to relate to her powerful metaphor—a common thought: "We, too, have wrecking ball thoughts."

Instead of turning away from the difficult, students of mindfulness learn that it is possible to establish a dialogue of mindfulness and tenderness with it. This makes affliction approachable and the habits of flight, fear, and avoidance cease to be so automatic. Rather than abandoning or defending against distress, we discover that this, too, can be befriended. It is a powerful lesson to learn that aversion and resistance are not life sentences, and that they only compound pain. We come to understand that aversion makes us a hostage to pain, tied to the difficult events and experiences through an aversive and fearful narrative. Thoughts such as "I just don't know if I can live with this pain for the rest of my life" and "I am a terrible parent" create and re-create suffering. These are understandable thoughts, but they are wrecking ball thoughts that we can step back from, see with curiosity and care, and allow them to pass through awareness without being knocked down by them. Exploring the possibility of befriending the difficult allows the difficult to be seen as a dynamic, unfolding process that can be approached and understood.

Regardless of whether mindfulness is taught in a traditional or contemporary setting, the shift from aversion to befriending is the most radical shift any student of mindfulness can make. Befriending is the primary attitudinal commitment that students learn to return to again and again in the midst of all of the difficult emotional habits that mindfulness reveals. It is a challenging lesson to learn, yet it is also a practice. At the end of 8-week mindfulness programs, many students report that in the beginning, their greatest learning was to develop kindness as an attitude of mind. It can be incredibly empowering to realize that we can find kindness—toward ourselves, others, and our experiences—in the midst of bodily pain, challenging thoughts and emotions, and seemingly overwhelming life situations. *Friendly curiosity* does not necessarily change the contents of our experience. The difficult is not automatically transformed into something pleasant. What is transformed, however, is the climate of our mind. The mind rooted in kindness powerfully impacts our experience. As aversion begins to soften, the difficult becomes approachable.

Sam, the young man in recovery from addiction, had always suffered from psoriasis, a skin condition. When Sam first did a body scan practice, he came face-to-face with a familiar aversion when he was invited to turn toward the itchiness that was a symptom of his psoriasis. The urge to scratch was powerful, but he knew from experience that scratching could exacerbate the condition. It was a powerful and understandable impulse, but also one he recognized in many areas of his life.

In those first weeks of practicing the body scan, Sam followed the invitation to recognize, allow, and turn toward the discomfort and urge to scratch. This was an unfamiliar way of being for him; his habitual mode was to be reactive. It enabled him to become more familiar with the sensations on his skin, the strong aversive tendency that was automatic, and the impulse to rub and scratch. Instead of reacting, he tried to meet the urges with curiosity, patience, and friendliness. The sensations were not pleasant. As he turned toward his discomfort, he discovered that the sensations waxed and waned, and even had epicenters and edges; beyond the edges there was no itchiness.

Sam came to learn that it was possible to relate to his body with friendliness, that the discomfort was not only part of him but also sat alongside the many other sensations in his body that were available during the body scan practice. He started to see that he could respond to unpleasant sensations differently. This was the beginning of a cultivation of mind that enabled Sam over time to meet the much more powerful—and potentially devastating—cravings to return to addiction. Here, too, he learned he could befriend these cravings, riding the waves with a friendly curiosity and noticing that they, too, waxed and waned, albeit with much greater force.

In time, Sam learned that he could extend these same qualities to his external life. In the 12-step program, further along in recovery Sam needed to make amends to the people who had been harmed through his addiction. This ability to befriend difficulty was a key to being able to repair his relationships. It gave him resources to be patient, tolerate difficult thoughts and feelings, and provided enough spaciousness to navigate misunderstanding and potential for arguments as he made amends to the many people he had harmed in active addiction.

An eighth-century Buddhist monk and scholar (Shantideva, 1997) speaks to the cultivation of befriending in ourselves and others:

> Looking after oneself, one looks after others.
> Looking after others, one looks after oneself.
> How does one look after others while looking after oneself?
> By practicing mindfulness, developing it and making it grow.
> How does one look after oneself by looking after others?
> By patience, non-harming, friendliness and caring.

People entering into mindfulness programs seek ways to address struggle and distress more skillfully, so that they can develop a capacity to live their lives with a greater wakefulness, joy, and wholeheartedness. Learning to befriend all moments and events places us firmly in the life we are living, rather than the ideal moment we are prone to lean toward where we envisage that all difficulties have ended and all vulnerabilities have been resolved. Like the development of attention, the development of befriending is an intentional cultivation.

It is possible to approach the difficult with a *cold glare of attention*. However, this can be disguised aversion or skepticism. It is possible to engage with the same difficulty with a genuine willingness to touch it with an attentiveness that is tender, interested, and kind. This *befriends* the moment and all it holds. As we saw with Sam, the cultivation of befriending enables us to recognize and uproot our deeply ingrained reactivity. Instead of aversion or trying to fix, befriending is a radically different approach, an "orthogonal" rotation of mind, a way of being with that enables a transformation (Kabat-Zinn, 1990). Our minds impact our actions and in turn, our actions shape our hearts and minds.

As Sam rebuilt his relationship with his older brother, at times his mind could fill with reactivity and aversion, "He just doesn't understand how hard this is for me; he is still an active alcoholic. Why do I bother? It's his fault I even became an addict." Befriending these thoughts enabled Sam to exercise restraint and hold his tongue. This restraint, which he wouldn't have managed before, created a calm space where trust could be rebuilt between him and his brother, so that Sam could make amends and find peace in his own mind.

Sam came to understand that befriending, in speech and action, are intrinsically interconnected. On his fourth 12-step anniversary in recovery, he made a commitment for a year to ensure his speech was rooted in understanding and kindness. He committed to avoid gossip, speaking ill of others, or lying, no matter how small or well-intentioned. He found that people started to trust him more and turn to him with their confidences and vulnerabilities. He found his own self-respect growing; holding his counsel was a powerful training in becoming more aware of his own intentionality and values. He realized gossip and untruths were often driven by aversion and ill-will.

There will always be opportunities for us to renew our intention to befriend. It is not as if difficulties or aversion will cease—there will be ample opportunities to practice befriending in life, especially as aging inevitably brings with it illness and physical limitations, and difficult events will continue to present themselves. Befriending is a capacity that deepens with practice—the intrinsic capacity to be friendly with our experience is reawakened and increasingly available to us in times of difficulty and in times of meaning, connection, and love. Try the exercise in Box 7.1.

Compassion

We have all experienced moments of compassion when the heart softens in the face of pain, distress, and suffering, and when we can be open to the vulnerability that is part of the human experience. These moments can be close to home—such as when a child in our family is sick, or an elderly relative becomes increasingly frail—or on the world stage, such as when we hear about a devastating natural disaster or an innocent bystander grievously injured in an act of senseless violence. In these moments, the divide between self and other softens, the narratives of criticism and blame fade, and we inhabit, perhaps for a few fleeting moments, a world infused with kindness and compassion.

Compassion is "an orientation of mind that recognizes pain and the universality of pain in human experience and the capacity to meet that pain with kindness, empathy, equanimity and patience" (Feldman & Kuyken, 2011, p. 143). Its roots in Latin (*compati*) are to *suffer with*; this is similar to the

BOX 7.1. Mindfulness Exercise: Befriending

Pause for a moment and sense what is happening in your body and mind, what is happening around you. Quite intentionally adopt a posture that has a sense of openness, care, and dignity.

Attending to your body, sense how your body feels touching the chair, the touch of the air on your skin, any sensations in the face and shoulders. You might begin to sense what your mood is—perhaps tired, restless, or calm. The background whisper of thoughts or images becomes discernible. You may discover yourself becoming sensitized to the sights and sounds of the moment. Take a moment to stand back, be still, turning your attention to the life of the body with curiosity, patience, and care. Sense how the air and your clothing are touching your skin, the sounds you are hearing. Sense the posture of your spine, the expression on your face, the placing of your hands. Be mindful of the places in your body that are well and sense the easefulness of those places.

Expand your attention to the places in the body that feel contracted or painful. Explore what it is to tend to those places with care, curiosity, and kindness.

Now, if it is helpful, say a few phrases under your breath—not trying to change anything—just saying the phrases and seeing how things are for you:

"Safe and well."
"Contented and peaceful."
"Caring and kind."

Continue with this for as long as it feels appropriate, with your body as an anchor. Be mindful of how sensations are moment to moment, ebbing and flowing. Explore what it is to steady the attention within the body—standing or sitting—the body sensing, breathing. When your attention is drawn elsewhere, bring the same simple knowing—a thought as a thought, an image as an image—returning once more to an awareness of the body of the moment, just as it is, without demand or expectation.

Sense what it is to expand your attention to include the thoughts, images, and mood present in this moment, including the difficult, unpleasant ones that you are prone to become lost in or judge. Explore what it is to be mindful of all of this with the same caring attentiveness. If it is helpful, again bring forward the same simple articulated intentions:

"Safe and well."
"Peaceful."
"Caring and kind."

Remember, this is not about changing what is present, but about cultivating our capacity to befriend what is present. It is not about having a particular feeling, but about strengthening our capacity to care for what is present.

As you bring the practice to a close, form an intention to continue to practice in the midst of your day-to-day life.

Buddhist tradition where it is described as *the heart that trembles in the face of suffering.* Its affective tone is deep care, connection, and responsiveness. It is not, however, an emotion—rather, compassion is an understanding imbued with intention. Its underlying intentionality is the "wholesome movement of the mind and body that seeks to alleviate pain and suffering of beings . . . it is the spontaneous response of an open heart" (Goldstein & Kornfield, 1987, p. 99). The *near enemy* of compassion is pity, because self and other are separated and there is a sense of "I am looking down on your suffering." Compassion's *far enemy* is the wish to see someone harmed, or outright cruelty.

Compassion can be traced in our evolutionary lineage (Darwin, 1871). Darwin wrote in *The Descent of Man, and Selection in Relation to Sex* that compassion[3] is our strongest instinct, sometimes stronger than self-interest, and he argued that it would spread through natural selection, for "the most sympathetic members, would flourish best, and rear the greatest number of offspring" (Darwin, 1871, p. 130). Frans De Waal (2009) uses the metaphor of a nesting Russian matryoshka doll to describe the layers of compassion. The layers are (1) recognition of suffering (in some species, even amoebae, this is simply resonance with another organism's state), (2) concern for others (seen in social species), (3) perspective taking (seen only in a few social species that are able to take the perspective of another [theory of mind]), and (4) targeted helping. In evolutionary and animal behavior accounts, compassion is deep in our nature as a caregiving response to vulnerable individuals. It was selected because it supports the fabric of the social group, including the vulnerable.

There is an interesting parallel in developmental psychology. In the first year of life, infants can sense the distress of others. They experience it somatically, but without differentiating self and other (Donovan & Leavitt, 1985). This differentiation emerges later in childhood as we become more able to know what others are feeling and thinking (Greenberg & Harris, 2012; Singer, 2006). We can see that parenting plays a key role developmentally as infants and young children develop empathy, the ability to differentiate what is their pain and others' pain, and the capacity to respond compassionately (MacBeth & Gumley, 2012). In healthy adolescence and adulthood, we see the development of a more nuanced ethical framework and learning history that support the capacity for compassion, both for ourselves and others.

Compassion is central to all of the great foundational spiritual traditions, including Buddhism, Christianity, Hinduism, Judaism, and Islam. Although it takes different forms, the intention to transcend self-centered concerns and the invitation to respond compassionately to pain and suffering is present in each. What is also present in each tradition is the notion that compassion can be trained and cultivated—that sustained and dedicated practice can educate and reeducate the heart (Armstrong, 2011). So although compassion is deep in our natures—present in us even as infants—education, cultivation, training, and practice can help us bring greater intentionality and a wider ethical framework to our compassionate response.

The Matrix and Process of Compassion

Compassion is a matrix and a process—that is, it is woven from a set of interrelated threads (matrix) and is a movement from pain toward the alleviation of pain (process). It involves recognizing pain and suffering, resonating with the suffering, understanding the universality of pain and suffering, being open to and accepting of it, and developing the capacity, motivation, and action to alleviate suffering (Strauss et al., 2016). Like a matrix, it is made up of these elements and, like an unfolding process, it moves through these phases.

As we learn to cultivate compassion in each moment and throughout our lives, we can also learn to differentiate the parts of a compassionate response. Compassion starts with recognizing and acknowledging pain and distress—with this quality of a *trembling heart* or *empathic resonance*—and being willing to see and turn toward the difficulty with stillness, wholeheartedness, and receptivity. For Mohammed, this involves recognizing the pain in his lower back; for Ling, the dark thoughts; for Sam, the addictive cravings; and for Sophia, her inner critic. But crucially embedded in this recognition of pain and distress is a willingness to engage with our bodily sensations, feelings, thoughts, and life circumstances with steadiness, kindness, and care: "I don't have to endure this pain for the rest of my life, nor let it rule me. I only need to meet it in this moment as a guest, and treat it, as best I can, with kindness and care."

So often we have demonized pain and sorrow to the extent that avoidance, flight, or fixing are felt to be our only options. These conditioned responses are, however, a major obstacle to invoking compassion. Worse than that, they maintain our suffering (as we saw in Chapter 5). Mindfulness teaches us to be still and curious in the midst of adversity, to allow for its presence, to explore its landscape, and to befriend it. This is befriending in action, but here the action is to invoke compassion in the face of pain and suffering. This requires patience, resolve, and courage. Initially, this might feel counterintuitive and *wrong*, since our patterns of avoidance or fixing the difficult are so familiar and understandable to us. In taking this first step, though, we stop allowing suffering to define our lives and who we believe ourselves to be. We learn instead to allow, meet, and even embrace vulnerability rather than fear it. Our recognition of pain and distress is now imbued with this empathic resonance: "Ah, here is pain; it's OK. I can be alongside this with kindness and care." It becomes clear that our willingness to be fully present in the midst of pain creates new opportunities for a compassionate response.

Mindfulness and Empathic Resonance

The next phase translates *empathic resonance* and understanding into thoughts, words, and acts intended to alleviate the pain and suffering. It is a courageous engagement with the small and large manifestations of pain, both our own and others. For Mohammed, this involved physical self-care around his chronic pain, including managing his activity levels, posture, and medication. Just as importantly, it involved mental self-care, seeing the moments when he was about to fire the *second arrows* of suffering that compounded his pain, and choosing instead to break the chain of reactivity in those moments ("I need only to be present to this moment, not fix or endure this pain in every moment"). Similarly for Ling, struggling with depression, her thoughts of "I feel awful, every fiber in my body wants to do a duvet dive" could be met with "Ah, here is my black dog. I know from experience I need to take him out and exercise him, not humor his destructive tendencies."

Mindfulness teaches us to calm the tendency to blame, shame, and judge others or ourselves for the pain or suffering in our life. Blame and judgment do little to alleviate distress, but compound it and disable our capacity to understand it. Blame and judgment generate endless narrative and rumination that cloud us from seeing alternative ways to ease our pain and distress.

Every single moment of adversity and distress in life is borne of a set of conditions, many of which we neither invite nor can control. Mohammed's nagging back pain competes for attention with his concerns about problems at work that he needs to address. Sophia's attention is drawn from the pleasure of a cuddle with her grandchild to the unwelcome reality that her physical health is deteriorating week by week. We tend to believe that suffering is a mistake, a failure or a punishment for something we have done wrong, and we are prone to blame, shame, and judge ourselves, others, and/or our situation.

Mindfulness teaches us the skill of calming the "It's not fair" narrative that plays in endless loops in our mind. This narrative serves only to disable our capacity to meet distress with empathic resonance. Sophia described a transition point in her relationship with her Parkinson's this way: "When I ceased to ask the question of 'Why did this happen to me?' and instead could say, 'Why would this not happen to me?' then the healing could begin." We learn that we can listen to the stories of judgment and shame and know that these, too, are expressions of suffering that are equally as worthy of compassion as the loss, the heartache, the pain, or the loneliness. Einstein framed this as a higher principle: "The true value of a human being is determined primarily by the measure and the sense in which he has attained to liberation from the self" (Einstein, 1956/1999, pp. 7–8).

To explore the landscape of compassion is to explore the dynamics of our personal relationship to pain, distress, and suffering. For many of us, the relationship we have to the painful and the difficult comes to define who we believe ourselves to be, shaping our sense of possibility and how we live our lives. When we start to fear our vulnerability to the pain and frailty that is woven into every human life, we are more likely to see ourselves as incapable, powerless, and unworthy. We engage in behaviors of agitation and avoidance that we believe will protect us from injury. Faced with the difficult, the uncertain, and the unwelcome, our tendency is to *get busy* and find solutions and ways to fix that which we feel unable to accept or embrace. We are dedicated doers and fixers, heroic in our efforts to make pain go away. Busyness becomes a substitute for meeting distress as it is, inhibiting our capacity to find an *empathic resonance* with the difficult in ourselves and in others. We disengage from our mental and somatic experience, from the present moment, and from the human family. A life of anxiety is borne. We live with a fear of being overwhelmed by pain. We hold a deeply embedded belief in our incapacity to find balance, strength, and compassion in the midst of life's greatest challenges.

As we cultivate mindfulness and turn toward the present moment just as it is, we come to understand that although there is not always a solution to suffering, there is always a possible response. Understanding that not all pain can be fixed is not a prescription for passivity. Instead, it is an encouragement for us to find a response that can care for even the direst pain. Finding the willingness to stop running from pain is the first step toward a compassionate response. Not all pain and affliction can be fixed, but all pain and affliction is eased when held with tenderness and compassion.

Developing a stance of care and empathy helps us understand suffering, its causes, and its end, even when the end is found in the midst of the continuing difficulty. This understanding does not in any way diminish or dismiss our present-moment experience, yet we come to understand that we are not alone, but part of a human family that has vulnerability at its core. As compassion is cultivated, we gain dignity and widen our concern to include the suffering of others—the suffering that is present in a wider common humanity. The matrix and phases of compassion loosen the sense of me and mine, you and yours; we glimpse a world where suffering and joy are seen as part of the human condition, to be recognized, met, and allowed. This creates the conditions for a more compassionate responsiveness. Without this understanding, compassion can falter because we limit it to the conditions and people we think are *deserving*—it becomes ideological and constrained, like a form of apartheid.

This sort of conditional compassion inevitably backfires, fueling fear and alienation. Divisions are created when we think "This pain is OK, this is not, this person is deserving of compassion, this person is not." Understanding and compassion arise together and mindfulness practices teach us how to care. Consider suffering where there is no blame, a sick child, those caught up in a natural disaster such as a tsunami, the elderly whose health is failing. Then consider the suffering brought on by perpetrators, the refugees escaping ethnic conflict, people who were victimized who go on to victimize others. These examples illustrate the mind's natural tendency to create a narrative that includes blame, perpetrator, and victim. When understanding and compassion arise together, though, we can respond with our hearts and minds. This protects us from habitual reactivity and enables us to respond with balance and care. It ensures that our responses are imbued with intentionality.

> As Sophia's Parkinson's progressed, she could see the suffering in her family and friends as they struggled to come to terms with the decline in her functioning. She could see in their eyes that often they didn't know what to say or do. On occasion this was also true with doctors and nurses, for whom treatment and cure are central to medicine. What should they say and do when everything that could be done had already been done, yet the disease marched on relentlessly? Sophia's years of mindfulness practice helped her to meet her family, friends, and caregivers with understanding and compassion. This tended to disarm their uncertainty and the aversion she sometimes saw flickering across their faces. This enabled both everyday conversations and real dialogue with family and friends.

Persistence and Transformation

Persistence is a key facet of empathy and compassion. Students of mindfulness learn to return their attention over and over to what is happening, just now, in the body and mind. Developing our capacity for sustained mindfulness in the midst of all things (e.g., pain, fear, or the desire to flee) reveals our growing ability for steadiness and resilience. We become more confident that we can meet distress with compassion. Persistence is not about gritting our teeth and stoically enduring pain. It is about caring and understanding how to meet the losses, unwelcome changes, and pain without fear.

We are affected deeply by the sorrows in our own lives and in the world that seem to have no end. An early teaching asks the question "What do we do with the life that doesn't go away?" We could reframe this and ask ourselves the question "What do we do with a heartache, a loss, an illness, a life that will bring afflictions that seem to have no end or solution?" Attending to this life and moment with compassion and care provides us with the key to freedom and balance. In committing our attention to the present, just as it is rather than being lost in the narrative of how it *should* be, we begin to develop resilience and courage, cornerstones in the development of compassion.

In mindfulness programs, this healing transformation is understood in a specific way. Transformation does not mean that distress and suffering disappear. There is little encouragement to delve into the past to dissect the conditions that have resulted in present-moment distress. Those conditions and events cannot be undone. Instead, in mindfulness programs, the learning is that when we transform the present, we can create a new relationship with our past. The transformation of the present is a process of changing our relationship to the narratives and somatic imprints of the past as they arise in the present, freeing us from the layers of anxiety, judgment, and narrative that compound distress. Compassion is central to that changed relationship.

Ling spoke of the early childhood trauma of an abusive, psychologically damaged parent that had overshadowed her life. As a young child, Ling had lived with a father who was so filled with rage it was like walking on eggshells on a daily basis. Later, his coercive abuse had corroded her sense of who she was. Her mother, also fearful, turned to alcohol and was often absent because she was intoxicated. The tremors of anger, fear, bewilderment, lies, and confusion rippled through the entire family. Ling's family was broken up, both literally and figuratively, when she went into care.

These experiences made Ling fearful of relationships, limiting her sense of possibilities, haunting her dreams. She sometimes got drawn into endless rumination: "Why me?; Did I bring this on myself?; Should I have done something differently?" She blamed herself. She felt rife with imperfections and anger for the rejection by her father. When she moved into foster and residential care she hunkered down, and these issues simply played out over and over again with peers and foster parents. An encounter with an authority figure, or being the recipient of an unfriendly look by another, would trigger waves of terror and helplessness, casting her back into the past. Even shows of love would engender suspicion and hostility. Reactivity was all that she knew; it was protective and made her feel safe.

Through her teenage and early adult years, Ling found herself doubting and blaming herself for being so unaware of her father's abuse of her cousin, asking herself, "Could I have done something to protect her and keep the family together?" She lay awake at night reliving gatherings with the extended family, wondering how she could have been so blind. She wondered why she had let his abuse of her go on for as long as it did. Her thoughts cascaded with all the ways she felt she had failed her cousin and herself. She blamed herself for the family disintegrating, even though she was only a child herself.

When Ling was in her 20s, two other people came forward to say Ling's father had abused them. He was charged and pleaded not guilty. She sat through the trial unable to disclose the abuse she had experienced even as she listened to the terrible story of abuse that was told in the courtroom. Her father died in prison before he was sentenced and with his death all possibilities of justice and resolution vanished. Living with a mind so burdened by guilt, shame, and anger, in desperation she sought help. She learned through personal therapy that there was not going to be a happy ending for anyone in the family. She used therapy to begin to make peace with and reframe her experience, enough to be able to live her life without continual shame, anger, and reactivity.

Following one-to-one therapy, in a more stable phase in her life, Ling participated in an 8-week mindfulness-based cognitive therapy (MBCT) program. Mindfulness practice helped her realize she could inch her way—with some compassion—toward traumatic memories and their effects. What had happened was always going to be terrible, but she described it as "a scar that could be touched and soothed with care." As Ling's practice began to deepen, she became increasingly sensitized to those trigger moments and began to develop the capacity to simply feel her feet touching the ground and the places in her body that were calm. She recognized the column of tightness and contraction in her torso that was fear and anxiety. Rather than react, she learned this was a sign she could use first to anchor herself, feel safe, and steady enough to then do what she needed to take care of herself.

Ling's body became a refuge. The thoughts and images of the past would often still arise, but now she was able to see them as simply thoughts and images, and increasingly, remain present rather than being lost in the thoughts and images. Ling began, she said, to glimpse the possibility of holding this little girl she had been and the woman she now was with a growing sense of compassion rather than with shame and judgment. It was, she said, a glimpse of freedom, a new beginning.

Critically, in time this capacity was something Ling could use as a parent herself. As she found herself less embroiled in her own shame and blame, she could be increasingly available for her own children. When she recognized her own shifting moods and impulse to reactivity around her children, she practiced, over and over again, recognizing, allowing, and, as best she could, responding. More and more she could hold steady in the midst of the inevitable challenges of parenting, but which for her were especially difficult, given that her childhood had been both abusive and largely devoid of stability.

Like all capacities, our capacity for compassion grows when we tend to it and nourish it. We are never short of opportunities to engage with this cultivation and need not wait for the dramatic moments of pain or distress. We can learn to mindfully listen to the small murmurs of distress in our bodies with tenderness and care. As we learn to recognize the thoughts and emotions of shame, anxiety, and blame—with tenderness rather than with judgment—we become more attuned to our inner life and the present moment. Our eyes increasingly begin to open to the world around us and we are touched by the vulnerability visible in so many of our encounters in a single day. We may open ourselves up to noticing, for example, the cries of a child, the cautious and faltering walk of an elderly person, the sight of someone begging on the street. In our noticing, we open ourselves to compassion and begin to sense, within ourselves, a heart that can tremble in the face of distress. Rather than turning away in fear or judgment, we start to find the courage and balance to embrace these moments with empathy and compassion.

How Compassion Is Cultivated in an 8-Week Mindfulness-Based Program

Just as mindfulness is woven into every part of the program, so, too, are the attitudinal dimensions of befriending and compassion. In fact, we defined mindfulness in Chapter 1 with these attitudinal dimensions as the heart of attention and awareness. In the second edition of *Mindfulness-Based Cognitive Therapy for Depression*, a new chapter on kindness and compassion was added because "one of the most important things people learn from an MBCT program is kindness and self-compassion" (Segal et al., 2013, p. 137). The same is true in mindfulness-based stress reduction (MBSR), where "the entire feeling in the clinic has always attempted to embody loving kindness" (Kabat-Zinn, 2005, p. 285).

The first way, therefore, that compassion is taught in mindfulness programs is through the embodiment of the mindfulness teacher. This embodiment can be witnessed, for example, when the teacher treats participants more "as guests than patients, with warm hospitality and respect for the courage that they show, even by turning up" (Segal et al., 2013, p. 137). Compassion is woven into every aspect of the program: how participants are treated, how the class is organized, how practices are introduced and led, and how participants' learning is supported and honored. In this sense, compassion is taught implicitly through the teacher's embodied teaching. This is intentional.

For people with a tendency to depression and other clinical disorders, a range of mental states are easily triggered: striving (e.g., "I need to conquer my depression"), aversion ("This is scary, I'd rather stick my head deep in the sand"), or a powerful inner critic ("I am worthless and don't deserve this"). A skillful mindfulness teacher is aware of this. Explicit invitations to be kind can backfire by reinforcing these preexisting beliefs and tendencies. Ling's history of living in an abusive household meant that if someone showed her kindness and care, she would back off, be suspicious, and sometimes even hostile. She would wear dark glasses so she could hide her vulnerability and reactivity. It takes great skill as a mindfulness teacher to create the conditions for someone like Ling to feel safe enough to access attitudes of befriending and compassion. The safety and the practices themselves helped Ling to cultivate befriending and compassion by giving her a safe space to move through the phases of recognizing, allowing, resonating with, and moving to heal pain and reactivity. The mindfulness practices and conditions of safety created by the mindfulness teacher are how she learned.

In the early stages of the mindfulness program, the body is used as the focus for attention. Participants learn to develop sustained attention and work with the inevitable attachment and aversion that arises. When they encounter pain, they are encouraged—through the mindfulness instructions and inquiry—to meet that pain with interest and kindness, to put out the "welcome mat" for pain and distress, so to speak, as best they can. Intentional attention, interlaced with kindness, is cultivated in the first three sessions using a range of core mindfulness practices: the body scan, mindful movement (stretching and walking), and mindfulness of the breath. As well as developing the *attentional muscle*, these practices highlight the impulsive and habitual patterns of thinking that are present and the associated aversion to negative mind states and judgments. Sam saw this in the practices where he met all the usual hindrances: with his psoriasis (where he met the understandable urge to soothe and make the itchiness go away) and the residual cravings that could easily be triggered during his recovery from addiction (where he met with aversive thoughts, such as "To hell with all this 12-step crap, I need a hit now").

With mindfulness, we become more able to withdraw power from our self-judgments and blame that only serve as fuel for depressive thinking. Then we see what happens when we intentionally step out of habitual patterns of thinking. Participants develop the capacity to be mindful of their breathing and body, cultivating a present-moment attentiveness and greater sensory awareness. The Pleasant Events Calendar that participants fill out in the second week reveals our sometimes hidden or unrecognized capacity for appreciation and connectedness with a world not colored by the bleakness of depression. The continual emphasis on curiosity, befriending, and kindness develops a skill and attitudinal base that can be brought to unpleasant events when they arise, either inwardly or outwardly. We find a new capacity for joy that we didn't know we were capable of. Mindfulness programs invite people to attend to pleasant and unpleasant events in their daily life, and note their sensations, emotions, thoughts, and impulses without trying to fix or change them in any way. This cultivates equanimity, which together with the rest of the program supports change.

In the second half of the MBCT for recurrent depression program, mindfulness and compassion are brought to bear on the person's unique signature for depressive relapse so that he or she can generate skillful responses. Participants come to see their habitual patterns of reactivity in how they think and behave. But now they are imbued with an orientation of befriending. The best example of this is the metaphor of the "black dog" that Winston Churchill used to describe his depression. His "black dog" was a dark presence, but also an animal that was, for better and worse, part of his life. Matthew Johnstone (2007) created the wonderful book *I Had a Black Dog*, which beautifully illustrates this changed relationship to depression. In a series of cartoons, he first shows how powerfully the black dog shapes all of his experience, but then goes on to show how he befriends the dog, learns to live with it, and, in time, comes to see it differently.

Throughout all mindfulness programs, participants come to have a sense of common humanity. The group inquiry that takes places in MBCT for people with depression, for example, reveals to every participant that depression is not a personal failure but an affliction that besets many human beings. The same is true of other groups, such as people living with chronic illness, people with cancer, and so on. The realization that what we thought was unique to us is also experienced by others can help us cultivate a strong sense of the universality of pain. We come to realize that we are not alone in our suffering. There have been recent innovations to enhance the explicit teaching of compassion beyond 8-week mindfulness programs (van den Brink & Koster, 2015) and evidence is emerging of its effectiveness to enhancing resilience through cultivating compassion (Schuling et al., 2018).

Two leading psychologists, Christopher Germer and Kristin Neff, have done a great deal to develop ways to teach self-compassion explicitly and have developed an 8-week program with this primary intention (Germer, 2009; Neff & Germer, 2013). They emphasize the importance of psychoeducation, which provides people with the background knowledge and understanding to help them know when they need to be discerning about when to open and close to pain and distress with compassion, when it might be possible to meet pain in a way that is healing, and when might it be overwhelming, counterproductive, and more discerning to close to it. They introduce the helpful metaphor of *backdraft*: if a door or window in a room with a fire is opened, oxygen can rush in and create a rapid escalation of the fire (i.e., the so-called backdraft). For those of us with strong aversive tendencies, for example, an aversive backdraft can be created when we open to kindness and compassion. There is a need, they argue, for psychoeducation and skillfulness in knowing when and how much to open to kindness and compassion. This fits with our own experience of teaching mindfulness around trauma.

Many mindfulness teachers are exploring working with these more explicit ways of cultivating compassion, some of which have a long lineage and all of which will require careful study and research to examine how best to develop this capacity that is fundamental to change and healing. Interested readers are directed to this work (e.g., Germer, 2009). Try the mindfulness exercise on compassion in Box 7.2.

BOX 7.2. Mindfulness Exercise: Compassion

Taking your seat and turning your attention to your present-moment experience, bring your attention initially to the places in your body that feel well and easeful. Perhaps attend to the palms of your hand or the sensation of your feet touching the ground. Attune your attention to a body of stillness, a body of restfulness, consciously softening any areas of tension. Sense what it is to cultivate a curious, caring attentiveness.

Then extend your attention to parts of the body that feel unpleasant or tight, with the same quality of mindfulness. With the same sense of befriending, alternate your attention between the experience of wellness and any part of the body that feels stressed. Sense what it is to listen deeply to distress with empathy and compassion.

When you feel able, extend your field of attention to include those you care for and the many people you meet each day who all have their own measure of joy and sorrow. Perhaps invite into your attention an image of a person struggling with uninvited life pain—loss, frailty, illness—and sense what it is to hold that person within an empathic resonance.

You might experiment with a few simple phrases:

"Allowing."
"Peace."
"Ease."
"Caring."

Joy

Joy is an intrinsic attitude of mind that includes gladness of the heart, soft-heartedness, and tenderness that supports a capacity for appreciation, contentment, and gratitude. Just as our hearts can tremble in the face of suffering, they can also tremble in the face of happiness and beauty. Its affective tone is gladness, aliveness, and vitality. It is associated with a range of emotions, including contentment, wonder, radiant pride, gratitude, and delight.

Empathy is as central to the cultivation of joy as it is to compassion. When we encounter pleasant states, empathy can blossom into appreciative joy, contentment, and gratitude. We discuss each of these in turn in this section. We also look at what can veil and obstruct joy.

The *near enemies* of joy are sentimentality and exuberance. We may be carried away by the idea of joy, rather than being truly alive to it in a given moment. For example, we denote days of the year to celebration, and it is possible to get caught up in a pretense of gaiety rather than being open to joy whenever it arises. Joy helps us befriend difficulties and meet suffering with equanimity and compassion. We have a capacity for joy and a capacity to find joy in others' happiness and success. Indeed, in the foundational teachings, the empathic, altruistic dimensions of joy are emphasized, creating the conditions for connection and harmony.

The *far enemy* of joy is resentment and the wonderful German word *schadenfreude*, where we take pleasure in someone else's failure. Finding joy in others' happiness is an antidote to resentment, lessening our own sense of inadequacy and tempering our tendency toward envy. When we free our minds and hearts from envy, resentment, covetousness, and continual judging, we can really appreciate our own and others' well-being.

Joy—like attention, befriending, and compassion—is an intention, cultivation, and a practice. Often neglected, joy is both a capacity we all have and a capacity that can be trained and developed. It is a primary component of psychological well-being, encompassing moments of appreciation, enduring contentment, and a sense of confidence and gratitude. It is an attitude of mind that can be cultivated through mindfulness practice and through how we live our lives. When we intentionally cultivate joy, we discover that it can be the *home where we reside*; we come home to joy. We withdraw from the tendency to orient to insufficiency that drives the elaborative judgment of distress and suffering.

Joy and Intention

The foundations of joy are simple: "thoughts, words and actions rooted in kindness and compassion" (Feldman, 2017, p. 94). Do our thoughts, words, and actions bring distress and suffering to an end? Do they support happiness and well-being? As we saw in Chapters 5 and 6, responsiveness borne of awareness and intentionality creates the conditions for joy.

For many years, Sophia's day had started with 30–60 minutes of mindfulness practice. This typically included bringing to mind the people she knew whom she would encounter that day, including herself, and wishing them well. This inclined her mind toward kindness in her interactions throughout the day, especially those that she anticipated might be challenging.

With every day that Sam stayed free of active addiction, his mind cleared and steadied. This made it easier for him to act in kind and compassionate ways both to himself and to those around him.

When Ling was separating from her children's father, she had to negotiate child custody, who should live in their home, and their finances. Many times there was the potential in unguarded moments to speak harshly and act punitively to her ex-partner. Through guarding her attention and resisting the impulse, Ling created the conditions for both herself and her ex-partner to enjoy a good relationship with their children and with each other.

Intention rooted in kindness and compassion creates the conditions for joy in ourselves and others. It also ensures that our mind does not carry the residues of regret and shame.

Appreciative Joy

It takes only a small step of mindful wholeheartedness to enjoy a piece of music, notice the stars in the sky, the sunlight glistening on the leaves, the people we love around us, a good meal, or all that is right in our bodies in any given moment. These moments are available all of the time. They offer a glimpse of a more enduring contentment. This step takes us out of automatic pilot and reactivity. Appreciation develops the capacity for responsiveness.

Appreciation involves a certain innocence of perception, in which we override our tendencies to judge or to rely on automatic, familiar ways of seeing the world. In mindfulness-based parenting, for example, parents are asked early in the 8-week program to find opportunities to be with their young children while they are asleep, and to bring full awareness to their bodily sensations, feelings, and thoughts in these moments.

Appreciation requires a certain orientation of mind, innocent perception, and discipline to see and experience these moments. We recognize them, allow them into our perceptual field, and experience them fully.

Sam lived in a house on a lake that his parents had gifted him. It was a house he had visited throughout his life, including many times while in active addiction. Only now in recovery from addiction, was he able to truly appreciate the lake house. One afternoon he tried to capture on paper his changed perception and appreciation:

"Long leisurely days. An outlook across the lake to a horizon of time-flattened mountains stalking eternity. The lake's surface chameleon-like, a myriad of personalities: frantic, rhythmic, a screaming child, lapping white tops, shivering, stiller and steadier than a Buddha's breath, a child settled at last, at dusk moon kissed, at night shimmering, thick oil covered, darker, unknowable.

"Smells of pine resin, charcoal, citronella, suntan lotion, an indefinable sweetness in the air. Sounds of leaves smattering, children's laughter, squeals, and shouts carried across the water, the loons' wail, cry, halloo, and clatter, insects' momentary whine. Sometimes stillness. The heart softens, trembles, and meets life with innocence.

"Sometimes an uncomfortable perceptual hijack; a memory of driving to the lake while high, harsh words spoken and then regretted, agitated impatience to step back into the oblivion of city life. Escorting attention back, with discipline and care, to summer, long leisurely days.

"Time stands still, and in each moment I am here for my life. The life I had lost momentarily reclaimed."

This form of appreciative joy loosens the link between underlying tendencies to judge and label our experiences and to go through our day on automatic pilot. It opens us to appreciate everyday moments with *innocent perception*. This may seem simple, but it requires an intention and discipline to be awake to our lives. To transform moments of appreciative joy into enduring contentment takes training and time. Try the exercise in Box 7.3.

Contentment

Contentment is more than transient moments of appreciation—it is a way of being. It is a place where our minds and hearts rest, an embodied understanding

---

BOX 7.3. Mindfulness Exercise: Appreciative Joy

Joy has its roots in a wholehearted appreciative attention. As you go about your day, bring your attention to seeing, touching, and listening wholeheartedly—mindful of how you are touching and being touched by the world. Take moments to pause—to feel the touch of the breeze on your skin, to hear the laughter of a child on the playground, to fully taste the food you eat. Reflect on all that goes well for you today—your ability to move through the world, to be fed and warm, and to care for yourself. See not only the trees but also the space around the trees, not only the stars but also the vastness of the sky that holds the stars. Sense the small moments of generosity you extend to or receive from others—the smile, the door held open. In every moment, sense what it is that holds the potential to gladden your heart when you are truly present.

Each day, intentionally bring awareness to something you do regularly and that you know you enjoy. It could be anything: a morning cup of tea or coffee, a walk, a favorite snack, an interaction with someone you appreciate or love, a person or a pet, or a spacious moment in your day while you travel. Commit to being wholeheartedly present, aware of your bodily sensations, feelings, and thoughts. Bring an innocent perception and sensitivity to the experience, to whatever is present in terms of sights, sounds, taste, and touch. Really sense how attention imbued with innocent perception affects the world of the moment. Allow your heart to *tremble* in the midst of the experience, gladdened by the simplicity of the moment.

that has deep within it a sense of contentment, an ease of being, a sense that all is well. Our brains evolved for survival and reproduction, rather than for happiness and peace of mind. This biological heritage seems to have left us with a natural tendency to give plenty of attention to what's wrong and to what might be a threat (Sapolsky, 2017).

Noticing and giving time to what is lovely doesn't come so easily for most of us, especially when we're under stress. However, there are steps we can take to train ourselves to bring awareness to the lovely and nourishing aspects of our lives and cultivate the conditions for enduring contentment. Raising and broadening our gaze can reveal many moments of appreciative joy in everyday life. Recognizing, seeing, and stepping away from our judging mind creates the conditions for enduring contentment.

The key to contentment is seeing and letting go of the relentless judging mind, and instead *resting* in our experience exactly as it is. It can be helpful to ask:

> *"What do I need in this moment to be happy?"*; *"What is lacking from this moment?"*

This practice is a great teacher, helping to reveal how the pervasive judging mind disrupts contentment and helping us rest in the moment, where we can be more open to contentment. A Chinese proverb speaks to this: "If we keep a green bough alive in our hearts, the singing bird will come."

Contentment does not deny difficulty or pain, nor the value of the judging mind if it is used judiciously. It is not some kind of Pollyanna positive thinking. In fact, contentment can mean recognizing and resting in a difficulty, letting go of the struggle that can, like a second arrow, perpetuate suffering. More than this, it can open our eyes to the goodness that often sits alongside any difficulty. Contentment in this sense opens to what is actually present in any given moment: the pleasant, the unpleasant, and the neutral, letting go of the striving for perfection, goals, and stability that simply don't exist.

Sophia, who had been practicing mindfulness for several decades when she was first diagnosed with Parkinson's, put it this way: "Even when the Parkinson's tremors are at their worst, I can access an ease of being, a sense of being alive. Don't get me wrong, it is not pleasant and I can be afraid, sometimes even terrified, but I can find and rest in a sense of peace in the midst of it all, and that includes all that is good in my life. When I first got the diagnosis of Parkinson's, I was shaken up for days and then weeks. My whole identity and future shifted—of course it did—I'd been given an awful diagnosis with a terrible prognosis.

"But through my mindfulness practice, I was reminded of the steadiness I can bring to my mind, and this brought back the friendliness and care to this new Sophia, the Sophia with Parkinson's. I got up and went into the garden with a cup of tea and noticed that the garden, the taste of my favorite tea, the birds, the sky, they were all the same, my mind and body were still the same, but now I had a diagnosis of Parkinson's. A certain ease of being came back to me."

Sophia is an example of how we can draw on what we learn in mindfulness practice to open to the pleasant and difficult, and let go of the judge that drives fear and discontentment. Contentment is a path of being awake to all that is lovely and challenging in our lives. Try the exercise in Box 7.4 to begin cultivating contentment.

Gratitude

Gratitude nourishes and supports appreciation and contentment. It is an active choice to identify all that we can be grateful for in our lives. We can be grateful for a seemingly trivial thing, like a moment of kindness a stranger shows us, or more seemingly profound things, like a loving relationship or our health. It is an antidote to the perhaps more natural inclination of the mind to identify everything that is lacking or imperfect in our lives.

There are many ways to develop gratitude, but one is to look at all the good things we often take for granted, and then look more deeply into them to acknowledge and extend appreciation to all the people and conditions that

---

BOX 7.4. **Mindfulness Exercise: Contentment**

Take a few moments to steady your attention. Take up a posture that communicates a sense of wakefulness and dignity. Steady for a few moments on your breath, anchoring your attention. Take note of any bodily sensations, feelings, and thoughts, allowing them to be as they are, with the breath as the anchor for your attention.

Bring into the practice the questions "What do I need in this moment to be happy?"; "What is lacking from this moment?" As best you can, stay very close to this moment. If you notice your mind wandering into judging or wider questions about your life, escort it back to *this moment,* back to "What do I need in this moment to be happy?"; "What is lacking from this moment?" Explore within yourself what it is to rest in this moment with ease, to rest in the small space between the ending of the out-breath and the beginning of the next breath, to rest in the quietude between sounds, to rest in the body.

brought them into being. As we read a book that we are enjoying, we can extend appreciation to the people who wrote it; the publisher who commissioned it and the large team that brought it to publication; the paper mill somewhere in the world that manufactured the paper; the printing factory that printed the book; the artists who created the cover illustration; the trees that were the raw materials for the paper; the sun, rain, and soil that enabled the trees to grow . . .[4]

Gratitude is neither sentimental, a denial of the difficult, nor necessarily easy. It is a training to incline the mind in a new direction, of appreciation, so that we can make choices about where to place our attention. When a friend has some good news, for example, we can allow envy to arise and entertain it: "Why does he get to have this (e.g., sporting or academic success, new car, new relationship)?" In that moment, we can choose to step back from envy and abide in an appreciation of our friend's happiness. This extends to difficulties as well, where the mind understandably wants to shut down or turn away. Even with the difficult, though, we can find a way to cultivate and train appreciation.

On the fifth anniversary of his last heroin and alcohol binge, Sam was asked to share his experience, strength, and hope in his 12-step meeting. He shared:

> "It is a strange thing to say, but I am grateful for my addiction. I feel more alive and connected to the people around me now than I ever did. I appreciate all that is good in my life in a way I never did before. I wouldn't wish what I have been through because of addiction on anyone, but I am grateful for the way the scales have fallen away from my eyes in recovery. Every day is an opportunity to practice appreciation and gratitude. I have friends who have died through addiction. Recently, a friend in recovery went on what he thought might be 'one last binge' and his body couldn't take it. It killed him and he was only in his 30s. I start each day with prayer and in my prayer I am grateful for each day of my recovery."

Gratitude can be cultivated in many different ways, in small everyday ways or in life-enhancing and saving ways, as we saw with Sophia and Sam.

Enablers and Hindrances to Joy

As we discussed earlier, joy is an intention, a cultivation, *and* a practice. Although we all have the ability to experience joy, this capacity can be trained and developed. This is particularly helpful because our capacity for joy can sometimes be depleted. Clinicians and teachers, for example, are exposed to an enormity of distress that can feel overwhelming. Some experience *compassion fatigue* that causes them to erect defenses as a way of protecting themselves. The intentional cultivation of gladness, appreciation, and joy, however, can help renew and replenish our inner resources, enabling us to sustain empathy. Joy inspires practice because it enlightens and is reinforcing. This intrinsic reward within joy naturally motivates our practice and supports positive change. In the midst of a lot of suffering we can be motivated to change, but once the suffering abates, we can rock back into our default position. Having the intrinsic reward of joy helps us to practice and grow in the absence of suffering.

When we experience joy, we are more likely to lift our gaze and broaden our field of awareness to notice pleasant experiences, allowing ourselves to fully experience them. The joy that is part of the path of awareness is not exhilaration or bliss, but more often a quiet gladness of the heart, a capacity for easefulness and appreciation. Nor is it a grasping at pleasant experiences, as this is craving that is most likely feeding a sense of lack and wanting (Chapters 5 and 6). Nor is joy about *me, mine,* or *my story*—rather, it is a more natural, intrinsic capacity that involves getting out of the way of the self, of *selfing,* where we create narratives in which we are the main actor.

As we know, much of our suffering stems from our discrepancy monitor, where we tend to continually see the discrepancy between how things are and how we think they should be. This is solidified by the stories we create. An example is believing that our happiness depends upon having the same successes and possessions as we think our peers do. Having acquired all of these, we achieve a moment of happiness, only to find it slipping away once more as we meet again the familiar discontented mind. At school and work, grades and performance reviews serve to feed our sense of inadequacy. They reinforce the tendency to continually strive to be the person we feel we should or ought to be. This insatiable cycle can be mistaken for the pursuit of joy, but in reality it disconnects us from our intentions, appreciative joy, and lasting contentment. Rather than look for joy within what we already have, we externalize it and make it contingent on owning things, achieving things, and reaching milestones. Stepping off of this hamster wheel and letting go of the impulse of compulsive wanting enables us to connect with our intentions, step into appreciative joy, and cultivate the conditions for contentment and gratitude. As we saw with the practice in Box 7.4, it can be helpful to *check in* with ourselves to ask, "What do I need in this moment to be content?"; "What is really lacking from this moment?"

For people living with depression, anxiety, chronic pain, and illness, the absence of gladness leads the mind to become increasingly despairing and bleak. Anxiety and depression leach joy out of our lives. In times of great challenge and difficulty, joy can seem like a distant memory or a faint prospect that hopefully will emerge after our current affliction, illness, or depression has ended. We become acutely aware of how the field of our awareness shrinks and contracts when faced with adversity, until our foregrounding of and preoccupation with adversity is the only feature in the landscape of our minds.

Cultivating joy involves a certain orientation of mind, a discipline, and a rigorous honesty. It requires that we need to lift our gaze to see all that is pleasant and right with our lives, discriminate joy from craving, recognize and step out of the stories that inevitably emerge, and have the courage to work both with the pleasant and the difficult.

Cultivating Joy in Mindfulness-Based Programs

Joy is cultivated through mindfulness-based programs in several ways. The first is perhaps the subtlest, involving the mindfulness teacher's embodiment and how he or she teaches the class. Rather like an orchestra conductor who can vary what musicians to bring in, and how to bring them in, the mindfulness teacher can work with the group to discover opportunities to cultivate joy and to know when this supports learning. The inquiry between Sam and his mindfulness teacher illustrates this:

SAM: About 20 minutes into the practice, my mind became really steady, all the clutter and noise seemed to stop, and I was totally at ease. Even the sounds of the heating clunking away were kind of interesting and enjoyable. It was nice. Then I had this thought: "Wow, I love this blissed-out state, I wish I could feel this way more of the time."

TEACHER: What followed this thought?

SAM: I got myself all tangled again. I tried to change my posture and get the breathing so I could get back into that blissed-out state. (*Laughs, recognizing his craving mind.*)

TEACHER: That's so interesting Sam, and so important, too. So, in the practice your attention steadied, and there was ease, even hearing the sound of the heating system was interesting. But then your thinking mind stepped in, it "loved this state," wanted to "feel this way more of the time." In that moment, the judging mind kicked back in, trying to fix and change things. These are moments to recognize your judging mind, and step back—with discipline and care—to the simple invitation to be with the breath and see what comes and goes. Can I ask you, Sam, to say a bit more about the ease you noted before this judging came in?

SAM: You know, it was as though my attention was a butterfly, resting in the palm of my hand. The endless chatter of my mind had settled, and my body sort of felt at ease. The sounds of the water system gurgling, the pipes creaking, sounds coming and going, the sense of heat in the room. I was sitting next to a radiator. I even reached out and put my hand on the radiator to feel the warmth through my hand. It was a contentment, I'd say.

TEACHER: Wow. So, your mind was like a butterfly that had settled on the palm of your hand, sort of at ease. (*Nods, and they both pause to let that sink in.*) Then what happened to the butterfly?

SAM: (*Smiles.*) I see where this is going. It was as if I tried to hang on to it, clasp it rather than just let it be—let it take off and land someplace else.

In this final segment, the teacher is bringing back simple appreciation of the moment, of ease and contentment. The lesson that the teacher is skillfully imparting is that we can, *with discipline*, come back to these moments. This intentional movement through different parts of awareness cultivates the capacity to choose greater contentment and ease of being. To use Sam's words, it is allowing the butterfly to rest on his palm. When he tries to grasp it, though, it changes and his craving mind sets in, but here, rather than drugs, he is craving a blissed-out state associated with his mindfulness practice.

In Week 2 of mindfulness-based programs, participants are asked to undertake a week's home practice in which they keep a record of pleasant events they encounter each day. For people in the midst of depression or anxiety, this initially is counterintuitive, as their attention is repeatedly drawn to the narrative of bleakness, hopelessness, or worry. During the week they intentionally undertake this task, they discover every day that there are events and moments of ease and loveliness that gladden their hearts. They are not dramatic moments—they are the simple moments of hearing the laughter of a child, the sensation of heat on our hands on a cold day, seeing a dog enthusiastically chase a stick, or the kind gesture of someone opening a door for us. When we intentionally *task* ourselves to be mindful of the pleasant, we open ourselves up to discovering much that can gladden our mind.

In the *Mindfulness: A Practical Guide to Finding Peace in a Frantic World* (Williams & Penman, 2011) curriculum, participants are encouraged each day to note five to 10 things for which they are grateful, things in their lives that they appreciate. They are encouraged to let the sense of appreciation be felt in the body, be breathed, be nourishing—"Letting the good things become good experiences." The intention of this practice is to encourage us to notice each day what we might normally overlook and then to actually take the time to experience it.

Toward the end of mindfulness-based programs, participants are encouraged to note what nourishes them in their day-to-day, note what gives them a sense of appreciative joy, and to become more aware of these experiences in their lives. In addition, they are encouraged to schedule more of these experiences into their lives. For Sophia, this was teaching mindfulness classes and preparing the reunion sessions for the many people who had attended her classes. Learning and teaching were moments of great joy to her. As her Parkinson's progressed, she noticed its impact on her motivation and feared that the tremors might be off-putting to the people in her reunions. Knowing how much this work was a source of joy and nourishment enabled her to ensure she kept it up; she recruited some help with the classes as a form of self-care. She started to self-disclose judiciously so that participants in her classes were aware that she, too, was using mindfulness to work with her illness, and that she, together with her co-teacher, would hold the mindfulness classes.

Powerful lessons are learned in exercises that are focused on savoring pleasant experiences, gratitude, and nourishment. We are reminded that we can choose what we attend to and how we pay attention. The Pleasant Events Calendar and gratitude exercise are exercises in choosing what is foregrounded in our field of attention. When the difficult or afflictive weighs upon us, we sense how the tendency to automatically foreground that pain banishes all that is well into the background to the extent that it no longer features in the field of our attention. In the midst of the difficult, we can intentionally foreground that which is easeful in the body or in our sensory world. Realizing this begins to widen and soften our attentional field.

> Even though Mohammed was no longer able to play football, he still followed his team by going to games or watching them on TV whenever possible. These were moments that foregrounded one of his loves (i.e., sports), and in so doing, backgrounded the pain. While walking out of the stadium with the crowds one time after a game and enjoying the collective sense of victory, Mohammed realized that for nearly 2 hours the pain had only occasionally come into his awareness.

Mindfulness practice helps lift us out of the contracted space of obsession and rumination so that we can see and listen wholeheartedly to a wider world. We learn that just as bleakness is a present-moment experience, so, too, are gladness and appreciation—our world of the moment is borne of how the mind and attention are inclined. We learn the lesson that sorrow and heartache do not exclude our capacities for appreciation and gladness—they coexist. Gladness and ease can be found and cultivated in the midst of the bleakest and contracted landscapes. We learn that when we remember our capacity for gladness and appreciation, we are less prone to define ourselves solely by the afflictive. Although we cannot contrive joy or gladness, students of mindfulness learn how to make room for gladness. A Chinese proverb encourages us to "write our sorrows in sand and our joys in stone." This is not a teaching in denial, but a recognition of our propensity to focus the difficult and the imperfect instead of on all that is well.

> When Ling's daughter was 7, she was diagnosed with a brain tumor. In the weeks Ling spent with her daughter on the pediatric oncology ward, she lived in a nightmare of worry and hypervigilance. She also began to see that her daughter and the other children on the ward did not share her world of fear. The children had many difficult moments going through procedures that were painful, yet they would bounce back. They would laugh together, play together when they could, and at times cry together. It was a ward of both sadness and smiles.
>
> Ling learned that she could choose to be stuck in her world of fear, or she could instead acknowledge the humanness of her fear and open herself up to be touched by and appreciate the moments of gladness. Now that her daughter was a teenager, she would sometimes slow herself down to see her in a snapshot moment. In that moment, she was able to access a sense of appreciative joy of her daughter's presence and life, the fact that she was alive having survived a tumor as a child, and that she had gone on to become a vibrant young person. "I slow myself down. I can sort of capture some of that, you know, joy of life that I would have lost by bulldozing ahead and not really taking notice."

Appreciation and gladness are not as far away from us as we often imagine. In the midst of rumination, heartache, exhaustion, and worry, mindfulness prompts us to widen the field of our awareness. It takes only a simple intention and a moment of mindfulness in the midst of pain or illness to notice the places in our bodies that are well and easeful. Gladness is not a reward for having endured or survived the difficult—rather, it is one of the key qualities that allows us to embrace the difficult without being overwhelmed by it, and to appreciate all that is well, lovely, and beautiful. A leading mindfulness teacher put it this way: "Peace is just one breath away." What he means is that in any given moment, we can steady the mind and orient to joy, one breath at a time (Thich Nhat Hanh, 1992). The expression "We're as happy as we make up our minds to be," also suggests this deliberate intention and action of mind to both reclaim and cultivate joy. Appreciative joy is much more than an episodic moment. It is an "ennobling quality of mind and heart," "a way of being," the "home of an awakened mind" (Feldman, 2017, p. 88). It is a quality and a capacity that can be cultivated, which can mature into contentment.

Equanimity

Equanimity, the fourth attitudinal foundation of mindfulness, describes a quality of inner balance imbued with awareness, care, and compassion. Equanimity is fully engaged with the events of every moment, both inwardly and outwardly. Its affective tone is cool poise and steadiness. Its underlying intentionality is to show how our experiences are far too often shaped by our discrepancy monitoring and learning history. The *near enemy* of equanimity is indifference, being remote and removed from life. Instead, equanimity describes a way of being relationally present in the midst of all things, responsive yet not overwhelmed. Equanimity is an intention, an attitudinal commitment, and a practice. The *far enemy* of equanimity is craving, where we cling to an idealized view of how things should be, and have a restless longing for belongings and life conditions that we believe make us secure and happy. Equanimity is in many ways countercultural. There are many cultural drivers for fame, praise, blame, the endless pursuit of happiness, material wealth, and success at school and work. These set up striving and craving, which are the antithesis of equanimity.

Every moment, our bodies experience an unfolding matrix of multiple sensations—thoughts arise and pass with rapidity. Interactions with people and events fill our days. We already stand in the midst of all of this. Equanimity teaches us a way of being present in which we are touched by all of this and we learn to touch the moment with stillness, receptivity, and steadiness.

Equanimity is infused with, and infuses, befriending, compassion, and joy by giving balance and selflessness to befriending, underpinning compassion with patience and courage, and guarding joy from sentimentality. Together, these qualities enable understanding (Chapter 5) and a path toward less distress and greater flourishing (Chapter 6). The four qualities of befriending, compassion, joy, and equanimity work together as a matrix.

Equanimity can be cultivated but it requires practice in the places it really matters. Equanimity is cultivated in formal mindfulness practice, in our day-to-day inner lives, and in our interactions with the world. Every moment of our inevitably changing minds, bodies, and lives is an opportunity to practice cultivating equanimity. Some of the most valuable opportunities to develop equanimity are when we get absorbed in narratives where we play every part (director, producer, lead actor, protagonist, antagonist, etc.), or where pain, pleasure, or our desires overwhelm us.

Equanimity and the Body

Developing equanimity is woven into every part of mindfulness-based programs. In fact, students of mindfulness learn the intention and practice of equanimity from the first step in their training. Mindfulness of the body, central to all mindfulness practice, is both a beginning and an advanced practice—the kindergarten and graduate school of equanimity. By exploring the landscape of the body, we encounter the spectrum of sensations present, including the pleasant, the unpleasant, and the parts of the body that are neutral. We encounter the body of agitation and the body of calm. The body scan, one of the key practices in contemporary mindfulness programs, teaches students to move their attention through the body without highlighting or giving preference to any one sensation over another. With mindfulness, we learn to be equally present with all sensations, stepping out of the attentional bias that prefers either pleasant or unpleasant, and dismisses the neutral. This is a powerful lesson for our lives. When we step out of attentional bias, we simultaneously learn to step out of the aversion, craving, and clinging that habitually appends itself to our preferences. Again we go back to the Buddhist teachings embedded in contemporary mindfulness: *to know the body as the body, to know sensation as sensation.* The primary understanding that begins to emerge is that it is not the *events* of the body that knock us off balance and lead us to be overwhelmed, but our *reactions* to those events.

Equanimity and the Mind

We can further develop our capacity for equanimity when we become more aware of the state of our minds in the midst of the cascade of thoughts, moods, and emotions that register in our present-moment experience. We have opportunities to practice equanimity wherever there is, for example, gain and loss, fame and shame, praise and blame, happiness and misery. Mindfulness helps us learn to stand in the midst of all of this, fully present and better able to recognize a mood as a mood, a thought as a mental event, an emotion as an emotion, and an impulse as an impulse. This present-centered awareness, this equanimity, enables us not only to *respond* rather than *react* in our usual ways but also to disarm the way we define ourselves in terms of achievements, fame, praise, and what we're told should make us happy. As the tendency to define ourselves through identification with our moods and thoughts abates, we become freer to meet our experiences and *ourselves* with care and compassion.

Mindfulness enables us to see the changing weather patterns of our minds. It helps us understand that when we don't cling to our usual patterns, aversion or anxiety will change and pass. We begin to understand that difficult moods and thoughts last longer when we react to them with aversion and identification. When we give up craving, there is no movement toward or away from the events of the moment, from the pleasant, unpleasant, and neutral as they arise and fall away, arise and fall away. A steely stillness emerges, suffering softens, and joy grows.

Sam put it this way: "When I was in active addiction, I knew all about balance, it was the place I glimpsed as I swung from one extreme to the other. [Laughs.] Now I see my mind wanting things, needing to be excited, desperate for an adrenaline kick. I try to anchor myself in my breath and body. I can see that great big pendulum swinging from one extreme to the other. Wow, it's powerful."

Equanimity is not a quality reserved for our inner life. Our health, the conditions of our lives, human relationships, and wider challenges in the world provide much *grist for the mill*. They change moment to moment. Other people don't always act the way we want them to, our lives don't run the way we anticipated. There are serious challenges in the world's changing climate, geopolitics, and migration. We have to find balance in our response, both internally, in our relationships, and in our lives. Each day we interface with a world that can be both delightful and challenging.

Sophia's Parkinson's disease demanded equanimity; its progression was both inevitable and distressing. When she was first diagnosed, she went through a period of frantic activity, researching the condition, getting second opinions, changing her diet, buying a fitness tracker, joining different support groups—hoping that somewhere she would find the key to unlocking her predicament. At the same time, her mind could be caught in a flurry of worry, resentment, and sometimes, outright terror.

One day Sophia was on the beach building sandcastles with her grandson, Noah. As they watched the tide come in, she held Noah on her lap and they enjoyed seeing the tide come in and reclaim the sandcastle. He fell asleep on her lap and they were together even as the sun set and the heat went out of the day. There was a quality of aliveness and reality to the moment. There was universality to the impermanence of the sandcastle. She realized that her frantic struggle to come to terms with her diagnosis was feeding her suffering. The qualities of befriending and care enabled her to begin to bring equanimity to the changed circumstances of her life, living with a progressive disease, just as inevitable and powerful as the tide.

Sophia started to deliberately bring an intentionality to her daily practice, and say to herself, "I care for you deeply, things are as they are. I take joy in all that is right with my body and life. I accept, allow, and embrace, as best I can, all that is deteriorating in my body." She would then end her daily mindfulness practice with a sense of purpose to carry these intentions into her day. She developed a deep sense of the impermanence that supported her equanimity:

"This, too, will pass." Having seen that powerful thoughts, feelings, mind states, and life conditions change, she came to embody and love this understanding.

Equanimity teaches us to navigate our way through this life, with all its unpredictability and uncertainty, without becoming lost. Building sandcastles on a beach is a delight, but we know that the tide will inevitably come in and wash them away, leaving only the sand and shells. The building and washing away are all moments that we can choose to be present to—with befriending, appreciation, and care—awake both to the appreciation and loss, with equanimity. Throughout our lives, we encounter moments of loveliness and have our own measure of sadness. We will be gladdened by the people we love and delight in the beautiful. We long to be happy and in caring relationships, yet we know that our worlds can crumble in a moment. Our care and love for people is not enough to protect them from distress and pain; another's care and love for us is not enough to shelter us from the vicissitudes of life. We will be touched deeply by both the lovely and difficult events in our own lives and in the world. As we learn to develop a sense of equanimity, we learn to engage with every aspect of our lives—the pleasant, the unpleasant, and the neutral; the evaluative elaboration—with awareness, care, and compassion. Try the exercise in equanimity in Box 7.5.

BOX 7.5. Mindfulness Exercise: Equanimity

Take a few moments to steady your attention on your breath, anchoring and stabilizing your attention. Take up a posture that communicates a sense of wakefulness and dignity.

Once your attention is stable, bring to mind a mountain you know well, its base, its flanks, the way it rises up from its solid base. Have a sense of yourself as a mountain, with a solid base where you're in contact with the ground, your body stable, and your head supported on the top of your body. Like a mountain through each day, through each of the seasons, through the years, having a sense of yourself sitting with dignity and wakefulness, your breath as your anchor, as experiences come and go, the mountain steady through it all. Like a mountain as weather patterns move through, so your body and mind are steady as thoughts, images, bodily sensations, impulses, and emotions come and go. Open to the sense of the steadiness and enduring nature of the mountain.

During the day, bring awareness to moments of the day, as best you can, meeting everything with a recognition and allowing that is poised and balanced. Bring this same attitude, as best you can, to experiences, whether they are pleasant, unpleasant, or neutral. Recognize, allow, and embrace caring for each moment of your waking day.

Wholehearted Responsiveness

With mindfulness, we are reminded over and over that even as we are touched deeply by delight and by sorrow, it is not the events themselves that make us feel overwhelmed and lost, but our resistance to those events. Our futile attempts to make life stand still only make us feel worse. The words *should* and *ought* can be considered red flags that signal when we have, on some level, dissociated ourselves from the actuality of the moment and begun to inhabit the narrative of denial and refusal.

We simply can't control many of the conditions we live in. We cannot guarantee that there will always be positive outcomes of the efforts we make. We cannot determine the weather or that only lovely people and events will frequent our lives. Yet we are not helpless to impact our inner and outer worlds. We have the ability to stabilize our attention and recognize the inner conditions (e.g., exhaustion, infatuation with narrative, busyness) that trigger our reactivity (Chapter 5). We begin to cultivate an inner climate of stable attention, new ways of knowing and being in an unpredictable life, to meet difficulty with balance and poise and the capacity to respond with discernment and skill (Chapter 6). The four attitudinal dimensions of mindfulness (befriending, compassion, joy, and equanimity) are foundations for this transformational work (see Figure 7.1).

The key insight is that mindfulness reminds us to return to the actuality of the present with an attitude of befriending, to establish a body of stillness and calm where we find the strength to meet the difficult with balance and compassion. The same attitude of

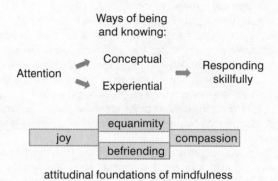

FIGURE 7.1. The transformational journey of change in mindfulness-based programs underpinned by the four attitudes of mindfulness.

befriending enables us to find contentment and joy in the midst of the lovely and the difficult.

Psychological Science

Of the four attitudinal foundations—befriending, compassion, joy, and equanimity—psychological science has focused most on befriending and compassion. Theoretical models and methodologically rigorous science to test these models are in their infancy.

This work has started with defining and operationalizing compassion, asking fundamental questions (Strauss et al., 2016), such as "How does human compassion build from what is seen in other species?"; "How do empathy and compassion relate to each other?"; "Is compassion toward the self and toward others the same or different?"; and "What domains make up the matrix that is compassion?" Given the matrix and process of compassion we set out above, perhaps not surprisingly, compassion has proven difficult to measure. The Self-Compassion Scale is a widely used questionnaire measure (Neff, 2003, 2016; Williams, Dalgleish, Karl, & Kuyken, 2014). Lately, innovative researchers have started to measure compassion across self-report (i.e., the person's subjective account), observer measures (i.e., what others are able to observe in a person's behavior), and biobehavioral measures (e.g., Lumma, Kok, & Singer, 2015; Weng et al., 2013).

This groundwork of psychological science has enabled researchers to ask important questions. For example, in charged situations, empathy, compassion, appraisal, and reappraisal are in constant interplay as people figure out how best to respond to a challenging situation (Kanske, Bockler, Trautwein, Lesemann, & Singer, 2016; Kanske, Bockler, Trautwein, & Singer, 2015). We have to recognize and see distress, understand it from a range of perspectives, and know when to respond with compassion.

There is now a large body of evidence that compassion is associated with better mental health and well-being (Krieger, Berger, & Holtforth, 2016; MacBeth & Gumley, 2012; Neff, Rude, & Kirkpatrick, 2007), as well as other key dimensions, such as emotion regulation (Engen & Singer, 2015) and positive parenting (Mann et al., 2016; Psychogiou et al., 2016). There is increasingly more compelling experimental evidence that compassion helps people respond more adaptively to distress (Diedrich, Grant, Hofmann, Hiller, & Berking, 2014; Karl, Williams, Cardy, Kuyken, & Crane, 2018). In addition, there is early promising evidence that compassion is associated with helping and prosocial behavior (Bornemann, Kok, Bockler, & Singer, 2016; Condon, Desbordes, Miller, & DeSteno, 2013; Leiberg, Klimecki, & Singer, 2011;

McCall, Steinbeis, Ricard, & Singer, 2014; Weng et al., 2013) and with biological markers, such as lower stress-induced inflammation (Breines et al., 2014).

In studies examining how mindfulness-based programs as a whole work, the development of compassion seems to be an important mechanism of change—that is, people learn compassion in these programs, and when the capacity for compassion increases, so, too, does mental health and well-being (Birnie, Speca, & Carlson, 2010; Kuyken, Watkins, Holden, White, Taylor, et al., 2010; Shapiro, Astin, Bishop, & Cordova, 2005). Although researchers are only just beginning to examine the constituent mindfulness practices that make up 8-week programs like MBSR, results are promising. Mindfulness trainings, such as the body scan, over longer periods of time can cultivate body awareness, and this awareness can support the way we use our embodiment to regulate ourselves (Bornemann, Herbert, Mehling, & Singer, 2015). Befriending mindfulness practices help us better manage our emotions and create the capacity for ease of being, joy, connection with others, and responsiveness (Engen & Singer, 2015).

The best is yet to come in this field of research. Psychologists such as Richard Davidson, Paul Gilbert, Olga Klimecki, Antoine Lutz, Kristin Neff, Tania Singer, Clara Strauss, and many others, including their students, have done much to begin to map out this field. Interested readers are directed to several reviews for an overview of this field (see Davidson & McEwen, 2012; Desbordes et al., 2015; Goetz, Keltner, & Simon-Thomas, 2010; Gu et al., 2015; Hofmann, Grossman, & Hinton, 2011; MacBeth & Gumley, 2012; Strauss et al., 2016).

SYNOPSIS

Befriending, compassion, joy, and equanimity are as essential to the deepening of mindfulness as nourishment is to the well-being of our bodies. These four attitudinal foundations help us *listen* to the tenor of our own mindfulness, so that we are better able to meet all moments with a mindfulness that is rich in kindness, compassion, gladness, and poise. This cools the fire of reactivity and creates the space for responding in ways that support our well-being and the well-being of those around us. This is not a surrender of intention, passion, or aliveness—rather, it is a wholehearted responsiveness, built from new ways of being and knowing that support us in leading our lives in ways that are meaningful, pleasurable, and rewarding.

CHAPTER 8

Embodiment

LIVING THE LIFE WE ASPIRE TO

> I think what people are seeking for is the experience
> of being fully alive, so that our life experiences on
> the purely physical plane will have resonances with
> our own innermost being and reality, so that we
> actually feel the rapture of being alive.
> —JOSEPH CAMPBELL (1991)

Sophia was overjoyed to visit her first grandchild hours after his birth. On the drive home, though, she received a call from her son telling her that the baby was seriously ill and in intensive care. Memories of losing her own child years earlier flooded back as if it were happening again right now. She had a palpable sense of nausea; she was reeling with shock and worry. She turned her car around and headed back to the hospital. As she drove back through the shock and nausea she prepared to launch herself into the project of her grandson's recovery.

Over the next week, she spent many hours each day sitting with the baby. "I started knitting, a cliché, I know. [Laughs.] I started by doing baby clothes for my grandson, but then I did them for other babies in the unit. Then I thought 'Oh, it's time to do something for me,' so I did a hat and scarf. It's strange, I know, but I loved it, being there with him, absorbed in my knitting."

The unit, she said later, started to become a place of sanctuary. Quietude prevailed, the babies were too ill to cry, and the nurses took care to speak in hushed voices, to close doors quietly, and to tend to the babies with an extraordinary care and love. She found herself drawn into the stillness, the present-moment responsiveness embodied by the nursing staff. They listened wholeheartedly to the family's worries, yet in the midst of all the heartache around them, the nurses moved with a calm dignity. Sophia learned that this is what she could also embody, and sat for hours simply stroking the baby's hand and quietly singing and whispering to him. It was, she realized, the greatest gift she could offer to herself and to those she loved: her son, his wife, and now her grandson. Even in the midst of this most challenging situation, she could be

183

fully present and alive with her grandchild. She could even be fully present and alive to the uncertainty and distress inherent in the grandchild's illness. She was even able, in the midst of it all, to meet the memories of losing her own baby with compassion.

The word *embodiment* conveys the resonance between our own inner experience and our outer world, where we feel the "rapture of being alive." Dictionaries define embodiment as the visible or tangible expression of a quality. From the perspective of Buddhist psychology, embodiment is the unification of body, mind, aspiration, intention, and attention in a present-moment focus that is informed by ethics and attitudes of kindness and compassion. The translation of this integration into our speech, actions, choices, and relationships completes the picture of embodiment. When we have embodiment in our lives, there is seamlessness among our values, understanding, and the ways we think, act, speak, and relate. Mindfulness trainings are the beginning of a path of understanding what it truly means to be an embodied human being, where mindfulness infuses our thinking, speech, acts, and relationships. Mindfulness, in its deepest sense, is not a set of practices or techniques but an illumination that guides us to be more present in our lives, with ourselves and with others, with clarity, kindness, and ease.

The path of mindfulness practice is a path of waking up to our lives, of learning to gather the mind, a transition from recognizing reactivity to responding to living with friendliness, care, balance, and joy (Chapters 6 and 7). As we explore our capacity for mindfulness, it becomes clear that there is a direct relationship between mindfulness and embodiment. Mindfulness is more than a skill, a theory, or an intention—it is a way of being fully present with kindness, care, and responsiveness. Mindfulness is more than a technique to be practiced occasionally—it is a way of living and seeing imbued with curiosity and compassion. Mindfulness is an exploration of what it means to be an embodied human being, living a life that manifests our deepest aspirations, intentions, values, and understandings.

In this chapter, we explain how change is a process of being fully alive, in the present moment, even in the midst of challenges, such as Sophia's first grandchild being in intensive care. We look at what it means to be embodied by exploring five dimensions of embodiment—namely, what it means to:

1. Be grounded in the body with mindfulness and insight;
2. Embody intentions and attitudes;
3. Embody insight and understanding;
4. Be an embodied human being; and
5. Be an embodied mindfulness teacher.

Embodiment can be challenging and even deeply troubling. We can be painfully aware of the discrepancy and dissonance in our lives between our values, intentions, and aspirations and the ways we act, speak, think, feel, and relate. We may sit down with the intention of being mindfully present, only to find ourselves lost once more in reverie or planning. We may counsel clients or patients to approach difficult experiences with kindness and curiosity, only to find ourselves snapping at our partner on our return home or seeking distractedness. We may start our day with the intention to be patient and responsive, only to find ourselves slipping into reactivity when our train is late or we meet a difficult colleague. Faced with these discrepancies, we are prone to feel discouraged or judgmental, a *failure* in mindfulness.

We can recognize that this dissonance between how things are and how our mind believes they should be is the classroom where we learn to develop our capacity for awareness, empathy, and compassion.

The "Body" in Embodiment

Mindfulness of the body is one of the five dimensions of embodiment. It is a direct way of bringing distress to an end. Mindfulness of the body provides an education from kindergarten right through to graduate school. This is why the body scan is normally the first formal mindfulness practice learned in mindfulness programs. The early teachings suggest that when there is no mindfulness of the body, there is no mindfulness at all. As we begin the process of training ourselves in present-moment awareness, we become woefully aware of how rarely we are embodied. For example, we walk down the street and in our minds we have already arrived at our destination. We engage in a conversation with someone, yet even as we partially listen we are planning our responses. We eat, yet we hardly taste, as our attention is lost in a reverie. We return from a walk in the countryside, but realize the beauty around us has hardly touched us, preoccupied as we were with planning tomorrow's meeting.

Our relationship with our bodies is part preoccupation, part dissociation, and part indifference. When the body is ill or in pain, when aging or frail, we see how automatically we can become anxiously preoccupied with the body. Our reactions of fear and aversion trigger rumination as we imagine a terrifying future, or find we can no longer ignore our mortality. Culturally, we absorb the message that our appearance is *who we are,* and as children we begin to assess our worthiness and lovability by how our bodies are assessed by others and by ourselves. Preoccupation takes the form of relentless discrepancy thinking of how the body *should* be and look. Preoccupation with the body triggers us into judging and striving as we seek for and devise strategies to *fix* pain or mold the body into the way we think it should be.

It is challenging to inhabit the body when there is a history of abuse, chronic pain, addiction, or illness, when we have an aversion to the body we have. We are understandably reluctant to be present with our minds when faced with difficult memories, moods, or afflictive thoughts. It is difficult to befriend or be compassionate with ourselves when we view ourselves as inadequate, unworthy, or unlovable. Faced with a life full of disappointment, loss, or struggle, we understandably are prone to flee rather than be fully present with what is. Equally, when we revert to automatic pilot, we lose contact with experiential being and knowing, with being fully present with things as they are.

In his classic story collection *Dubliners,* James Joyce (1914/1996) wrote about how many people live their lives without much awareness of their bodies. As we discussed throughout this book, there are many ways that we distance ourselves from our heart, mind, and our body. We resort to dissociation when we feel we cannot tolerate what the body or mind is experiencing. We become adept at distracting ourselves from present-moment experience through thought, fantasy, planning, substance abuse, and numbness. We live within the world constructed by our minds, avoiding the life of the body. For people with histories of abuse, addiction, or physical distress, dissociation is often a survival mechanism, protecting the mind from the intolerable. Dissociation equally arises in the face of chronic or extreme pain or illness. The fear of being overwhelmed by the distress of the body triggers the impulse to flee or to seek solace in numbness or distractedness. The body can be seen as an "enemy," the source of struggle to be escaped from. In the journey of cultivating a mindful, connected life, we are asked to understand that our habit of dissociation is an impulse that only compounds our feelings of helplessness and despair.

The body is our enduring companion in this life, easier to befriend when young, well, and vital. The body is a much more vexed companion when we are in pain, ill, or dying. These are the moments when we face the reality of our mortality and vulnerability, the times we most want to flee from the body and from a present-moment experience that feels terrifying and too much to bear. Jon Kabat-Zinn (1990) taught: "The time to weave your parachute is not when you are about to jump out of the plane."

In bringing mindfulness to the body, students turn their attention toward not only the loveliness of the body but also to its vulnerability, frailty, and mortality. A nurse who worked many years in hospices spoke of caring for those close to death and the spectrum of ways that different patients met that inevitability. Some people, he said, found "an unexpected grace and peace."

For others, the patterns of denial, anxiety, and control mechanisms—so well practiced in their lives—became their default responses. He remarked,

> As medical staff, we accept dying and hope to communicate that acceptance to those in our care. Yet it is still extraordinary to me to witness how many continue to see dying as a battle they are failing to win. All that we can do is help people meet what is present in this moment with compassion and care. This is all we can offer and embody, and trust that it can make some difference.

When our body is not sending us powerful messages of pain, hunger, lust, or thirst, we are prone to be indifferent toward it. We move through our days intent on our busyness, our goals, and plans, rarely noticing the life of the body. The excitement and drama of our thoughts engrosses us—our moods and narratives captivate us to the extent we barely notice their impact on the body. We lean into the past and the future; by ignoring the body, we ignore the present moment. Our attention becomes externally focused, seeking the stimulation that excites and makes us feel alive. We become desensitized to somatic experience, feeling it to be unworthy of our attention. Mindfulness presents an alternative, where we can open to the possibility of cultivating and inhabiting a body of calm, a body of mindfulness, and a body of sensitivity in the midst of agitation, anxiety, and dissociation.

Mohammed had lived with chronic pain for years before he began the mindfulness-based stress reduction program. He spoke of the steep learning curve he undertook to step out of the dissociative patterns he had constructed to protect himself from being overwhelmed by the 24/7 pain. Sleep and fantasy had become primary escape valves, but offered only temporary relief. He spoke of how completely counterintuitive it was to turn toward a body he had learned to fear.

As he began to do so, though, he became acutely aware of how much anxiety had embedded itself in and around the pain in his body. With careful encouragement he began to explore the landscape of his body and notice the places that weren't in pain, such as his ear lobes, the palms of his hands, his feet, and his face. He also became aware of how much sensation there was in his hands and face.

Foregrounding those pain-free places with mindfulness, he began to appreciate his capacity to rest within a body of calm and ease in the midst of the pain. The pain did not disappear, but there was a marked decrease in the anxiety and dread. He noted that when he focused on the pain, this triggered tension and tightness in his face, shoulders, and back, which would exacerbate the pain further. This body of calm, he remarked, became a much more reliable place of refuge and ease than the patterns of fantasy and tuning out he had previously relied on.

Both early and contemporary teachings of mindfulness suggest that when we do not inhabit the body fully, we rarely inhabit the present moment or our life fully. It is no surprise that in both ancient and contemporary teachings of mindfulness, foregrounding the body is the primary sphere of mindfulness. Alternatively, when we are disconnected from our bodies, we are barred from understanding some of the most profound life lessons that mindfulness of the body offers us. The *satipatthana* discourse encourages "whether standing, sitting, walking or lying down, whether moving or still, establish mindfulness within the body. This is the most noble way of living in the world" (Bhikkhu Analāyo, 2003). Exploring this invitation is the first step in liberating ourselves from being governed by impulse, habit, and distress.

The body is always a present-moment experience. Mindfulness of the body is the first step to bringing discrepancy thinking to an end, because it helps us learn to meet the body as it *is* in this present moment, and not as we think it *should* be. Developing mindfulness of the body is to develop curiosity, friendliness, sensitivity, care, and responsiveness, rather than automaticity, indifference, and reactivity. Being mindful of the body, we begin to discover the many ways that the mind, heart, and somatic experience are in constant communication, continually sending signals to and shaping one another. Messages of dullness, sadness, and anger imprint themselves upon the body, just as messages of calm, well-being, and kindness leave their imprint in the body. Without mindful awareness of the body, this exchange among mind, heart, and body leads to a closed feedback loop in which distress becomes increasingly solidified. Mind and body are intimately united in an enduring marriage, for when one suffers, the other will sympathize.

As we learn to inhabit our body more intentionally, we can begin to unify our mind, body, and present-moment experience. We can begin to develop the courage to embrace the reality of change and mortality. As our attention becomes increasingly sensitized to the ever-changing nature of the body, we understand how little we are in control of many of those changes and learn to embrace unpredictability. Finding greater stability in our capacity to inhabit the body, we are less prone to be lost in the world of thought and rumination. Inhabiting the body more fully, we learn, see, listen, touch, and sense more wholeheartedly and our sense doors become portals for a deepening appreciation of the world of sensory impressions. We discover that pain can be met with compassion rather than with fear and avoidance. When we are intentionally present within our body, we find that our habits of craving and reactivity begin to calm.

Early and contemporary teachings of mindfulness encourage us to *know the body as the body,* decentralizing the sense of *self* within somatic experience. This encouragement is not a more sophisticated mechanism of dissociation, but a direct way for us to establish a relationship to our body that is attentive, curious, kind, and caring—qualities that tend to disappear when the *self* and conceptual ways of knowing *get in the way.*

The key insight is that when we inhabit our bodies with mindfulness, we become acquainted not only with the fluctuations of our own bodies but also with the universal story of all bodies— vulnerable, changing, mortal—deserving of compassion and care. Everything there is to learn from mindfulness can be learned in mindfulness of the body.

The Embodiment of Attitude and Intentions

The second dimension of embodiment is the embodiment of attitude and intentions. Mindfulness is rooted in clear ethical and attitudinal foundations: "What supports my and others' well-being in this moment?"; "What does this moment need?"; "Can I bring attitudes of sensitivity, befriending, compassion, and care?" These ethical and attitudinal foundations give mindfulness its transformative capacity.

At the end of 8-week mindfulness programs, participants sometimes learn for the first time the transformative lessons of kindness. Being fully listened to by the teacher and fellow participants—without fear of judgment and with sensitivity and compassion—models how to apply the same qualities of listening to ourselves. The psychological and emotional attitudes that underpin mindfulness—in both ancient and contemporary teachings—invite radical shifts in how we relate to life and ourselves. They are attitudes that bring depth, richness, and meaning to our lives; we are asked to learn to embody them in the present, in our relationships with others, and in ourselves.

In his work, Kabat-Zinn (1990) emphasizes the attitudinal foundations that are intrinsic to understanding mindfulness. Nonjudgment, patience, beginner's mind, nonstriving, acceptance, letting go, and intentionality are all aspects of mindfulness practice. We learn to welcome present-moment experience rather than to layer aversion-based judgments upon it. We begin to understand the ways in which aversive judging is symptomatic of dissonance and discrepancy thinking. Judgment is countered by the conscious cultivation of a friendly curiosity. Practitioners of mindfulness begin to understand the depth of patience and practice this journey requires. Rather than being a *quick-fix* answer to affliction, mindfulness is a journey of a lifetime. We begin to sense that impatience is yet another form of aversion, the demand that something goes away in order for us to be well and easeful. As our mindfulness deepens, we begin to discover our capacity for *wellness* in the midst of imperfection. We begin to embody the essential qualities of kindness, compassion, joy, and equanimity explored in the previous chapter.

Throughout this journey of mindfulness—which is a lifetime endeavor—we learn the value of being willing to *begin again* in each moment, rather than despairing at the repetitive nature of our thoughts, distractedness, and reactivity. Practitioners of mindfulness recognize that striving to *get somewhere* other than where we are, *to become someone* other than who we are in this moment, is a recipe for all of the distress associated with failure. *Nonstriving* is not a relinquishment of the effort that is required to be fully present—it is a relinquishment of the ideology that tells us that peace and well-being lie elsewhere. Acceptance is not passivity or *giving up*. It is a willingness to meet ourselves and this moment, even in the face of affliction and adversity. It is the letting go of the aversion and fear that tie us to affliction and adversity. It is the forerunner of change.

There are other qualities and attitudes woven into the fabric of mindfulness. Curiosity, kindness, compassion, empathy, and unconditional positive respect and regard are indispensable foundations of transformative mindfulness. They are qualities that help uproot the emotional habits deeply implicated in the creation and re-creation of struggle and suffering. The path of learning to embody these qualities is not linear, yet students of mindfulness begin to discern when they are present and when they are absent. They learn to develop the skillfulness to recall these attitudinal foundations into their present-moment experience and begin to embody them.

As we become increasingly mindful of our present-moment experience, it becomes evident that we embody something in every moment through our speech, our body language, our mental states, and our thoughts. We can embody anger, confusion, agitation, dullness, or fear. Equally, we can embody calm, sensitivity, care, or compassion. All are borne of intention. Our life exemplifies our intention of the moment whether conscious or unconscious, skillful or unskillful. Intention is the bridge linking past, present, and future experience. There is an adage: "If you want to know about your past, look at your mind now. If you want to know about your future, look at your mind now." Intention draws upon our moods and emotions, both the helpful and unhelpful. It is mirrored in our actions, speech, thoughts, and choices, powerfully shaping our present-moment experience.

Our thoughts, acts, speech, and choices are not random but have roots in our psychological habits and self-views. The concept of intention is so central to mindfulness practices because it shapes our body, mind, and world of the moment. For example, we could pause and explore how aware we are of the intentions and attitudes that are shaping our body just now—impatience or calm, boredom or curiosity, restlessness or ease. When we go to lunch or go home, are we aware of the intentions that shape how we speak to our partner, how we sit in the traffic jam, or the choices we make over how we use our time? To be mindful is to be conscious of each moment. To be conscious of our intentions is to have choices. Intention translates the foundational attitudes of mindfulness into our speech, thought, and acts.

It is a basic principle of life that whatever is fed will grow. Whatever we consistently practice—the helpful or the unhelpful, habit or responsiveness—we will become more adept at. Embodiment is one of the core aspirations of mindfulness. Even though we emphasize that mindfulness is a present-moment cultivation, it also has a direction. We are learning to assimilate and naturalize some important intentions: to bring suffering to an end, enable our potential to be realized for our mind and heart to flourish, and to enable us to live a mindful life. We do not live in a random or accidental world of experience. Although we are not always able to control the range of conditions and events we find ourselves in, the responses we are able to bring to that world are rooted in intentionality. Our intentions shape our present-moment experience and they shape our thoughts, speech, and actions.

Our entire life experience has taught us that the unconscious intentions of discontent, aversion, and confusion can lead to more distress. When we are mindful of this, we learn that we can meet these patterns with conscious intentions of kindness, interest, and compassion. It becomes clear that mindfulness and habit cannot coexist and that unconsciousness and conscious intentionality cannot coexist. We can experiment with this. Try to tie your shoelaces habitually *and* mindfully at the same time. Explore whether it is possible to walk down the street, or to speak habitually and mindfully, in the same moment. Mindfulness enables us to make conscious choices about the attitudes we foster moment to moment—attitudes we increasingly learn to embody in our thoughts, speech, and actions. Kindness, compassion, empathy, and sensitivity can only be fostered in the present moment, woven into the fabric of mindfulness practices, attitudes, and intentions.

When Sam was discharged from an addiction rehab unit following his rock bottom, his recovery from addiction required a transformation that took many years. Early on, the support of his 12-step meetings and sponsor were the mainstays of his recovery. The meetings were places of compassion and common humanity. His sponsor, also a recovering addict, embodied recovery, and with great patience and care would know that these moments of agitation, craving, and potential relapse needed restraint, patience, befriending, and compassion. In mindfulness programs for addiction, this is called "surfing the waves of craving," knowing that they peak and feel powerful and overwhelming, but will eventually break down (Bowen & Vieten, 2012).

During his long walks on the beach with his sponsor, Sam began to learn to bring these attitudes to his agitation, negative self-views, cravings, and impulsiveness. As the space between stimulus and reactivity grew, Sam became able to ask, "What does this moment need?"

Sam took up running. "That was the only time I could release my emotions. I had to hold it together the rest of the time but I could go for a run for an hour and that would just be when I would melt down and cry the whole time. I used to see exercise as something I had to do, otherwise something terrible would happen. [Laughs.] But now I'm much kinder to myself and think I'm actually really physically tired and the reason I'm physically tired is because I did a massive run—so that's OK. I'm less compulsive in my exercise." [Laughs again.] He started running without music. "I just think about my body and what's happening now while I'm running. So, I'm not in a bubble running, I'm just, you know, there more, enjoying the actual run, taking in everything." After his mindfulness program, Sam continued with the mindful movement through finding a yoga class. "It helps me see things more in my body . . . that are there, if you know what I mean."

Sam's regular 12-step meetings started with a moment of silence for reflection. Early on, he would use this moment to recall the horrors of where his addiction had taken him, and form an intention: "Please don't let me go back to that rock bottom ever again." A few years into his recovery, Sam noticed a transformation in these moments, and a new intention arose: "Please let me enjoy the life I see in those people further along in recovery, like my sponsor, who have a life with friendship, ease, love, and usefulness." He started to sponsor other people who were earlier in recovery as a way of embodying this intention, helping them as he, too, had been helped. This cultivated his intentionality to live a useful life and the attitudes of curiosity, sensitivity, and care both for himself and others. Later he trained as an addiction counselor. "I have the feeling that I am more alive; my emotions aren't 'leveled out' anymore. I can be sad, angry, calm, like normal people instead of swinging from extreme to extreme like a wrecking ball. I finally have a normal love life again."

The key insight is that a mindful life is an intentional life that fosters the underpinnings of the ease, peace, and responsiveness we aspire to and long for. Kindness, compassion, joy, and equanimity are not distant goals to be strived for, but present-moment attitudes that color and shape our experience. Intention, central to all mindfulness practice, translates the foundational attitudes of mindfulness into our speech, thoughts, and acts.

The Embodiment of Insight

The third dimension of embodiment is the embodiment of insight. Reactivity on automatic pilot in busy lives is where so many people live and is a cauldron for distress and suffering. The first waypoint on a journey of learning mindfulness is beginning to recognize this, and then to understand more deeply how it creates distress and suffering. Learning to respond with mindfulness to these moments is a major waypoint because it opens up a new repertoire of possibilities, both in our experience and also in our lives. This understanding enables us to begin to make different choices, borne of clear intentionality, that have inevitable downstream consequences. Not only can we learn to respond differently but a whole new repertoire of responses can become available to us.

Mindfulness brings into the light of awareness the times we slide into the same patterns of reactivity. Practitioners develop a growing capacity to know these familiar patterns, navigate their way around them, and in time even develop a new repertoire of responses. It is a journey from habit to embodiment; from helplessness and despair to the capacity to make wise choices in the midst of cravings and habits. It is equally a journey from conceptual knowing to a naturalized living of that knowing, an embodied insight that integrates conceptual and experiential knowledge.

Many people who begin mindfulness training bring with them a considerable wealth of self-knowledge. This self-knowledge is gleaned from lessons learned from our life experience and from our familiarity with the patterns of thinking and behaving that cause us suffering and pain. We know about impermanence, our whole life has taught us the lesson of the unarguable nature of change—sometimes welcome, sometimes unwelcome. Change is ever present, reflected in the seasons of our years and the seasons of our life. We know that we cannot make life stand still for us. Every moment we sense the changing nature of our bodies, our thoughts, our moods, and everything around us. We know the landscape of loss. Loved ones who are no longer part of our lives, friends who are no longer friends, the loss of roles, status, relationships—the sorrow of loss has touched us all. We know about uncertainty and instability, and all the ways our world can crumble in a moment. We know we cannot find enduring stability in a world of changing conditions that we cannot control. We know about pain—physical, emotional, and psychological—and know that as vulnerable, relational beings we will not be exempt from our own measure of distress in life. We know that a life governed by craving, fear, and aversion has only one outcome (i.e., emotional and psychological pain, defensiveness, and ill-will). It is a pattern of reactivity we have run off many times. We know that grasping and clinging leads only to agitation and contractedness.

We know, too, the power of generosity, kindness, and compassion in our lives. We have been touched by the kindness and generosity of others and have touched the lives of others with simple gestures of kindness and care. In the most difficult moments of our lives, it is not advice or strategies that sustains us, but love.

However, there is a point in everyone's journey of mindfulness when they realize there is a gap between their knowing and how they are living, speaking, thinking, and acting. It is the most challenging part of the path, and one that easily invites judgment and despair. Yet this is the classroom of the practice, where we learn to *inch* our way toward embodiment. We begin to ask the challenging questions of what it is that makes us forgetful. It can be a long list of answers—fatigue, busyness, and the absence of support—yet much of it may be distilled down to our patterns of self-doubt and psychological habit. As we persevere with practice, it becomes clear that one of the most radical shifts that any student of mindfulness makes is the shift from self-doubt to self-confidence, from a sense of helplessness to a growing sense of capacity. We begin to learn to live in the light of what we know as our knowing turns into a *felt understanding.* It is this felt understanding that becomes the foundation of our thoughts, acts, speech, and ways of relating to present-moment experience.

Familiar patterns of repetitive thought may make themselves known, the nagging voice of self-judgment may arise, and habits of anxiety and aversion may appear. However, mindfulness practitioners discover that they can look at these repetitive thoughts directly with a new understanding that thoughts are not *facts,* and they do not define who they are. The possibility of walking down a different street, in that moment, is available—there is a clear understanding that the path to ending distress is a path that can be taken only in the moment that distress arises. Mindfulness offers the freedom to choose where and how we establish our attention. As our confidence and capacity for insight deepens and becomes more available to us, we can choose to live in the light of what we know sustains our well-being and happiness, rather than remain stuck in the destructive habits that undermine our well-being.

The key insight is that through mindfulness practice and an examined life, we come to internalize a route map for change. Our new-found shift in perspective enables us to live a more mindful, embodied life.

Being an Embodied Human Being

The fourth dimension of embodiment is what it means to be an embodied human being. It is a unique journey for each of us, full of twists and turns, and requiring perseverance and a compassionate willingness to be open to our inner and outer experiences. This journey begins from the moment a group of strangers walks into a room at the beginning of an 8-week mindfulness program. Their stories and histories will vary widely, but their common bond is distress, a motivation to find a way to heal that distress, and a wish for happiness and ease of being. Throughout the 8-week program, they will become familiar with their minds and bodies, with some of their strengths and frailties, and witness others in the group going through the same learning. This is an unfamiliar classroom for many people, a different way of learning. In 8-week programs, people discover the willingness to be open and present with their deepest vulnerabilities.

As participants enter into mindfulness training, they bring with them the often unarticulated longing to be an embodied human being. They long to be rooted in the present moment, awake, creative, and free of the distress that dissonance and dissociation engenders. One way of seeing mindfulness training is as a journey from dissonance to embodiment. This is not a reliably linear journey—there will be many moments of forgetfulness, of relapsing into familiar patterns of reactivity. Yet people learn again and again to refrain from adding the second arrow of judgment and blame. Practitioners also begin to taste the happiness that moments of embodiment bring, when they truly sense the alignment of their deepest aspirations and intentions and the ways that vthey interface with their inner and outer worlds. Mindfulness, which is often initially experienced as a somewhat laborious task, begins to offer the balance, responsiveness, and sense of aliveness that has been longed for.

Kindness and compassion can truly underpin our thoughts, words, and actions. Increasingly, we discover that in inhabiting the body more fully, we can live a more wakeful and responsive life (i.e., a more embodied life). Rather than being governed by habit, there is a growing awareness of our psychological and emotional processes where there is the freedom to choose our response to the moment. Mindfulness, we experientially understand, is not an end in itself, but an open doorway to understanding and transformation.

The Embodied Mindfulness Teacher

> The principal art of the teacher is to awaken
> the joy in creation and knowledge.
> —ALBERT EINSTEIN (1956/1999)

The responsibility for creating a safe, containing environment in which course participants can learn lies with the mindfulness teacher. People embarking on mindfulness training will inevitably look to the teacher for clues of what it means to be mindfully present with kindness, curiosity, and compassion. How the teacher is present is a primary factor in shaping how clients learn to relate to themselves and to the others in the group. Presence means body language and tone of voice, the vocabulary that teachers use, and their capacity for attentive listening, acceptance, and warmth. Course participants will anticipate that the teacher embodies the lessons he or she is offering. This is an enormous and often intimidating expectation for many mindfulness teachers—yet their capacity to embody the teaching they are offering will have a profound outcome on how the group develops and deepens.

In offering mindfulness programs, teachers quickly discover the need to continue to be students of mindfulness. In supporting participants' learning, teachers need to embody a sustained, empathic attentiveness that gives equal respect to the student who reports a minor irritation as to the student who speaks about facing his or her greatest fears. Mindfulness teachers are asked to embody the acceptance and warmth that welcomes all experiences nonpreferentially—the difficult and the lovely. They are asked to embody the curiosity in clients' experiences—the same curiosity that clients are learning to cultivate in themselves. Teachers set the tone of kindness through the personal warmth, interest, and welcome they embody in leading sessions. In the presence of the sadness, anger, despair, and resistance that may be raised in inquiry sessions, it is the teacher who embodies the balance that is able to meet layers of pain without floundering, judging, or personalizing the distress. Participants in programs report remembering not so much what is said in the classroom but how it is said and how they are met with compassion.

Like anyone, in my mindfulness practice I (WK) have sometimes encountered impatience, busyness, fatigue, and agitation. Once I was on a mindfulness retreat around the time my father was terminally ill, my wife was pregnant with my eldest daughter, and I was negotiating a trans-Atlantic move. I found that my mind was a torrent of restless activity. During an interview, the mindfulness teacher leading the retreat said, to my great surprise and relief, "Perhaps this is not the place for you just now, maybe now you need to be at home taking care of what you need to take care of." She said it with enormous steadiness and care. It was how she said it that enabled me to really hear it and take it on board. It was a moment in which I could recognize the torrent of restlessness and do what was necessary.

This was a lesson that has enabled me as mindfulness teacher to embody the same steadiness when people come with a lot of challenges, like agitation, doubt, or anger. I remember a particular client, someone not unlike Ling, who in the body scan met enormous aversion. She looked like she wanted to be catapulted out of the class. During the inquiry about the practice, I could see what was happening for her from her body language. I started by making sure my feet were firmly planted on the ground, my posture was upright and digni-fied, that I was embodied. As she described her experience, I could hear what she was saying and feel the resonance in my own body, alongside a worry and urge to fix it for her. Anchoring in my breath and body enabled me to support her to find a place in her body where she could be present: her toes. This gave her a focus where she could begin to work with the aversion.

Kindness, compassion, empathy, warmth, attentiveness, and interest are difficult, if not impossible, to contrive. Mindfulness teachers learn these les-sons in the classroom of their own practice and vulnerability. When people train to teach mindfulness, they are not always aware that two simultane-ous journeys are taking place. On the one hand, we are learning the skills of teaching. Simultaneously, we are embarking on an inner journey, where we learn to be intimate and present with our bodies, emotions, moods, and thoughts.

It is possible to learn the theory that underpins mindfulness programs, even the procedural skills of teaching the program, yet be unmindful. It is our capacity to sustain an empathic attention, developed in the classroom of our own practice, that enables a therapist or teacher to establish rapport and empathy with the clients who participate in the program they are offer-ing. Embodied mindfulness teachers have learned about self-compassion through meeting—with understanding and acceptance—their own frailties and imperfections. They have learned to be more accepting and less critical and judgmental of themselves. These primary lessons enable them to see their clients as whole human beings, with all their strengths and vulnerabilities, capable of change. This is in stark contrast to a model in which we see just the clients' pathology and adopt a model of curing, remediating, or fixing this pathology. Through our own personal practice and development, we learn as mindfulness teachers to let go of attachment to outcomes. This enables us to communicate to our clients and patients the patience and nonstriving that are essential to learning to be present in the midst of seemingly intractable patterns that create distress.

Mindfulness practice values not only our capacity to sustain attention in the midst of present-moment experience that can be fraught with difficulty. Mindfulness practice also equally values the *how* of our attending. Warmth, interest, and kindness form the essential foundation for all mindfulness development. Many clients have little or no background in these essential qualities—they are far more familiar with the landscape of blame, judgment, and shame. An embodied mindfulness teacher has learned to develop a *safe* learning environment in which clients and students feel able to disclose these most difficult emotions without fear of being judged. They learn from the

teacher that even these most challenging emotions can be met with acceptance, care, and compassion.

Mindfulness teachers frequently become acutely aware of the dissonance
between the advice and guidance they are offering their students and how
they are living their own lives. Mindfulness teachers can often feel like *frauds*.
There are moments in every mindfulness teacher's life when he or she realizes
that dissonance is optional and that it may be time to renew the connection with his or her personal practice to cultivate greater self-compassion and
stability. Mindfulness teachers know that to be able to meet and tolerate the
pain and distress disclosed in teaching sessions, they need to be able to access
inner stillness, calm, and balance. Embodiment is challenging, yet it is the
reason why mindfulness teachers continue to be motivated to be mindfulness
students—for their own well-being and the well-being of their students.

Embodiment will not look the same for every teacher or student of mindfulness. It is not a quality that can be contrived, and there is no single tem-
plate of embodiment. Embodiment is not learned in a teaching classroom,
but in the classroom of our own mindfulness practice and life experience.
Every teacher of mindfulness learns to find his or her own voice and way
of communicating rather than endeavoring to emulate a teaching style of a
senior teacher whom he or she respects. Mindfulness teachers offer programs
in different settings—a mindfulness course offered in schools to teenagers is
likely to look different from one offered in a clinic for people being treated for
cancer. A program offered to clients with a depressive relapse history will have
a different shape from one offered to executives dealing with stress. In some
mindfulness programs, a teacher will offer comprehensive instruction, and in
others there may be much more silence and stillness. Mindfulness can have
many different flavors and presentations. But the embodiment of the teacher
is central to all this teaching, regardless of the context. It may manifest in
different ways in different contexts, but the teacher teaches the mindfulness
curriculum from his or her own lived experience of the practice.

Adaptability is one of the great arts of a mindfulness teacher—it is rooted
in present-moment responsiveness. An awareness of what is needed and what
is helpful in differing situations is borne of a teacher's confidence, capacity
to listen, and to not be identified with the "right" way or the "right" model.
The intentions that endure through the range of client groups that teachers
encounter are kindness, care, and compassion. Being an effective mindfulness
teacher means finding an inner authenticity rooted in one's own experience.

As mindfulness programs are taught in an ever-widening range of settings, we are seeing tensions arise between maintaining the integrity of
designed programs and adapting those same programs for diverse participants.

One teacher, for example, mentioned that the language of the program was alien to the language of the residents of the South African township where she taught. A teacher working with gangs in inner-city London said that if the program was going to be useful to his young clients, it would need to be set to rap music. Mindfulness in school programs adapt both the language and structure of the teaching to the age groups participating. Mindfulness teachers learn the need to attune themselves to the cultural, social, and ethnic roots of those they teach, rather than feeling obliged to import a model of teaching that is alien and inaccessible to clients participating in their groups. Maintaining the integrity of mindfulness programs, while enabling them to be adapted for diverse groups, is an ongoing and evolving discussion.

As teachers, we can never assume that our view of the world, life experience, or values are the same as those participating in our training. We may be teaching from a position of privilege so normalized that it is unquestioned for us. People learning mindfulness may be simultaneously swimming against two tides. One tide is their own experience of distress, depression, lack of self-worth, or anxiety. The other tide may be the reality of living in a disadvantaged or discriminatory society and culture where they have been told and retold the story of inadequacy and impossibility. Those who reach out beyond the comfort zone of their more privileged worlds frequently become aware that they need to be trained not only in mindfulness but also in all of the complex issues of diversity. In any group of mindfulness teachers, embodiment will take as many forms as there are teachers.

Sophia was a warmhearted person with a great sense of humor; she had a way of making her students laugh. She started her journey as a mindfulness teacher using her humor, but it soon became apparent that the humor functioned, at least in part, to mask her inner critic. It could at times make her teaching edgy. When she felt uncomfortable, or out of her depth ("I don't know what I'm doing, they'll see I'm a fraud"), she would make people laugh, often with a self-deprecating joke.

For Sophia, learning to be a mindfulness teacher involved really seeing her inner critic, meeting it with friendliness and compassion, and responding to it with the question "What does this moment need?" As she softened as a teacher, the edge was softened and eventually eroded away, and her warmth and potential started to be realized. She used humor less, and when she did, it had a common humanity and compassion to it that had not been there before. She became a more authentic, engaging, and potent teacher.

Mindfulness teacher training programs provide feedback to teachers, often asking teachers to video record themselves. Having our vulnerability captured on video for others to see powerfully evokes any inner critic. It can be intimidating and discouraging for us to see—and to have others see—all of the inevitable stutters and flaws in our teaching, particularly in the early stages of learning to teach. This was Sophia's experience:

> "At first I just could not bear to watch myself on video. It was paralyzing and cringeworthy. But over time, I softened and, by the end, I was able to watch the videos, even staying with my experience of discomfort as I watched, with a bit of distance but also love. Last time I watched video of myself, I found myself saying, 'Ah, bless, look at Sophia, she is doing the best she can [laughing], but not sure about the dress.'"

For most teachers, the journey of learning to teach involves recognizing, allowing, and befriending the inner critic that can kick in when we learn anything new, especially when it is something important and impactful. This work is not easy, not saccharine, and likely exposes some quite challenging thoughts and beliefs. However, when we look hard into the self-critic, it is possible to find the wholesome intentions that underpin its architecture. Often it is something like "I want to be the best teacher I can," or "I'd like to really help people enjoy the transformative journey I've had myself," or "I'd like to support people through some of the challenges with compassion." When this linchpin is identified, the structure of the self-critic collapses.

Sophia's path of mindfulness practice included first really seeing and looking into the thick crust of negative thinking and self-views (inept and worthless), with generalized memories (e.g., freezing in front of a class of students as a student teacher) and imagined scenarios of failure. When she looked deeply, she could see that beneath the crust were feelings of fear, with a sense of contraction in her belly and chest, and heat in her face. She learned to open and soften to these experiences.

Even when Sophia suffered further episodes of crippling anxiety and life-sapping depression, she saw this not as a failure but rather as further learning of the territory of anxiety and depression, and the paths through and out of it. The inner critic softened enough for her to really turn toward it and befriend it. As she opened to this profound insight—of turning toward and befriending—Sophia could see that beneath the inner critic was a wholesome intention to be a good teacher and, importantly, to be of service in her life. This understanding, when known both conceptually and experientially, helped dissolve the inner critic. It enabled her to teach from a place of service, where her performance was not the issue but rather the learning of her students. Self-views of worthlessness eroded as Sophia connected with how to best help and support her students' learning and enjoy teaching.

SYNOPSIS

The human longing for meaning, health, and well-being, our desire to be respected and honored, to do good work, and to help and not harm ourselves or others, can come to be embodied. Embodiment starts with coming to inhabit our bodies with awareness. This broadens to include our intentions, attitudes, insight, and understanding. Like a willow tree, we can be firmly rooted in intentionality and understanding, yet bend with the wind of changing conditions. Embodiment is seamlessness between our values, understanding, and intentions, and the ways we think, act, speak, and relate. It is fundamental to teaching and learning mindfulness.

CHAPTER 9

Ethics and Integrity
in Mindfulness-Based Programs

Only the individual can think, and thereby create
new values for society—nay, even set up new moral
standards to which the life of the community conforms.
Without creative, independently thinking and judging
personalities the upward development of society is
as unthinkable as the development of the individual
personality without the nourishing soil of the community.
—ALBERT EINSTEIN (1956/1999)

It is not difficult for us to act in ways that are harmful to
ourselves and others. It is far more challenging to live and
act in ways beneficial to ourselves and others.
—ACHARYA BUDDHARAKKHITA (1996)

If you go into a large bookstore to peruse the contemporary psychology section, you will find many books on mindfulness. But if you look in the indexes of these books for the terms *integrity* and *ethics*, you will rarely find them. In the same bookstore, in the sections on philosophy or religion, you will find entire shelves dedicated to the discussion of integrity, ethics, virtue, values, and wisdom. In Blackwell's bookshop in Oxford, United Kingdom, for example, psychology, religion, medicine, and law are all located in the cavernous Norton reading room. In the middle of the room there is a lower level, a sort of open basement, with all the philosophy books, with shelves dedicated to sophists—Hume, Kant, Russell, and others—many discussing ethics and integrity. Why are ethics prominent in philosophy, the contemplative traditions, religion, law, and medicine, but absent from contemporary mindfulness books? Is it irrelevant in contemporary mindfulness? Does an emphasis on ethics introduce something potentially problematic into *secular settings,* perhaps because the subject of ethics is often associated with religion or particular schools of philosophy? What do we mean by ethics and integrity anyway? What does integrity look like for a participant in a mindfulness-based program, for a mindfulness teacher, and for the field as a whole?

In this chapter, we look at:

- What are ethics and integrity;
- Ethics and integrity in mindfulness-based programs: the challenges;
- Ethics and integrity in mindfulness-based programs: the response (from the *inside out* and *outside in*); and
- Safeguarding the integrity of the wider field.

What Are Ethics? What Is Integrity?

Ethics are the moral principles and values that govern our behavior. They are our understanding of what is right and wrong. They help us understand and navigate dilemmas that we regularly encounter—particularly ones that challenge our values—so that we can figure out how best to respond. In Buddhist psychology, the words *wholesome* and *unwholesome* are used rather than *right* and *wrong*. The difference between wholesome and unwholesome is whether our thoughts, words, and acts lead to the end of suffering (wholesome), or whether they lead to the suffering of ourselves, others, or both (unwholesome). We are further encouraged to inquire whether our thoughts, words, and acts obstruct understanding and lead away from freedom (unwholesome), or whether they support understanding and lead toward freedom for ourselves and others (wholesome). These considerations firmly place mindfulness in the relational world, where we are asked to consider not only the intentions that guide our thoughts, words, and acts but equally, the imprint and consequences of those thoughts, words, and acts upon others and ourselves.

Consider the scenarios depicted in Boxes 9.1 and 9.2. These are the sorts of questions that can arise in mindfulness training, both for teachers and participants. We refer to them later in the chapter as we discuss specific themes and practice regarding ethics.

Integrity is the ethical alignment of our state of mind and actions. Integrity can be cultivated when we live and act in ways that are in alignment with our ethics—that is, integrity involves both enacting wholesome states of mind (i.e., being aware of how actions are shaped by and in turn shape our state of mind) and undertaking training that supports and develops integrity (see Figure 9.1).

BOX 9.1. Examples of Ethical Dilemmas for Teachers of Mindfulness-Based Programs

- As you teach an MBSR program, you are diagnosed with a serious health condition and you feel scared and worried. Your stress levels suddenly seem as high as that in some of your participants.

- You teach MBCT in a health care setting for people at risk for depressive relapse. Your manager tells you that resources are tight and you need to run the MBCT program in fewer sessions, no more than four, and that one-to-one orientations are definitely not possible. She also asks whether you could open it up to more people on the waiting list who have other common mental health problems.

- You are a mindfulness teacher teaching an all-day retreat. After one of the practices, a participant describes experiencing frightening dissociative experiences and hearing voices telling her to hurt herself.

- You are a mindfulness teacher teaching mindfulness-based programs in the community. You receive a call from someone who has signed up for your next 8-week program, who tells you he has lost his job and is a single parent. He would like to attend your program, but cannot afford your fees and needs child care during the classes. Do you have any arrangements for people who cannot afford the full fees?

Students and participants in mindfulness programs—whether seeking ways to bring acute distress to an end or to enhance well-being—discover that mindfulness does not deepen or thrive in a vacuum and that facing ethical and life dilemmas provides opportunities for learning and change. In other words, mindfulness gives us the opportunity to be aware of and reflect upon our wholesome and unwholesome thoughts, words, and actions, so that we can then respond with integrity. Consider the examples in Box 9.2.

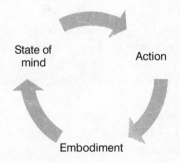

FIGURE 9.1. State of mind and action.

Ethics are as fundamental to humans as the more primitive instincts and drives that can determine behavior.[1] It is easy to understand the natural drives for food, physical comfort, and sexual gratification. However, deep in our nature, we also have the capacity for awareness, experiential and conceptual understanding, and compassion. These provide a deeper framework for integrity.

We often sense ethics quite intuitively; we have a sense of the *right* response. Ethics can spark a sense of discomfort or unease, which may alert us to some misalignment among our principles, a situation, and our behavior. At these moments we know something is not quite right, and our embodiment can help us recognize this unease. It is an invaluable invitation to reexamine our state of mind and intentionality so that we can consider how to respond.

The key insight is that ethics are the moral principles and values that govern our behavior. It is our understanding of what is right and wrong, wholesome and unwholesome. Integrity is the ethical alignment of our state of mind and actions. Integrity can be cultivated when we live and act in ways that are in alignment with our ethics. Ethics and integrity are foundational for teachers and students of mindfulness.

BOX 9.2. Examples of Ethical Dilemmas for Participants in Mindfulness-Based Programs

- Mohammed's Muslim faith is very important not only to him spiritually but also as a way of life and a community. His imam questions his participation in the mindfulness class and how it sits with the tenets of Islam.

- Through the mindfulness program, Ling becomes increasingly aware that her reactivity can make parenting teenagers a real challenge; sometimes she worries she may be abusive. She also came to reflect that when she was her daughter's age, she had used her sexuality to get the attention and care she craved. Ling wants more than anything that her daughter doesn't repeat some of the mistakes she made while growing up.

- As Sam's recovery from addiction and mindfulness practice progressed, he became more acutely aware of the pain and destruction his addiction had caused not just to himself but others, too. He has stolen from his mother, been unreliable and fired from several jobs, and has shared needles with people.

- Sam finds the mindfulness program transformative and his teacher inspiring. He idealizes his teacher, flatters her, and has fantasies about being her special student.

Ethics and Integrity in Mindfulness-Based Programs: The Challenges

When Jon Kabat-Zinn began teaching mindfulness in the 1970s in the Stress Reduction Clinic at the University of Massachusetts Medical Center, there was a single coherent approach: mindfulness-based stress reduction (MBSR). It was taught by a relatively small set of teachers who were all trained and mentored by Kabat-Zinn. Mindfulness teachers were operating in health care situations where there was a commitment to the Hippocratic principles of doing no harm and putting the needs of patients above any self-interest (Kabat-Zinn, 2014).

In the early years of contemporary mindfulness, it was assumed that anyone teaching MBSR would take personal responsibility for his or her conduct, intentions, and motivations in teaching. There was an assumption that anyone teaching mindfulness would be deeply rooted in a pathway of personal contemplation and development that would be embodied in compassionate and caring relationships with his or her clients. It was also assumed that the practice and application of mindfulness would, implicitly, be imbued with deeply ethical attitudes of care and compassion. Moreover, there was a reluctance to develop higher authorities or regulators who would have the power to approve or endorse ethical standards. There was no need to *police* the mindfulness world if mindfulness teachers embodied integrity (Kabat-Zinn, 2011, 2014).

Since the 1970s, though, the landscape of mindfulness-based programs has changed dramatically and the concept of mindfulness itself has taking on myriad meanings. Moreover, there has been a proliferation of mindfulness-based programs (Crane, 2017). At first, the arena for mindfulness programs was primarily behavioral medicine. Today, we see mindfulness taught in schools, physical and mental health care settings, and within corporate entities, the military, and the criminal justice system. There has been an exponential rise in the amount of scientific research being undertaken, which has not always evolved programmatically (Dimidjian & Segal, 2015).

The United Kingdom is a good example of this proliferation of mindfulness and mindfulness-based programs. The UK's National Institute for Health and Care Excellence (2009) recommends mindfulness as a treatment in preventing depressive relapse, available through the National Health Service. October 2015 saw the publication of the *Mindful Nation U.K. Report*, written by the Mindfulness All-Party Parliamentary Group (2015). It recommends the funding and implementation of mindfulness training in health care, education, the workplace, and the criminal justice system.

As the landscape of mindfulness trainings has expanded, so, too, has the spectrum of trainings available. In the early years, mindfulness-based programs were primarily taught by a small group of people who were deeply established in their own mindfulness and contemplative pathways, who had a passion for the practice and a commitment to serving others. They had been trained in contemplative traditions that included comprehensive teachings on integrity. Out of a clear intentionality and deep commitment, many sacrificed good careers and economic security to engage in teaching this ancient training in secular situations. They had to carefully examine what to retain and what to leave behind from Buddhist psychology, which is rooted in rigorous inner development and training. The search for happiness, peace, well-being, and freedom was the fundamental human quest. Religious or esoteric overtones or rituals were not needed. The early teachers undertook the challenge to speak in a language that everyone could relate to and to retain the core motivation to minimize distress while maximizing their own and their clients' capacity to thrive. Teaching mindfulness in those early years was not a career choice but a passion rooted in compassion and an embodied integrity.

As interest in mindfulness and the field itself have grown, so, too, have the range of trainings. There are comprehensive university master's degree programs available that take years to complete. These programs require students to understand the theory underpinning mindfulness-based programs, establish a personal mindfulness practice, learn how to teach the programs and teach them with supervision, and finally, commit to ongoing personal and professional development. It is also possible to obtain a certificate to teach mindfulness in a short period of time, or even through an online course. In addition, while some mindfulness teachers have a professional identity that includes professional codes of conduct that govern their relationships with their clients, there are teachers who do not have ties to any professional ethical framework. There is sometimes pressure to abbreviate mindfulness training for clients, even though most of the research evidence is based on evaluating the full 8-week programs (Dimidjian & Segal, 2015). Evidence suggests that there is a direct link between long-term change and the amount of time spent immersed in mindfulness practice (Parsons, Crane, Parsons, Fjorback, & Kuyken, 2017). As mindfulness trainings are increasingly offered in diverse cultures and communities, there is considerable adaptation needed in the language and the presentation of the program for them to be meaningful. In all of these developments, the commitment to ethics and integrity safeguards the participants, mindfulness-based programs, mindfulness teachers, and the field more widely.

Perhaps inevitably, following the intense growth in the interest and practice of mindfulness, there has also been significant backlash. Questions have been raised about standards, including accusations that mindfulness training is *value-less*, that charges levied for mindfulness programs exclude the economically disadvantaged, what qualifies a person to be a mindfulness teacher, and what constitutes a comprehensive mindfulness program. These are important ethical questions. In the absence of any regulatory body, there is little to safeguard the development of the mindfulness field or the participants who undertake mindfulness training—apart from individual mindfulness teachers' personal commitment to integrity.

Mindfulness research and training centers around the world have concerns about the risks incurred by the rapid and unregulated growth of mindfulness. Aspects of the core training can be *cherry-picked* and combined with a range of other disciplines. Mindfulness can be presented as simple attention training, stripped of its underpinnings of intention, attitudes, and ethics. Participants undertaking a mindfulness program may be new to mindfulness practice and have vulnerabilities; they have the right to be assured that the course they are undertaking is being taught by a well-trained teacher able to hold that vulnerability, minimize the risk of harm, and maximize the likelihood of benefit. Many research and training centers are deeply aware of the ethical underpinnings of the teaching of mindfulness. They typically take the position that this includes mindfulness teachers taking responsibility for their own personal and professional development and the degree to which they are able to embody the practice in compassionate and mindful teaching.

As mindfulness training is adopted by health systems and workplace settings—ostensibly to support the well-being of employees—there is also the risk that the burden of mindfulness is transferred to the employee without the organization itself being willing or able to undertake the necessary changes to make it a mindful employer. In other words, mindfulness can be utilized with the intent to make an employee better equipped to handle unsustainable workloads and pressure, or serve the economic objectives of a corporation. The question of personal mindfulness and organizational mindfulness is rarely discussed.

The key insight is that as the field of mindfulness has grown and evolved, it has raised important ethical questions around training and standards that require a response.

Ethics and Integrity in Mindfulness-Based Programs: The Response

Understanding and promoting integrity require both an *inside-out* and *outside-in* approach. Many contemplative traditions, including Buddhism, teach us that integrity is a practice of examining our intentions, mental landscapes, and actions: *inside out.* What is the impact of our thoughts, speech, and acts upon ourselves and others? This is a key point: Mindfulness is inherently ethical. It is a path of understanding and a way of being and acting rooted in nonharming and beneficence. If it is not rooted in this intentionality, it is not mindfulness.[2] There is also a collective responsibility to create frameworks for ethics and integrity to support the field that will encourage integrity and safeguard people doing this work: *outside in.*

First we consider the inside-out work (i.e., the work of mindfulness practice for developing integrity and embodiment). We then consider the levels of mindfulness-based programs, teacher training, mindfulness teachers, and finally, principles and practices for the field as a whole.

Ethics and Integrity in Mindfulness: From the Inside Out

"Everything Rests on the Tip of Intention"

The expression "The mind is the forerunner of experience" is key to any understanding of ethics in the wisdom traditions and world religions. A mind that is rooted in wholesome intentions will support ethical action and create the conditions for a good life. A mind rooted in unwholesome intentions is vulnerable to destructive action. Bringing awareness to our minds allows intentions and actions to be examined and understood. It creates the conditions for wholesome intentions to be cultivated, so that we can act in ways that affect ourselves and other people positively. Integrity is at the heart of healthy relationships, societies, and communities. The collective commitment to integrity is seen to be the key element that safeguards the well-being of families, communities, and societies. Integrity places collective wellness above personal gratification. The commitment to ethical guidelines sets a moral compass inwardly that not only protects the well-being of our own mind but also helps us positively impact those around us. Integrity is seen to be the foundation of psychological health and central to the deepening of understanding and inner freedom.

Ancient and contemporary contemplative traditions place ethical guidelines as the foundation for contemplative practice. Ethical guidelines are presented as trainings, investigations, and commitments. There is typically no assumption that a student beginning a contemplative training will start from an ethical base. Conversely, it is assumed that students beginning a contemplative training would bring with them the spectrum of confusion, distress, views, and mental and behavior patterns that had beset them prior to beginning their training. Traditionally, behavioral commitments are set in place, not as rules or measures of *right* and *wrong* but rather as ways of establishing an intentional way of interacting with the world that does no harm and protects the well-being of all beings. Moreover, these commitments are set up as trainings and investigations.

"How can you expect to deepen in this path without integrity? In its absence you simply create the conditions for afflictive states of mind to govern your mind" (Sayadaw U Pandita). Enmity darkens our minds. Harsh self-judgment creates waves of guilt and shame, or worse, self-loathing. When we lose our ethical compass, we act, speak, or think in ways we regret or which are harmful to ourselves and to others. As we set out in Chapters 2–5, the afflictive nature of these mind states generates unhelpful patterns of thought and behavior that undermine our well-being, creating and perpetuating distress.

Buddhist psychology emphasizes the cultivation of right, skillful, or wise mindfulness, but equally points out that there is wrong or unskillful mindfulness. For example, clear perception and focused attention can be important to someone playing computer games, pickpocketing, or in a more extreme example, a sniper. In reality, these are examples of perception and attention, but not mindfulness. It is ethics that protect us from subverting clear perception and attention into unwholesome actions. When attention and perception are on the tip of an ethical intentionality, wholesome thought and action become more possible. In fact, a mind grounded in understanding and the attitudinal dimensions of mindfulness lends itself more readily to attention and clear perception.

Ethics Are Intentional *and* Relational

None of us survives or thrives alone. We are relational beings constantly impacted by the world around us and impacting the world and the lives of others through our thoughts, words, and actions. Buddhism sought to safeguard this interdependence and interrelatedness through the commitment to integrity. It describes integrity as being thoughts, words, and acts of kindness and compassion. With mindfulness, we learn to live in an intentional way, sensitive to the kind of footprint we leave on the world with our thoughts, words, and acts. The protective element of mindfulness, discussed previously, has a deeply ethical nature—committed to protecting the well-being not only of our own mind but equally committed to safeguarding the world with which we interact. The protection offered by mindfulness is through the restraint of the impulses of ill-will that will harm others and ourselves. Our relatedness is the place of our greatest vulnerability, our greatest disappointments, and our greatest happiness. We cannot control the minds or actions of others we interact with, however hurtful or harmful they may be. We can only learn to be aware of the roots of our own actions, speech, and thoughts. When we develop our capacity for sensitivity, mindfulness, and compassion, we find that these qualities are more likely to influence how we lead our lives. A friend and colleague put it this way: "We create a path by walking it" (Crane, 2017), both through steps imbued with wholesome intentionality and the avoidance of steps that are harmful or imbued with ill-will and potential for harm.

"Making the Path by Walking It"

Many contemplative traditions take the radical position that integrity is trained; that we make the path by walking it (Crane, 2017). This training starts with the scaffolding of key ethical guidelines. In the early teachings, five primary ethical guidelines are offered to anyone beginning to practice or to teach, as listed in Box 9.3. They are offered not as commandments, but as trainings that incline the mind toward relationships of health, both inwardly and outwardly. They are the roots of profound transformation. The invitation is to use the principles to embody respect and compassion, as gifts that we offer to ourselves. They are *not* rules to create shame, guilt, and judgment, or a puritanical or punitive way of relating to others.

Integrity is presented as a pathway of understanding that begins with commitments that *rest on the tip of intention.* The first guideline—refraining from harm and committing to honoring and respecting life—is the compass for the other four precepts. The primary commitment to nonharming infuses our speech, actions, our sexuality, and our thoughts, even though we know that we cannot move through life without unintentionally harming living beings. For example, on occasion, speaking honestly may be hurtful to others.

BOX 9.3. **Primary Ethical Guidelines in Buddhism**

- Refrain from harming living beings; commit to honoring and respecting all living beings.
- Refrain from taking what is not freely given; use what we have with care and commit to generosity with our time, our belongings, and our actions.
- Refrain from false or harmful speech; commit to speaking honestly, with care and respect.
- Refrain from sensual and sexual misconduct; use our sexual energy with sensitivity and respect.
- Refrain from the misuse of substances that cloud the mind and lead to heedlessness; commit to training the mind in awareness and clarity.

Although we know this, we can continue to foster a commitment to protecting the well-being of others and our own minds. For attention to be *mindful* means it is nonharming and respectful at its core. This first guideline of nonharming and kindness is the bedrock for the attitudinal dimensions of mindfulness and embodiment. Indeed, this precept has infused the whole map of the mind and path of mindfulness that we have considered so far (Chapters 2–8). Befriending and compassion, in particular, are fundamental to integrity, as they involve a deep understanding of and resonance with distress and suffering, as well as action to alleviate suffering, both our own and others' suffering (Armstrong, 2011).

What Supports Personal Integrity?

When we live with integrity we are able to ask the question "How does this state of mind and action (speech and bodily action) affect me and others?" We can use the answer to shape our response in any given moment and to recognize and respond to ethical dilemmas.

Buddhist psychology suggests the following three levels of training to support the development of integrity:

1. *Restraint and protective mindfulness* involve recognition of and restraint in the face of habitual impulses and reactivity. Restraint is a mindful pause inserted between the arising of an unwholesome impulse and carrying it out. When our recognition and restraint are imbued with befriending and care, we learn the kindness and transformative power of renunciation. The more we practice this, the more natural it becomes. Over time, our attention and awareness become stable and spacious enough for us to see impulses and reactivity with a much broader and larger mindscape. When we learn restraint, we are better able to see our impulses and reactivity like whirlpools in a large river into which we don't need to get drawn—in fact they can be places where, like a skillful kayaker, we can rest to consider a skillful response.

Restraint and renunciation can be confused with a number of *near enemies*. Renunciation can mistakenly be associated with suppression, deprivation, or punitive withholding. It is not well-disguised aversion, a reason to disconnect from what we don't like, rationalization for simplistic notions of *de-cluttering*, or worse still, a sort of nihilism. Instead, renunciation is an act of kindness that arises when we stop acting on impulses that create distress inwardly and outwardly, to ourselves and others.

As our well-being improves, we see that renunciation and restraint are potentially transformative in wholesome, positive ways. For example, if we want more time to be present with our children, we may need to let go of other things in our lives; if we let go of compulsive busyness, we can access greater spaciousness. The difference between restraint and suppression is that the impulse of suppression is one of aversion and the unwillingness to fully acknowledge what is occurring in our thoughts and our emotions. Restraint, on the other hand, is grounded in mindfulness. It is a genuine willingness not only to really see patterns of mind as they arise but also to be unwilling to engage in patterns that lead to harm and distress. Having this greater understanding of our mind helps us develop protective awareness and restraint (as we set out in Chapter 5), because we have learned that we have a choice to respond rather than react (as we set out in Chapters 6–8). It requires steadiness and spaciousness to really see and respond, remembering what is important and what we value. It is a discipline imbued with kindness and investigation.

2. *Cultivating and enhancing our values, intentions, and positive behaviors.* Mindfulness training can initially feel counterintuitive. We have to learn to walk a different pathway rather than automatically getting sucked into our habitual patterns of thinking, reactivity, fear, and aversion. Mindfulness training helps us learn to replace those habit patterns with curiosity, attentiveness, intentionality, and kindness, so that we can cultivate more wholesome states of mind.

When we become absorbed in narratives of *me, mine, and self*, distress and suffering arise as our beliefs are activated ("I am a good person" or "I am a bad person"). Our elaborative judging mind, driven by a discrepancy monitor, kicks in ("If only I were more generous, I would be a better person"). Alongside an understanding of our universal and particular vulnerabilities and resilience, we come to see these views as just that: thoughts and not facts. We come to see the discrepancy monitor as just that: a mental process, not a fixed part of our mental landscape. Our views, like seismic changes in a landscape, shift.

Generosity is an important part of cultivating appreciative joy, ease of being, and equanimity—it is an antidote to self-absorption and fear. It opens the heart, connects us with others and ourselves, and rises above self-absorption. It plays from a chord in the heart that responds to connection, and with both joy (as appreciative joy) and suffering (as compassion). Generosity says to fear: "Fear is the cheapest room in the house, and I would like to see you in better accommodation."[3] It is also an antidote to insufficiency. It is imbued with a sense of abundance, that there is enough to go around, and to be generous is not to use up some limited resource. It sees the beautiful and lovely, with care and an understanding of impermanence that eschews attachment: "I see you, like a butterfly on my palm."

Integrity and generosity are conjoined—generosity is informed by integrity even when the gesture of generosity is uncomfortable or unpopular. Socially, when a group turns against an individual or subgroup, social norms can dictate that everyone follows to shun that person. Generosity is to continue to extend friendship at these times. At primary school, my (WK) daughter was a keen sportswoman. In her last years of elementary school, the boys became more identified with sports and the girls with socializing and games; all the girls who were "tomboys" gave it up, except for her. It was only a few of her friends who extended their friendship to her sovereignty, to do what she loved, and none of the boys did, even though she was better at sports than most of them. The hardest part was for her to extend generosity and kindness to herself, to honor her own sovereignty, and to not give in to the prevailing and powerful gender stereotypes perpetuated in so many ways in her life, including through her school.

Generosity and kindness can be mirrored at every level, from our own hearts and minds, to social groups, to institutions, and to larger movements, such as those that counter a rise in hatred toward a whole group, be that Jews or Muslims, refugees and asylum seekers, or on the basis of gender, race, and sexuality. Within Buddhist psychology, generosity is a precursor or stepping stone to greater understanding, renunciation, patience, befriending, equanimity, and care, including to that which is different and unpopular. It is a key to integrity and embodiment. It enables us to create a path by walking it (Crane, 2017).

3. *Dedicating our lives to the welfare of others.* When kindness, compassion, and generosity imbue our thoughts, words, and actions, we can discover a deeper sense of relatedness, trust, and well-being. Dedicating our lives to the welfare of others supports this cultivation. Integrity is a set of mutually reinforcing concentric circles, starting with our minds and behavior, extending to the people around us who we relate to immediately, and then outward to wider communities and the world we live in (see Figure 9.2). Many mindfulness teachers have chosen this work because of a deep commitment to service and the welfare of the people they wish to serve.

These Buddhist teachings were originally taught through a long and repetitive recounting of instructions, which served to communicate the sense that this practice requires repeated and ongoing training. For example, the discourse on wholesome and unwholesome action sets out the process of intention, action, and reflection, and illustrates the layers of training (Thanissaro Bhikkhu, 2017). The extract[4] below sets out the training for speech:

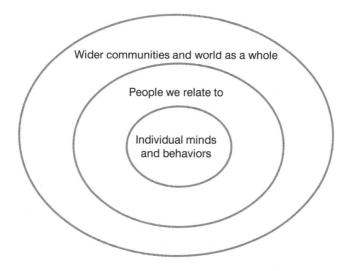

FIGURE 9.2. Integrity as a set of mutually reinforcing concentric circles.

Whenever you want to speak, you should reflect: "These words—will they lead to my suffering, to the suffering of others, or to both? Would it be an unskillful verbal action, with painful consequences, painful results?" If, on reflection, you know that it would lead to suffering; it would be an unskillful verbal action with painful consequences, painful results, then any verbal action of that sort is absolutely unfit for you to do. But if on reflection you know that it would not cause suffering . . . it would be a skillful verbal action with pleasant consequences, pleasant results, then any verbal action of that sort is fit for you to do.

While you are speaking, you should reflect on it: "This verbal action I am doing—is it leading to my suffering, to the suffering of others, or to both? Is it an unskillful verbal action, with painful consequences, painful results?" If, on reflection, you know that it is leading to suffering . . . you should give it up. But if on reflection you know that it is not . . . you may continue with it.

Having spoken, you should reflect on it: "This verbal action I have done—did it lead to my suffering, to the suffering of others, or to both? Was it an unskillful verbal action, with painful consequences, painful results?" If, on reflection, you know that it led to suffering; it was an unskillful verbal action with painful consequences, painful results, then you should confess it, reveal it, lay it open to the teacher or to a knowledgeable companion. Having confessed it . . . you should exercise restraint in the future. But if on reflection you know that it did not lead to suffering . . . it was a skillful verbal action with pleasant consequences, pleasant results,

then you should stay mentally refreshed and joyful, training day and night
in skillful mental qualities.

The structure and content of the discourse repeats the instructions above
for our thoughts, our bodies, and our speech, as well as our actions; it is long
and repetitive, giving a sense of the need to train in integrity persistently and
systematically across each domain.

Ethics Require Discernment

While wholesome intention is the forerunner and foundation for integrity, we
also need discernment to ensure that we make good choices and use our understanding and judgment to choose what speech and actions are likely to be helpful (see Figure 9.1). Discernment is knowing what response a situation needs and
knowing what intentions underpin this response. Integrity is a commitment to
discern—within our thoughts, speech, and acts—what is unwholesome and
leads to distress and what is wholesome and leads to ease of being and freedom.
In Buddhist psychology, the unwholesome is ill-will, craving, and ignorance
(greed, hatred, and delusion). This finds its expression in our thoughts, words,
and actions, and leaves a trail of distress both inwardly and outwardly. The
wholesome is befriending, generosity, and wisdom. This, too, finds its expression in our thoughts, words, and actions, and creates the conditions inwardly
for ease of being and joy, and outwardly for a mindful life and making a positive
impact in the world. In Buddhist psychology, this is expressed in our mind,
body, speech, and actions, and discernment involves being able to differentiate
the wholesome and unwholesome intentions and actions (see Table 9.1).

Most ethical challenges involve a complex range of factors that require
us to adopt a holistic view so that we can discern how best to respond. As we
discussed, integrity and discernment support our ability to respond (Chapter
6). Being able to draw on both experiential and conceptual understanding
also increases our ability to understand and then respond.

In contrast, a more narrow perspective, with little or no awareness of
intentionality, typically drives reactivity (Chapter 6). It is a compassionate
response to someone suffering versus seeing the person as *other* and blamewor-
thy. For example, when we encounter an asylum seeker, do we see him or her
as someone fleeing persecution or as a threat to our own security?

When discernment is combined with a compassionate motivation, we have
the two components of a comprehensive approach to ethics. . . . Compassion, by reducing fear and distrust, creates a space in our hearts and minds
that is calm and settled, and this space makes it much easier for us to exercise discernment. (Dalai Lama, 2011b, p. 81)

TABLE 9.1. Wholesome and Unwholesome Intentions and Actions

Wholesome	Unwholesome
Mind	
• Attention and awareness imbued with befriending, empathy, and care • Equanimity • Understanding and wisdom	• Ill will • Covetousness • Lack of awareness, ignorance, fear, and anger
Speech	
• Speech that is true, kind, helpful, timely, and not harmful • Based in and builds trust and respect	• Gossip • Speech that is untrue, harsh, slanderous, self-aggrandizing, and/or harmful
Action	
• Actions that have neutral or positive outcomes for ourselves and others • Actions that arise out of and mutually reinforce wholesome intentions	• Actions that have negative outcomes for ourselves and others • Actions that arise out of and mutually reinforce unwholesome intentions

In Buddhist psychology, integrity is a commitment to well-being and leading a good life that impacts positively in the world. We don't have to wait for a perfectly ethical mind to be achieved for us to live in an ethical way. We don't have to feel kind to act with kindness, we don't have to feel generous to be generous, and we don't have to feel compassionate to act with compassion. This challenges the prevailing ideology that *how we feel and what we think is true* and that it has an unquestioned authority to be enacted. Rather than investing authority in transient emotions and thoughts, mindfulness reminds us to return again and again to the question of what benefits our well-being and the well-being of others, what protects, and what cultivates the wholesome. When we choose to commit to thoughts, words, and acts of kindness and compassion, our minds begin to learn the liberating power of awareness, kindness, and compassion.

We turn now to the first of the ethical challenges from Box 9.1: teachers teaching mindfulness when they themselves have a serious health condition.

After Sophia had taken in her diagnosis of Parkinson's disease, she sat with an ethical dilemma, including it lightly in her morning mindfulness practice over several weeks. First, she became deeply aware of her sense of service and commitment to the participants in her 8-week mindfulness programs. In a way, since receiving her diagnosis, her sense of service to and common humanity with her participants felt deeper, for there were often others with Parkinson's in the classes.

She also became aware of her need to take care of herself, allow herself to learn to live with her new health status, and get the treatment she needed. She took the questions to her mentor and, afterward, sat with what they discussed. She decided to recruit a co-teacher to help her teach her 8-week courses. When she introduced herself to participants at the start of each course, she briefly included her health status and explained that she now taught with her co-teacher alongside her. The sense of common humanity and shared journey was palpable at that moment and enabled Sophia to be there for herself and the other participants, but in a different way. Later, Sophia transitioned with the support of her co-teacher to being a participant in her monthly mindfulness classes for graduates of her 8-week classes. Knowing her illness was now so advanced that it was not possible to teach, she let go of being a teacher and allowed herself to be nourished by being a participant.

Each of the ethical dilemmas we set out for teachers and participants can be considered from the inside out (see Boxes 9.1 and 9.2). Take a moment to consider each dilemma in turn, using the dimensions of personal integrity and discernment to reflect on each.

The key insight is that our intentions, state of mind, and actions (speech and bodily action) are interwoven, affecting our well-being and the well-being of those immediately around us, as well as the wider world in which we live.

Ethics and Integrity in Mindfulness: From the Outside In

Having considered integrity and ethics in mindfulness from the *inside out*, we now consider how mindfulness-based programs, teacher training, mindfulness teachers, and principles and practices for the field as a whole support ethics and integrity, from the *outside in*.

Mindfulness-Based Programs

The explosion of interest in and proliferation of mindfulness-based programs requires clarity about what is, and is not, a mindfulness-based program. There has been much innovation, but we have also seen innovations that are parodies, such as mindful dog walking, mindful surfing, and mindful coloring books. The developers of mindfulness-based programs outlined the intentionality, program content, and program structure, as well as sequencing of their programs (Kabat-Zinn, 1990; Segal et al., 2013). We summarized a paper that outlined the essential features of mindfulness-based programs (see Chapter 6, Table 6.1; Crane et al., 2017). The best scientific evaluations of these programs' acceptability, efficacy, and effectiveness take care to ensure program fidelity (Weck, Bohn, Ginzburg, & Stangier, 2011). This means that the research is actually evaluating that those programs are taught as intended, and delivered competently and adherently (Dimidjian & Segal, 2015). Therefore, integrity at the level of mindfulness-based programs means respecting the integrity of mindfulness programs, rather than adapting them to suit teachers' personal interests or preferences.

Respect for program integrity coexists with innovation with integrity. There are many excellent examples of innovation, including mindfulness-based cognitive therapy (MBCT) for recurrent depression (Segal et al., 2013) and mindfulness-based approaches for people with substance dependence (Bowen & Vieten, 2012). What characterizes these innovations is that there is a clear need for the innovation; careful attention given to intention, population, and context of the innovation; and a commitment to evaluating the benefits and potential costs of any innovation.

We turn to the second of our ethical challenges set out in Box 9.1:

You teach MBCT in a health care setting for people at risk for depressive relapse. Your manager tells you that resources are tight and you need to run the program in fewer sessions, no more than four, and that one-to-one orientations are definitely not possible. She also asks whether you could open it out to more people on the waiting list who have other common mental health problems.

This mindfulness teacher first noted the unease she experienced when asked to offer MBCT in ways contrary to the manual, the evidence base, good practice guidelines, and her own training. She began a dialogue with her manager and learned that cost and targets to reduce the waiting list were driving the manager's directives. The manager herself was worried about the service and her own job but felt she needed to respond to the wider service pressures. She was intransigent on the need to shorten and open the MBCT service to people on the waiting list.

The mindfulness teacher sought supervision and consulted colleagues in another service. She identified a service that had innovatively adapted MBCT to fit these service demands, taking great care with the adaptation and ensuring everything they did was evaluated to ensure evidence of intended benefit alongside monitoring for any unintended harm. She learned that they also offered staff mindfulness groups, and they often had positive impacts on staff and services. With this wider understanding and supervision, she was able to negotiate a phased widening of the program and staff groups, but resisted the demand to abbreviate the program, explaining to her manager that a lot was being asked of participants, and that an 8-week group intervention is already a relatively brief program. She also ensured an evaluation of acceptability and outcomes.

In fact, she found the program proved to be acceptable and helpful to those on the waiting list, many of whom then went on to use what they had learned to engage more fully with other evidence-based psychological therapies offered within the service. The rates of full recovery for the service were enhanced. As with the original service, the group improved staff understanding of MBCT, improved staff well-being for some, and in several cases helped staff to recognize life changes needed to respond to stress, including in a few cases people who decided to leave the health service, including her manager.

Mindfulness-Based Training Programs

As the field has developed, consensus and good practice guidelines have evolved about how best to train mindfulness-based teachers (Crane, Kuyken, Hastings, Rothwell, & Williams, 2010; Segal et al., 2018), as well as how to support ongoing supervision and mentoring (Evans et al., 2015). Teacher training recognizes that learning to teach mindfulness-based programs is a pathway that includes certain prerequisites, foundational training, basic teacher training, and an apprenticeship with supervision and mentoring. Even when a teacher is competent to start teaching a mindfulness program, there must be a commitment to ongoing learning and development.

Crucially, there is a consensus that the teachers' embodiment of mindfulness requires the development of a personal mindfulness practice. This includes a sustained and regular mindfulness practice alongside retreat opportunities to deepen understanding (Peacock et al., 2016). Moreover, the training curriculum cultivates and trains integrity in the ways envisaged in the foundational teachings as well as teaching ethics more formally. The MBCT training pathway articulates one of its learning outcomes as "Reflect on the ethical framework of Mindfulness Based Cognitive Therapy teaching and apply this to complex issues arising in clinical practice" (Segal et al., 2018, p. 7). The pathway also suggests that foundational training includes "Teaching on delivering Mindfulness Based Cognitive Therapy safely and ethically, with attention to appropriate Mindfulness Based Cognitive Therapy inclusion/exclusion criteria, participant assessment, screening (and appropriate referral when needed) and orientation, outcome monitoring and risk management/referral/clinician back-up" (p. 9). MBSR programs similarly include ethics at the heart of their training.

Psychological therapies (such as cognitive therapy) and psychosocial programs (such as MBSR and MBCT) involve working with people who are in mental and physical distress, and who are often quite vulnerable. The cognitive-behavioral techniques and mindfulness practices used reveal and transform the mind. The training required to carry out this work has parallels to a surgeon. In the same way that a surgeon needs the training to do his or her work with the body safely and effectively, a mindfulness teacher also needs a thorough training. Undertaking a high-quality training is an extraordinarily important and rewarding investment of time and energy, as the rewards will be reaped many times over throughout a career. It is not unusual to hear experienced teachers say that each time they teach a new course they learn something new, as myriad individual and collective mind–body states present themselves. With the development of their personal mindfulness practice, teachers' embodiment deepens and their teaching evolves. In this sense, learning is lifelong.

As of yet, there is no universally agreed mindfulness teacher certification or accreditation. Transparency and openness means that anyone embarking on mindfulness training is entitled to know the level of training and competence of the teacher. For their own well-being and protection, teachers of mindfulness are best served by being open and honest about the extent and limitations of their training.

Mindfulness Teachers

Each mindfulness teacher is asked to be responsible for his or her own ethical development and the quality and integrity of his or her teaching.

Because the ethical basis, the value system, and the philosophical underpinnings to the programs are implicit rather than explicitly visible within the teaching process, the teacher takes quiet personal responsibility for holding the integrity of the process. There is a lot of unseen work taking place. The teacher is carrying frameworks of theoretical and practical understanding of the human mind, and of how these interface with the practice of mindfulness meditation. These are held in readiness so that they can be used to help participants make sense of experiential observations as they emerge. These frameworks are drawn from a range of settings—primarily from contemporary psychology and aspects of Buddhist psychology. The teacher is also holding the ethical codes of his or her profession and of the institution. This is one reason why so much emphasis is placed on the teacher—he or she sits at the fulcrum point conveying the authenticity of the teachings, while also skillfully ensuring that the process is held and embodied in a context-appropriate ethical framework (Crane, 2017).

In the same way that mindfulness-based programs have several defining characteristics, so do mindfulness teachers (Chapter 6, Table 6.1). The defining characteristics of mindfulness teachers who teach with integrity largely ensure that teachers have the requisite training, competencies, and experience, and that they keep updating their learning. This applies to each domain of teaching competencies, theoretical knowledge, professional training, and embodiment (see Table 9.2).

Teaching with integrity requires mindfulness teachers to maintain a mindfulness practice, to *walk the talk*, teach what they know conceptually and experientially, and for embodiment to be a practice. We do not ask our clients to undertake or commit to anything that we are not personally willing to undertake and commit to.

Teaching and practicing mindfulness can reveal an unsettling dissonance between our intentions and the actualities of our lives. We require students to commit to a daily practice, yet this may have lapsed in our own lives. We encourage students to bring mindfulness into every area of their life, but our own life may have been overtaken by *busyness* or relationships that are anything but *mindful*. We encourage clients to develop the capacity both to appreciate the lovely and to turn toward the difficult, yet may find ourselves engaging in acts of avoidance with the difficult and skating over the lovely.

Dissonance Is Not Negative

Dissonance does not have to produce judgment and blame. It can describe a moment of creative tension, of *waking up*, and living a life that embodies our

TABLE 9.2. Essential and Population/Context-Specific Features of Mindfulness-Based Teachers

Essential features	Population/context-specific features
• Has the competency to effectively deliver the mindfulness-based program. • Embodies the qualities and attitudes of mindfulness in their teaching. • Has engaged in appropriate training and commits to ongoing good practice. • Is part of a participatory learning process with their students, clients, or patients.	• Has the knowledge, experience, and professional training related to the specialist populations to whom they will be teaching the mindfulness-based program. • Has the knowledge of relevant underlying theoretical processes that underpin the teaching for particular contexts or populations.

Note. Reproduced from Crane et al. (2017, p. 993).

deepest aspirations and values. Dissonance as a teacher may well be a call to examine our own embodiment in as honest a way as we can. Committing ourselves to ongoing practice and to supervision from peers is a profound gesture of integrity that recognizes that being a teacher of mindfulness means being a student of mindfulness. As we saw in the earlier chapter on embodiment (Chapter 8), our longings—for health and well-being, to respect and love others, to help and not harm—are the wholesome intentions that can lie beneath a powerful inner critic, that can create the dissonance between how things are and how we would like them to be. In this sense, teachers' integrity is a path, part of their training, and ongoing personal and professional development.

Mindfulness practice is often a transformative part of mindfulness teachers' lives, perhaps linked to their ideological values and beliefs or their spirituality and religion. Mindfulness-based programs, however, are not vehicles for teachers to impart their personal, spiritual, or religious values. Integrity means that teachers need to find a way to teach authentically, while ensuring that they offer their mindfulness programs in a way that is accessible to people from all faiths and backgrounds, including those from faiths that may have concerns about other faiths, and those people with no faith (Crane, 2017). Some participants who find the mindfulness program transformative may then integrate what they learn with their spiritual and religious values and practices, but this is not an intention or a requirement.

One of the ethical dilemmas we set out in Box 9.2 was of Mohammed's Muslim faith. This was important to him spiritually, but also as a way of life and as part of a community. His imam questioned his participation in the mindfulness class and how it sits with the tenets of Islam.

What are the ethical issues here? How might the mindfulness teacher respond?

In this case, the mindfulness teacher worked carefully with Mohammed to make clear that the mindfulness program is secular and it was for him to find ways to apply it to his chronic pain and life more generally. Mohammed described how he prayed five times a day and that this had become rote, a habit. He learned to use mindfulness in his daily prayer and be more present for his prayer. Explaining this to his imam reassured the imam and opened a door for Mohammed to develop his prayer and service. His imam, aware how prayer could become rote for many Muslims, was intrigued at how mindfulness enabled a greater presence with God during prayer.

Ensuring Participant Safety in Mindfulness-Based Programs

Ethics and integrity play out in multiple ways for those participating in mindfulness-based programs. First, the principle of nonharming means we need to ensure the safety of participants. Ruth Baer and I (WK) set out a framework in which we considered three levels to ensure safety: the vulnerability of the participants, the intensity of the program, and the competence of the teacher (Baer & Kuyken, 2016). More vulnerable participants and more intensive practices require greater teacher competence and skill (which all mindfulness-based teachers should have acquired during their training).

In MBCT for depression, for example, one aspect of ensuring safety is the requirement for potential students to attend an orientation session prior to beginning the program. In that orientation, it is mutually determined whether or not it is appropriate for the student to begin the program. People who are dealing with active posttraumatic stress symptoms, are experiencing dissociative states, misusing substances, or are in the midst of major life changes, may not be in the right place in their lives to undertake a mindfulness program. Indeed, it is a gesture of integrity, dedicated to protecting the well-being of the program's participants, to ensure we have the training and processes to safeguard our participants.

Another ethical dilemma we set out in Box 9.1 was of a mindfulness teacher teaching the all-day retreat. Following one of the practices, a participant described experiencing frightening dissociative experiences, and hearing voices telling her to hurt herself.

What are the ethical issues here? How might the mindfulness teacher respond?

Clearly the safety of this participant is paramount, and the context is key. Is the teacher already aware of the person's vulnerability to these experiences? Is the teacher a qualified health or mental health professional? Does he or she have the competencies to assess and work with the person's experience? How do the others in the class respond? Is the teacher able to maintain steadiness and embodiment to enable a skillful response, or is he or she feeling reactive?

The answers to these contextual questions will determine the skillful response. A clinically qualified and experienced mindfulness teacher—who was aware of and had already worked with this person's proneness to dissociation—may feel able to offer enough support for the participant to work with these mental states safely and constructively, providing requisite support and careful ongoing evaluation. A mindfulness teacher without these competencies might ask the person to step back from mindfulness practice at times like this and instead find ways to manage and maintain mental health and safety. The teacher might seek supervision. He or she might refer the person on to someone able to better help him or her. In each case, the well-being of the participant is paramount and the teacher works within his or her competency.

There must always be a match between a teacher's competence, understanding of the distress or psychopathology he or she may encounter, and knowledge of the working context to safeguard participants' well-being. Mindfulness is not a panacea, and teachers are not able to work with every mental state.

Integrity and ethics infuse every aspect of learning and teaching mindfulness. We provided a few illustrative examples in Box 9.2. What are the integrity and ethical issues in these four cases? The first example is of a participant who, through mindfulness, begins to see how agitation and impulsiveness are the forerunner of destructive words that damage her relationship with her daughter. As she learns to exercise protective awareness and restraint, she starts to see the positive effects on her relationship with her daughter and her own state of mind.

One morning, Ling hadn't slept well and had woken up feeling irritable. She noticed that her teenage daughter was eating her breakfast, watching a show on her laptop computer, while also texting a boy. It was 10 minutes until she would need to head out the door to catch the bus to school. Ling noticed that the bathroom light was on and there was a wet towel on the floor, the fridge was ajar, a container of milk out on the counter, and a cereal box left open.

Seeing what to her mind was a "trail of destruction" in the bathroom and kitchen initiated a wave of irritation and an impulse to nag her daughter. The words formed in her mind: "You have 10 minutes to eat your breakfast and then I need you to clean up after yourself in the bathroom and kitchen." When Ling was the same age as her daughter, she had been living in foster care. Somehow, irritation morphed into a feeling of anger and the impulse to nag went up a notch into an impulse to lash out verbally: "What the hell do you think you're doing? I am not your slave, you're not leaving this trail of destruction for me to clean up when you go to school!"

What are the issues here, what is the potential for harm and for benefit? How might Ling use what she has learned to respond skillfully?

These feelings of irritation are not unfamiliar to any parent of teenage children. Parenting adolescents involves navigating their self-centered behavior and riding the waves of their moods and emerging identities. It is a time where parents need to show constancy, boundaries, and steady love. However, many parents understandably find their teenage children's words and behaviors hard to bear. It is easy to be reactive.

Pausing, Ling noted her impulse and reactivity. She noted the nag on the tip of her tongue, the angry words beginning to form in her mind, and the impulse to lash out. From previous experience, she knew the likely scenario that would unfold. Her daughter would roll her eyes, say something rude under her breath, make a half-hearted attempt to put a few things away, and then head out the door without a good-bye, leaving a black cloud of anger and resentment behind her. Ling would be left feeling helpless and in the grip of a downward spiral of negative thinking: "It's not their fault they've got a mental mother," "I am a terrible parent, she hates me," "Why don't I just stay home and get back into bed?" Ling restrained herself from saying anything on the grounds that this was not a fight worth picking. As her daughter headed out the door she said, "Have a good day, I love you," and her daughter looked back and smiled, saying, "Thanks, you too." Her daughter was oblivious to what Ling had been thinking or the mess she was leaving behind. But in the space after her daughter left Ling felt relief she had not lashed out: "I know I have a tendency to snap at the children, especially if I'm down or worn out, but it doesn't help and I just feel bad afterward."

That evening, after school, Ling gave her daughter a ride to a friend's house. In the car, her daughter opened up about how a boy was pressuring her to have sex, but she did not feel ready, that she wasn't even sure whether she liked him, but he was very popular at school and her friends said they all thought he was great. They talked together and during the conversation, Ling shared her own experience of how she had used her sexuality to get the attention and care she craved. They came up with a plan together for how her daughter should handle the situation with the boy. Ling reflected that if she had lashed out in the morning, her daughter might not have come to her with this problem. She felt pleased that her daughter was so much more together and resilient than she had been at her age.

This example shows how Ling's awareness of her thoughts and impulses gave her a choice to respond, rather than react. "If I don't fly off the handle, you know, suddenly get angry and lose it, I can do a breathing space and just center, and then um, not fly off the handle and think a bit more." Later in the day the same reflective awareness enabled her to reflect on the positive downstream impact of that restraint, of "not flying off the handle." These sorts of examples of alignment of intentionality (to support my daughter's development), thoughts (I am aware of the impulse to nag, but will bite my tongue), and action (in this case, restraint) are examples of the ethics of intentionality in mindfulness-based programs that support participants in leading better lives.

Sue was in one of our (WK) MBCT classes. Like Ling, Sue had a history of abuse and two children; she was prone to angry verbal outbursts. Sue deeply misunderstood the mindfulness teaching and said, "I give my kids a real verbal lashing, my tongue can be like a razor sometimes, and afterward I can feel bad. But now I say to myself, "No, you are not a bad person; let these regrets go. It is quite understandable that I lash out at my kids, everyone does it." Clearly, regret over actions that are damaging can be helpfully corrective; it is what appears in the space between stimulus and reactivity. In this case, however, Sue needed help not only to be self-compassionate with the thoughts and feelings that create irritability and anger but also needed help with some practical parenting skills to ensure her behavior toward her children is not harmful and destructive. This would enable her to have greater awareness earlier in the chain of reactivity, so that she could respond with wholesome intentionality.

The third example we gave in Box 9.2 was of Sam's recovery from addiction and how in recovery he became more acutely aware of the pain and destruction his addiction had caused not just to himself, but others, too. He had stolen from his mother, been unreliable and fired from several jobs, and had shared needles with others.

Sam had crossed numerous ethical lines during his active addition. His mindfulness practice generated a strong dissonance between his actions and his wholehearted wish for peace of mind for himself and the well-being of the people he loved. As we've already discussed, 12-step recovery programs—in the later steps—include making amends. Sam's mindfulness practice enabled him to explore his intentions and actions here with great care so that he could know better when and how to make those amends. His mother had heard so many excuses and apologies when Sam was in active addiction. Sam knew that his actions to rebuild trust would be a more powerful form of amends than any words, and over the years the words were no longer needed, as his actions restored his relationship with his mother.

Ethics, in the sense of intention, thoughts, actions, and their effects, are at the heart of each of these examples. They apply both to participants and teachers of mindfulness-based programs.

The Relationship between Teachers and Participants of Mindfulness Programs

The relationships between mindfulness teachers and those learning mindfulness demand clarity and some delicate balance. Teachers provide teaching, instruction in mindfulness practice, and a safe container for learning. They have trained as mindfulness teachers and have a body of knowledge and experience. In this sense, the teacher has power because his or her greater expertise enables participants' learning.

The intention in mindfulness programs is for participants' learning to be primarily participatory, experiential, and emancipatory. Good mindfulness teachers inspire this kind of learning—that is, the teachers try to offer the teaching in a way that participants learn for themselves via the practices and their own inquiry into what comes up for them in the practices, over and over again. The teacher's role is simply to make the learning from the program and the mindfulness practices themselves available to the participants. This is another asymmetry and teachers can be perceived as *gurus*.

On the other hand, the vehicle (i.e., mindfulness practice) is the same for the teacher and the participants—both are on the same journey; the teacher is teaching what he or she has learned. In this sense, the relationship is equal. Great care needs to be taken to build teacher–participant relationships that support learning and minimize teachers being seen as *experts*, or gurus. Yes, they have knowledge and experience that can be of service to participants, but teachers are primarily seeking for participants to unlock their own learning. Participants can find themselves idealizing teachers or romantically or sexually attracted to the teacher. Teachers can similarly be romantically or sexually attracted to the participants. Teachers should understand the power differential in the teacher–student relationship; it is always the responsibility of the teacher to appropriately maintain the boundaries of the different roles.

It is not uncommon for mindfulness teachers to say that if they set up an 8-week class well and teach the first few sessions well, then midway through, the class starts to teach itself—that is, the structure of the program, the participants' mindfulness practice, and the sense of common learning among the participants take on a life of its own. However, the particular role of a mindfulness teacher—and the normal processes that can take place in any group—can create dependency, idealization, and teacher power dynamics.

Integrity concerns itself solely with the best interests of the participants in mindfulness programs and not with material rewards, praise, or dependency. Mindfulness practice and embodiment provide potent signals and guidance that teachers can heed. If we find ourselves drawn into roles of guru or sense praise, dependency, or sexual attraction to participants, these are moments for pausing and responding with care and understanding. In the example below, Sam praises the teacher in quite an effusive way in the homework inquiry. The teacher feels herself reacting with a sense of feeling flattered and *puffed up*.

SAM: Last week in the class you said something that was so helpful to me about the body scan practice, thank you. I am going to learn so much from you—you are so wise.

TEACHER: [*Recognizes Sam attributing the wisdom to her and notices a pang of self-importance. Having noticed the impact of his words on her, adjusts her posture to feel steady and steps back from her own feelings. She then tries to help Sam take responsibility for this practice and the learning that will come from it.*] What was the learning for you?

SAM: You know I was so agitated.

TEACHER: What did you do in the body scan at home to work with that?

SAM: Like you said, I tried to see the agitation for what it was, and maybe stay with it for a moment, noting how it was, before coming back to the body. You had said it was like training a puppy, and because I had dogs growing up, that was so helpful to me.

TEACHER: Ah, good for you. So, what qualities from your puppy training did you use with your mind? [*smiling*]

SAM: [*laughs*] Well, being firm and kind, and patient; you know it takes time, and that is how it was with my mind as well. It wasn't easy, but I did it 6 days out of 7 like you asked, and by the end of the week, I can't say the puppy was trained, but I wasn't wanting to jump up every time I started.

TEACHER: Thank you, it's great to see you developing this capacity for firmness and kindness with your mind, and using what you know about training dogs to train your own mind! What I hope you'll all learn [*includes the whole group here*] is that the main teacher is your mindfulness practice. I will be here to help you unlock some of that learning, but you will do the work and reap the rewards.

Peer support, supervision, and community all support the integrity of mindfulness teachers. Within the Buddhist traditions, choosing people whose judgment can help you develop integrity is seen as key. Supervision and peer support are also parts of the good practice guidelines for mindfulness teachers (Crane, 2011).

We encourage mindfulness teachers to take time to practice mindfulness before each class, to stabilize the mind, and cultivate the attitudinal dimensions of mindfulness. If each participant is then brought to mind in turn, this can support effective teaching because it can highlight issues teachers can or need to attend to. This can include inevitable thoughts and feelings, as well as reactivity: "I really like her, she is such a star," "I hope he doesn't come, he is so skeptical," and "I'm scared of her anger, I won't know how to help her and I'll be exposed as a bad teacher." Bringing awareness to these thoughts and feelings is key to teaching with embodiment and integrity.

The Wider Mindfulness Field

The widespread interest in mindfulness in different contexts such as health, education, criminal justice, and workplaces have rightly led commentators to question the intentionality, ethical framework, and impact of this work (Baer, 2015; Cook, 2016; Monteiro, Musten, & Compson, 2015). This has led to a response that the field as a whole needs to put safeguards and frameworks in place (Crane, 2017). We have argued that the long view demands that we attend to ethics and integrity, by taking a series of intentional steps (Kuyken, 2016).

There are those who have argued that professional bodies, such as the American Psychological Association and British Psychological Society, can provide the ethics and integrity for the mindfulness field; these professional bodies have carefully considered and evolved ethical guidelines through many decades (Baer, 2015). Such professional guidelines tend to take a three-pronged approach: (1) expositions about ethical principles underlying codes in preambles, (2) codes of conduct (which provide a bottom line of *dos and don'ts*, below which standards should not fall), and (3) guidelines (which are exhortatory, rather than mandatory). At ground level, ethics codes provide us with guidelines for our work, enable us to resolve ethical dilemmas, transmit standards from one generation to the next, provide a yardstick against which to judge those whose behavior has been questioned, affirm the integrity of a profession, and protect professions from the need for sociolegal guidelines, enforcement, and policing. They are helpful and good practice guidelines for mindfulness teachers to advocate adherence to the ethical framework appropriate to the teacher's professional background and working context (Crane, 2011).

However, there are mindfulness teachers who do not have a professional background and in these cases, guidelines tend to advocate that if they do not have such a code, they should adhere to codes set out by the most relevant professional body to safeguard and to promote good practice (Segal et al., 2018). We have argued that while immensely helpful, such guidelines are just one part of the fabric of integrity.

In several contexts, consensus statements of good practice have been instructive processes, co-creating consensus and providing important guides for teachers and the contexts in which they work (Crane, 2011). In the United Kingdom, for example, the good practice guidelines first built a sense of community around shared ownership of these guidelines and then were helpful as guides for people training and establishing mindfulness services in the health care system and elsewhere (Mindfulness All-Party Parliamentary Group, 2015).

Baer (2015) has argued cogently that *how we communicate mindfulness is key to the integrity of the field.* This includes mindfulness teachers knowing and communicating the limits of mindfulness-based programs, knowing whom it is suitable for and not suitable for, and knowing whom we are trained or not trained to teach mindfulness to. Honesty and integrity are needed to acknowledge that mindfulness may not be the most appropriate pathway for all people in all situations. If a client is in imminent danger of harm, at risk of a psychotic break, or unable to undertake the rigor of the training, this needs to be acknowledged and the person supported in accessing appropriate help. This sort of honest and informed communication can prevent some of the legitimate critiques of the mindfulness field as overclaiming the benefits of mindfulness-based programs.

Money and power can be enormously seductive and compromise integrity. In the early days of contemporary mindfulness, the economic dimension of teaching mindfulness was acknowledged and many mindfulness teachers taught on a model of generosity to safeguard their integrity. In other words, they taught without expectation of payment, but people gave donations for the teaching in a spirit of generosity. This supported an ethical livelihood. In some countries, insurance and health care systems cover the costs of a student's or patient's participation in a mindfulness program. It is a harsh reality that this is not universal and many cannot afford access. Those suffering from psychological distress, whose capacity to earn a livelihood may be compromised, are far too often excluded from participation.

The final example we provide in Box 9.1 is of a mindfulness teacher teaching mindfulness-based programs in the community. She received a call from someone who had signed up for her next 8-week course. The caller tells her that he has lost his job and is a single parent and would like to attend the program but cannot afford the fees and needs child care during the classes.

Integrity in the development of mindfulness asks us to address the question of how to include people who do not have the funds to pay for a program. There are no easy answers. There are numerous mindfulness teachers who offer time and availability generously, without compensation, yet who also need to have a livelihood. Some teachers commit to offering a subsidized place or places on all their courses for those on low incomes, or arrange manageable payment plans. Some teachers will arrange their course fees so as to have some scholarship money available for people unable to afford the cost.

The question of economic integrity is profound and raises many issues about access, inclusion, power, and intentionality. How to respond ethically to economic questions is a key question for any mindfulness teacher.

Respect for diversity of values and cultures. As mindfulness takes root in our society, we have to recognize how diverse our society is and how mindfulness fits into this diverse landscape. What steps are required to make mindfulness available to people of any faith or none, to adapt the language of teaching to make it appropriate and accessible for diverse communities, and to cross the economic and social barriers that lead people to see mindfulness trainings as the domain of the white, educated middle class? It is important to listen carefully to people from different social backgrounds, educational backgrounds, and ethnicities. Mindfulness teachers will need to learn how to speak and deliver the program in ways that are inclusive and appropriate, without compromising the core teaching. This is a challenge for the present and the future. It is also an ethical challenge as we remind ourselves of the many shapes distress can take and the range of ways it can be expressed.

The examples and issues we have raised can each be applied to diversity, accessibility, and inclusion. Mohammed's Muslim faith and Ling's history of abuse were both potential barriers to a path of mindfulness, but also rich learning opportunities. Our own views and learning histories are the same; they can be barriers or opportunities. Working with diversity is an inside-out and outside-in inquiry.

> *The key insights are that high-quality mindfulness teaching is enabled through the integrity of mindfulness programs themselves, combined with high-quality teacher training and teachers who embody integrity and who continue with ongoing learning and supervision. Integrity should be imbued at the level of the mindfulness programs, teachers, and the wider field.*

SYNOPSIS

Questions of integrity and ethics are an ongoing investigation. This inquiry involves us personally and as a community of mindfulness researchers and teachers committed to the highest levels of teaching and learning. At the root of this investigation is the primary ethical commitment to *do no harm* and to promote the well-being of all. Mindfulness teachers learn where there is a convergence between integrity from the *inside out* and *outside in* and where there are tensions. This is part of the ongoing investigation and learning.

Even though ethics and integrity don't feature much in contemporary mindfulness books, we have argued that they are part of the fabric of teaching and learning in mindfulness programs. Ethics and integrity are not comfortable topics and there are no easy answers to ethical questions. A colleague remarked, "If the question of ethics does not make us uncomfortable, we haven't understood the question properly." There is a growing acknowledgment within the mindfulness community that ethics are not only a personal responsibility but a collective responsibility.

As a community of practitioners and teachers we need to be brave enough and ready to ask probing questions. Clearly, it is not appropriate to question a client's personal ethics in a mindfulness class, but mindfulness practice does intrinsically raise these questions. Moreover, it may be deeply appropriate for us to question our personal and collective understanding of integrity. Ethics is more than simply having good intentions—it includes being aware of the consequences of those intentions. We may have a well-meaning intention to help others by teaching mindfulness, but if we are undertrained or underskilled, the consequences may be deeply harmful. We may personally be undergoing a challenging period in our lives where our personal practice falls by the wayside and we enter a teaching situation carrying an embodied tension that is readily communicated to clients. Integrity might mean periods when we stop teaching and focus instead on resourcing ourselves, as we saw with the case example of Sophia when her health deteriorated to the point she no longer felt able to teach.

Ethics is a complex landscape. It includes an investigation of the intentions underpinning our choices, acts, thoughts, and speech. It includes discernment, as well as restraint and responsiveness in our speech and actions. The words *wholesome* and *unwholesome* can have burdensome associations of *good* and *bad*, or they can lead us to examine the ethical quality of how we engage with the world and ourselves (i.e., Do our psychological and physical acts lead to distress or the end of distress?; Do they lead toward freedom or away from freedom?; Do they lead to a greater compassion or a greater harshness?). Honesty, courage, respectfulness, and restraint are qualities of ethics that are not grand ideals but ways of being present and living a good life.

Service providers and organizations that seek to incorporate mindfulness training into their services are calling for greater regulation and recognized standards of competence. There are reservations and concerns within the mindfulness community, however, about regulation. Who decides

standards of competence? Who would regulate? Given the spectrum of trainings and presentations of mindfulness available, it is probably impossible to
provide overarching regulation. A broader commitment to integrity and ethical guidelines may be the answer to these concerns. Integrity is not only a
personal responsibility but is deeply concerned with our relationships, our
work, and our engagement with the world. It protects, safeguards, and provides the framework for positive change and evolution that lies at the heart of
mindfulness-based programs.

CHAPTER 10

A Final Word

Can we envision a world
where we live with understanding, compassion, and responsiveness;
without the devastating effects of depression; and
where children learn how to be and to flourish?

We have suggested that mindfulness deepens our capacity to embrace the inevitable vicissitudes of life; it strengthens our resilience. As we develop our capacity to cultivate a mind that is not so easily gripped by agitation, anxiety, or depression, our capacity for effective responsiveness and action is enhanced. We open to joy.

- Mohammed was able to live a good life, with chronic pain.
- Ling was able to make a life for herself, and find joy within it, despite the devastating effects of depression and abuse.
- Sam was able to live a life in recovery from addiction; embracing it so his life work became serving others with addiction.
- Sophia wove mindfulness into every aspect of her life.

Essentially, mindfulness practice cultivates a mind that we can experience as a friend who supports us in the face of challenge, joy, and service. It is a friendship that guides us as we navigate through each moment of our life.

Using our understanding of Buddhist psychology, psychological science, and our own mindfulness practice and teaching we have offered a map of the mind for teachers and students of mindfulness. The map not only sketches the mind's landscape but also enables us to find the routes from suffering to ease and even flourishing. Any journey requires certain skills. A kayaker needs basic kayaking skills, but also skills in navigating safely through rapids. This combination of a map, route map, and skills is equally applicable to the journey that is mindfulness training.

We summarize the key insights from the book:

• Buddhist psychology and modern science together provide a helpful perspective on some of the major challenges in the contemporary world and the question of how to live well in the contemporary world.

• The dialogue among Buddhism, contemporary mindfulness, and psychology is not always easy. There are tensions that include underlying assumptions and central intentions, use of language, professional identity, and ethics. But looking for bridges and synergies is more constructive than building fences and creating silos.

• We define mindfulness as a natural, trainable human capacity to bring attention and awareness to all experience; it is equally open to whatever is present in a given moment with attitudes of curiosity, friendliness, compassion, discernment in the service of suffering less, enjoying greater well-being, and leading a meaningful, rewarding life.

• Mindfulness has several key functions: simple knowing, protective awareness, investigative awareness, and reframing perception and views.

Psychological science has mapped some of the key features of the mind in instructive ways for teachers and students of mindfulness.

- Our mind spends much of the time on automatic pilot, which has many advantages but also some costs.
- Our minds wander much of the time and an untrained wandering mind tends to be an unhappy mind.
- While perception starts in our sense organs, it is a constructive and creative process of the brain.
- The kind of attention we pay alters our experience of the world (i.e., we actively create our experience).
- Our experience can be separated into body sensations, emotions, behavior, and thought.
- The mind is dynamic and ever changing.
- Appraisal, judgment, and discrepancy monitoring are present at every level of perception and attention, powerfully shaping our experience.

- The mind can be trained and transformed through mindfulness practice.
- We have different ways of knowing and being in the world, and we highlighted two: experiential and conceptual modes of mind. They serve us in different ways at different times.
- Our minds are continuously constructing meaning out of our moment-to-moment experience. They are inclined to look for patterns. Context is important, both the context outside us and the internal context of our current state of mind. It shapes how we make sense of our experience.

Buddhist psychology has also mapped some of the key features of the mind.

- Suffering is like two arrows: the first arrow is pain, ill health, and ultimately dying (which is part of life); the second arrow compounds pain with worry, resistance, avoidance, and catastrophizing (which is optional).
- Everything changes, nothing stays the same.
- Struggle, denial, attachment, and aversion fuel distress and suffering.
- There are four ways of establishing mindfulness, called the Four Foundations of Mindfulness:
  o Mindfulness of the body (i.e., somatic experience)
  o Mindfulness of feeling tone (i.e., the primary appraisal of experience as pleasant, unpleasant, or neutral)
  o Mindfulness of mental states and mood (i.e., the cognitive and affective realm of experience)
  o Mindfulness of our experience of the world (i.e., the cognitive, discursive aspect of our experience, including what supports well-being and the factors that obstruct well-being)
- Through mindfulness practice, a greater sense of resilience and equanimity begin to emerge as the mind steadies and calms.

We can synthesize and distill these insights from psychological science and Buddhist psychology in ways that provide a route map for mindfulness teachers and students.

The mind can be described and understood, at least in part, and to a degree that helps us. Much of the time we process the many stimuli that make up the landscape of our lives automatically and rapidly. We are often not even aware of our reactions. Awareness and understanding opens a space between stimulus and reactivity, and in that space we start to have a choice to respond more flexibly, creatively, and skillfully. The direct path from stimulus to reaction is through the experience of a stimulus as a bodily sensation or mental state (the first arrow), which then triggers an immediate reaction. We react in understandable ways that serve us and can provide short-term relief from pain and distress. But some of these reactions add to our suffering, which can be described as the second arrow(s) of suffering.

The ways distress and suffering are maintained and exacerbated can be divided into "what" and "how." The what refers to deconstructing our experience into sensations, emotions, thoughts, and behaviors. The how refers to the labeling (pleasant, unpleasant, or neutral) and subsequent elaborative evaluation of our experience. This is driven by craving for pleasure, an ideal of ourselves and our lives, and sometimes a wish for oblivion. Reactivity stems from a difficulty recognizing and allowing experience to be as it is—an inability to meet challenging experiences with radical acceptance. We all use reactive ways of coping that at one level are completely understandable. However, when examined carefully, we see that they often loop back in ways that inadvertently maintain the problem.

Health and mental health are borne of understanding how distress is created and re-created in our mind, so these processes can be seen and transformed—it becomes possible to respond in new ways. We learn to stabilize and harness our attention, intentionally and effectively. We access new ways of knowing and being, both experiential and conceptual, and know when to use them. Mindfulness training opens a space that enables greater discernment, wisdom, and responsiveness. Mindfulness training cultivates the conditions for living our lives with greater friendliness, compassion, joy, and equanimity. These four attitudinal foundations of mindfulness help us listen to the tenor of our own mindfulness, cooling the fires of reactivity and creating the space for responding in ways that support our well-being and the well-being of those around us.

Embodiment starts with coming to inhabit our bodies. This broadens to include our intentions, attitudes, insight, and understanding. Like a willow tree, we can be firmly rooted in intentionality and understanding, yet bend with the wind of changing conditions. Embodiment is seamlessness between our values, understanding, and intentions, and the ways we think, act, speak, and relate. It is fundamental to teaching and learning mindfulness.

Integrity is not only a personal responsibility but is deeply concerned with our relationships, our work, and our engagement with the world. It protects, safeguards, and provides the framework for positive change and evolution that lies at the heart of mindfulness-based programs.

The Long View

All that we are now is a result of all that we have been, all that we will be tomorrow will be the result of all that we are now. This is true of us individually and it is true of us collectively as the community that will shape how mindfulness will develop over the coming years. Mindfulness is finding its place in the mainstream in a range of contexts, including health, education, the criminal justice system, and the workplace. Although this brings exciting possibilities for new applications for mindfulness, it also raises important questions. In the long view, what will support sustainable development of this field? We close with a reflection on the long view and what is needed to support the sustainable evolution of mindfulness and mindfulness training in the contemporary world.

First, any mindfulness-based intervention needs to be clear about its intentions, aims, and context. When Jon Kabat-Zinn (1982) had the extraordinary insight to develop mindfulness-based stress reduction (MBSR), he was clear that ancient meditative practices might have much to offer people suffering with long-term health conditions. He then carefully considered how best to offer mindfulness in mainstream North American hospital settings. The result was the 8-week MBSR program that has now been taken by tens of thousands of people. Segal, Williams, and Teasdale (2013) were equally clear when they developed mindfulness-based cognitive therapy (MBCT) for recurrent depression. Their theoretical account of depression, articulated and refined through experimental work, is the focus of MBCT. The teacher conveys the MBCT themes in all aspects of the course, so that participants have opportunities to learn to respond resiliently to those pivotal moments that can spiral into depressive relapse. These mindfulness-based programs have a clear intention and theoretical integrity. Each carefully considers the population for whom it is intended and has selected a pedagogy that matches the context in which it is offered. New innovations should similarly attend carefully to the map of the particular landscape they are navigating, develop a customized route through that landscape, and then consider how best to support the traveler in navigating it.

Second, any bridging of different perspectives inevitably involves tensions. An almost universal human tendency is sectarianism, where different camps claim supremacy and disdain others. Mindfulness can help us see when we get involved in unhelpful judgment, taking things personally, and feeling ill-will. The heart of all transformation rests in learning to take the self out of the center of experience. We need to learn lessons of respect and dignity. Mindfulness can be seen as a therapeutic tool for managing life, or it can be seen as part of a transformative pathway concerned with understanding, uprooting the causes of distress, and cultivating the conditions for greater well-being. There are those in more traditional meditative lineages who see contemporary mindfulness as a movement that has abstracted one aspect of the path from the training in liberation and is presenting that fragment as being the whole of the teaching. There are those in contemporary mindfulness who feel misunderstood and judged by the traditional Buddhist communities that are unaware of secular mindfulness's ongoing investigation into ethics and the whole of the path of awakening. We have suggested that deeply understanding mindfulness relies upon deeply understanding the core psychological processes outlined in both Buddhist psychology and modern psychology. There are also voices that suggest that understanding the origins of mindfulness in the ancient teachings is irrelevant.

The perspective of mindfulness as a skill and an attitude that helps us to navigate our way through life and the perspective of mindfulness as one significant feature of a path of transformation are not mutually exclusive. There is an immediacy to mindfulness, and there is the long view. Any of you who have undertaken the serious path of cultivating awareness, stillness, calm, and understanding know this is the work of a lifetime. Eight-week courses are offered to people who often come to a startling understanding and changes in a short period of time. Yet it is a beginning, just as it is for someone doing an introductory course in meditation or a weeklong retreat. We have yet to fully develop a comprehensive way of sustaining and supporting people over the long term. In traditional meditative communities in the West, we were good at establishing centers and offering retreats—we have also come to understand the need to provide a means for people to feel supported and inspired in their lives when retreats come to an end. Following an 8-week course, how do we continue to encourage people not just to survive but also to thrive and build upon the learning that has taken place in the 8 weeks? It is a work in progress, and developing a stepped path for people to follow will be another significant step in developing contemporary mindfulness in our society. We envisage widely available, accessible introductions to mindfulness, accessible mainstream 8-week programs, and more intensive programs and retreats.

Third, let's develop the science of mindfulness and be mindful of the evidence base. In a seminal paper reviewing the current state of the science, the field was characterized as a large body of promising preliminary and foundational research that needs to be pulled into well-designed, robust, large-scale studies that answer key questions about the effectiveness of mindfulness training, how mindfulness training works, for whom and when mindfulness training might be indicated, and how best to scale and implement mindfulness in the real world (Dimidjian & Linehan, 2003). Any field of inquiry goes through stages of progress and maturation, and in this sense mindfulness is no different. Most scientists are aware of how much we don't know and how extraordinary and mysterious the mind and the world are. For example, Einstein (1956/1999) said about the mysterious: "It is the fundamental emotion which stands at the cradle of true art and true science. He who knows it not and can no longer wonder, no longer feel amazement, is as good as dead, a snuffed-out candle" (p. 5). The Dalai Lama (2005) has long had a reciprocal view of science: "Although my own interest in science began as the curiosity of a restless young boy growing up in Tibet, gradually the colossal importance of science and technology for understanding the modern world dawned on me. Not only have I sought to grasp specific scientific ideas but have also attempted to explore the wider implications of the new advances in human knowledge and technological power brought about through science." While noting some important cautions he concludes: "I believe a close cooperation between these two investigative traditions can truly contribute toward expanding the human understanding of the complex world of inner subjective experience that we call the mind."

There is an emerging but promising science around mindfulness, mindfulness training, and mindfulness-based programs. A body of scientific research suggests some encouraging insights about the role of mindfulness in mental health, resilience, and the realization of human potential. We need to report the science responsibly, recognize its limits, and try to answer the many remaining questions as best we can, using robust methods. Unexpected findings should be welcomed and reported transparently. They can often point to something far more interesting than the expected. Science can help us build theory, develop effective interventions, consider optimal ways of training mindfulness teachers, and reach the people who might benefit.

Fourth, it is important to have leadership around integrity. The last 25 or so years have seen centers like the University of Massachusetts Center for Mindfulness, the Oxford Mindfulness Centre, the Bangor Centre for Mindfulness Research and Practice, and the University of Exeter build a consensus about how best to train MBCT teachers, to decide when they are ready to teach MBCT, and when they are ready to train others to teach MBCT. Let's honor these standards. Let's safeguard the public so that they, too, will know whether a teacher meets these standards. Training centers in Europe, Asia, and North America offer trainings. We estimate that a teacher in his or her early 30s might teach MBCT to 4,000 people over a career, so a cohort of 20 teachers might teach 80,000 people. Investing in high-quality training seems worthwhile. The impact of these teachers is and will be profound.

Finally, let's keep learning through our own mindfulness practice, training, and the science. Throughout history contemplative traditions have faced true difficulty when teachers have forgotten to be students—instead becoming identified with a role and forgetting that this is a journey of a lifetime. They can forget, too, that the capacity to embody this teaching is directly linked to the aliveness of their own practice. Mindfulness is something much deeper than a technique we learn solely as a means to teach others. In developing and deepening our understanding of mindfulness, there are two simultaneous journeys being made. One is the journey of learning and developing the skills that support the development of mindfulness-based applications. The second journey, equally if not more significant, is the journey we make inwardly in understanding how our own world of experience is shaped and understanding what it means to find a freedom from habitual patterns that create personal distress. Through dedicated and sustained personal practice we begin to develop an inner awareness of our own mind and heart that is the root of the compassion, warmth, acceptance, and understanding we bring to being with others. This work is invitational, empirical, participatory, and democratic. It is the work of a lifetime.

If the mindfulness field is to flourish, it needs clarity of intention and a basis in robust science; it needs us to be willing to consistently examine our embodiment and integrity. We can all do our best to take personal responsibility for our own teaching and practice. Yet if mindfulness is truly to be embedded in our culture, the services and organizations we work for will ask us to take collective responsibility for good practice and competence.

Mindfulness is a rigorous training, developed in the midst of confusion and adversity. We can take responsibility for the comprehensiveness of our own training and practice and quality of our work. We can take care to root our teaching and research in the deepest motivations of service and compassion. We can widen the circle of our concern to include those in our world who would or could not walk easily through our doors. We can commit ourselves to learning the craft, the art, and the science of mindfulness that allows the seeds of understanding, empathy, integrity, compassion, and care to deepen in others and ourselves. We can commit to being students and teachers of awakening and compassion. Let's see what unfolds.

APPENDIX 1

Definitions of Key Terms

Capacity: The potential, faculty, or ability to do, understand, or contain/hold something. For example, the capacity to recognize and tolerate states such as discomfort or joy.

Discernment: The process of discriminating, understanding, and making judgments that are based in insight and wisdom. Discernment implies *good judgment* based in wholesome intention and an ethical framework. It means knowing not only what thoughts, words, and actions lead to distress but also what thoughts, words, and actions are wholesome, that end distress and suffering, and create the conditions for well-being and flourishing.

Distress: Any state that involves a sense of *unsatisfactoriness*. It can range from a low-key sense of unease through to excruciating pain. It can be physical, emotional, mental, or some combination of all of these. We use the term *distress* for this spectrum of experience.

In Pali, the word *dukkha* is a partial synonym for distress as we use it here, but its meaning is broader, connoting a sense of unsatisfactoriness. We sometimes use the term *dis-ease* to connote this particular meaning. In psychology, it encompasses negative emotions and states, such as sadness and pain, but is broader in scope to encompass worry, anxiety, and more mainstream terms such as *angst* or *despair*.

Feeling tone: The primary texture of experience, it is also known as *vedenā* in Buddhist psychology and primary appraisal in scientific psychology. It is the simple evaluation of an experience as pleasant, unpleasant, or neutral.

Health: We adopt the World Health Organization's (2011) definition as set out in its constitution—namely, "a state of complete physical, mental, and social well-being and not merely the absence of disease or infirmity." We recognize that it is an aspirational definition, and chose it because it is consistent with the thesis we developed in this book.

Intention: Intention orients attention, cognition, and behavior. It determines how we relate to experiences and how we act. Intention and ethics are intertwined—actions that come out of discriminating intentionality will lead to positive outcomes. Intention can lead both to renunciation (i.e., giving up negative thoughts and inclinations) and/or to positive actions.

This maps most closely to the Pali word *cetanā*. The expression "Everything rests on the tip of intention" gives a good sense of how central intention is in mindfulness-based programs. It maps onto theoretical ideas of what is involved in maintaining distress and suffering, as well as what can lead to mental health and well-being in psychological science.

Investigative awareness: A function of mindfulness that recognizes distress, investigates the origins of the distress, and identifies the pathway to the end of the distress. It provides discernment and choices.

Meditation: Major religious traditions all offer forms of meditation—contemplation, prayer, reflection, and ritual are among them—that take different forms and serve different intentions. In the Buddhist tradition, there are a range of techniques and practices to cultivate calmness of mind, one-pointedness of attention, and to develop qualities of heart, such as kindness, compassion, joy, and equanimity.

Mental health: Positive psychological and emotional states of being, which include the range of positive emotions (e.g., happiness), psychological states (e.g., contentment, optimism), and functions (e.g., ability to regulate emotions in the face of changing circumstances). We use it to describe a mind that is not imprisoned by reactivity—rather, mental health connotes a mind that has integrity and capacity for peace and creativity, and enables us to form relationships of trust and respect where we can better respond with discernment, understanding, and skill to the world around us.

Mental health often has the word *problem*(s) tagged on to describe psychiatric disorders.

Mind: The states, processes, and functions that make up our mental experience. This is made up of both conscious awareness and also the processes and functions that are not in awareness. Our mental functions are located in both the structure and function of the brain and nervous system, and the bodily organs and systems that shape mental experience. In psychology, *embodied cognition* refers to the way the body is implicated in cognition, where the mind arises from the nature of our brains, bodily experiences, and functioning, plus our experiences in the physical world (e.g., "This beautiful spring day is making me smile from ear to ear; even my eyes are scrunched up with joy").

The Pali word *citta* is a much broader word than *mind* in psychology. *Citta* connotes intuiting, knowing, and awareness, as well as the energetic quality of mind, in some ways paralleling the idea of *embodied cognition*. It also includes the large body of awareness that is energetic/active, even when attention is not focused on it. In short, while there are parallels between how the word *mind* is used in Buddhist and modern psychology, there are also important ways in which they diverge. When we use the word *mind*, we use the definition "states, processes, and functions that make up our mental experience."

Mindful life: A life lived with awareness, open to whatever is present in a given moment. A mindful life is one imbued with attitudes of curiosity, friendliness, and discernment in the service of suffering less, enjoying greater well-being, and leading a meaningful, rewarding life. This refers not just to the person but also his or her interactions with others and the world. It does not mean *every moment* is lived with awareness, since this would be exhausting—rather, we mean the capacity to choose when and how to deploy mindfulness in the service of living a good life.

In contemplative traditions, religion, and philosophy, there is a large body of work on the *good life*—the idea that certain understandings and practices will lead to a range of positive individual and societal outcomes. For example, Aristotelian philosophy refers to leading a *good* or *ethical* life. Terms such as *eudemonia* and *arete* connote happiness, welfare, and virtue. Contemporary practical philosophers, such as William MacAskill and Richard Rorty, offer pragmatic ways to live such a life.

Mindfulness: A natural, trainable human capacity to bring attention and awareness to all experiences. It is equally open to whatever is present in a given moment with attitudes of curiosity, friendliness, compassion, and discernment in the service of suffering less, enjoying greater well-being, and leading a meaningful, rewarding life.

Reactivity: The tendency to react automatically, relying on deeply ingrained, often learned ways of perceiving and acting. There is no gap between stimulus and reaction, leaving no space for choice. While it can be functional, it can also be dysfunctional.

Resilience: The capacity to respond to challenges in ways that are adaptive and lead to health and well-being. The challenges can be either minor (e.g., some mild physical discomfort) or major (e.g., a terminal disease). They can be internal (e.g., worry) or external (e.g., losing one's job). Resilience describes the process of adapting to challenges that enables the person to manage and, if possible, resolve the difficulty. If the difficulty cannot be changed or resolved (e.g., a chronic illness), resilience refers to learning to live with the difficulty.

Shape: The process of giving a particular form to our experience of creating, molding, framing, and carving it out. For example, we might say mindfulness practices shape the mind because the mind becomes better able to choose what and how it attends to experiences. In a passive sense, this can be likened to the way a river shapes the mountainside through erosion, but in an active sense, the sculptor shapes his or her sculpture. Here this might refer to habitual reactions shaping the mind (passive) or intentional responses based on insight and wisdom shaping the mind actively and in turn cultivating insight and wisdom.

Suffering: A word that describes the process where distress is created, maintained, and possibly exacerbated, as well as the endpoint itself. It encompasses pain, distress, hardship, and inherent challenges of life, such as illness and aging. Crucially, when we use the term *suffering*, we add the dimension of the mind getting involved with the primary experiences of direct sensing or life events, the *discrepancy thinking* that things are different from how they should be, have been, or might be in the future. It connotes first that there is a universality of experience—that is, we all age and get sick, struggle with these experiences, and we are all subject to suffering. Second, it begins to connote that there is a way of understanding and, therefore, a potential method for responding to suffering that can alleviate and even end the psychological dimensions of suffering. Some suffering is optional!

Reactivity to distress causes suffering.

Understanding: The body of knowledge and mental/behavioral capacities/competencies that enable good judgment and skillful behavioral choices. In short, when we use the word *understanding* we refer to insight that helps us to lead a good life. It refers to understanding that is both experiential and conceptual.

In Buddhism, the word *wisdom* is used to refer to *right view*, *wise attention* (*yoniso manasikāra*), and *right understanding*. It arises through clear intention alongside the investigative work of mindfulness practice. This in turn supports clear intention, mindfulness practice, and everyday living.

Well-being: A broad, multidimensional construct that connotes positive mental and physical health, social relationships, and life functioning. It covers both the state and the healthy functioning that enables people to live and lead fulfilling lives.

What Is Mindfulness Training and a Mindfulness-Based Program?

Mindfulness is an innate, universal capacity of the human mind. It is a way of being present in the moment and a fruition of understanding rather than something that we do. It helps us understand how our experience is constructed moment to moment, maximizing our capacity for healing and transformation, and for living a compassionate, ethical, and meaningful life. We define mindfulness fully in Chapter 1.

What Is Mindfulness Training?

Like a garden in the care of a skilled gardener, mindfulness can be cultivated and developed with the right conditions. Mindfulness practices, such as meditations, are tools used to cultivate mindfulness. This cultivation is in the service of greater understanding and responsiveness so that we can live a good life, well.

There are many different types of mindfulness practices, each with somewhat different aims. Some practices aim to stabilize attention. Others aim to develop understanding and insight, and still others to cultivate particular attitudes. A skillful mindfulness teacher knows what will support the cultivation of particular effects, for a particular individual, at a particular time. Contemplative traditions use a variety of ways to train mindfulness. Many include the possibility of more intensive "retreats," where people can dedicate periods of time to meditative and contemplative practice, often with a teacher who guides and supports. The meditative practices are framed within the aims and intentions of the contemplative tradition—for example, to be closer to God.

Christianity, Islam, and Judaism use devotional prayer, while certain forms of Buddhism use meditation to focus attention and cultivate particular qualities of mind. Most religions encourage the adoption of ethical precepts and codes of living.

Within each religion there are lineages, each with their particular training methods. For example, in the third-century C.E., Christian Desert Fathers would retreat to the Scetes desert in Egypt to monastic lives of silence and prayer to cultivate God's presence. This is similar to what was happening in India and Tibet with Buddhist monastics at about the same time where groups of monastics would practice together to cultivate attention and insight. While we acknowledge the rich and varied methods for training mindful attention across religions, that is not the subject of this book. Instead, our main focus is on mindfulness training in secular settings. Important research from Tania Singer's group has started to demonstrate what the Buddha hypothesized: that these different practices affect the mind and body in different ways (e.g., Kok & Singer, 2017).

There has been a proliferation of mindfulness trainings in mainstream settings, including digital mindfulness (apps, websites, and videos), self-help books, workshops, and mindfulness introduced through the arts. These approaches have brought mindfulness training into the mainstream and have, without any doubt, made mindfulness training available to millions of people. These approaches tend to be brief, low-intensity approaches. They introduce mindfulness and provide ways for people to learn about mindfulness and begin to build it into their lives.

Finally, there are several *mindfulness-informed* programs—such as acceptance and commitment therapy (Hayes, 2004), compassion-focused therapy (Gilbert, 2014), dialectical behavior therapy (Linehan, 1993a, 1993b), and mindful self-compassion (Germer, 2009)—as well as developments in the field of positive psychology that include mindfulness practices (Seligman & Csikszentmihalyi, 2000). These programs each have their own aim, theoretical framework, structure, and program of research evaluating effectiveness. They use mindfulness training as a tool within an array of other tools and integrate it into their understanding of distress and how to effect change in particular ways. However, these programs are not our focus in this book.

What Defines a Mindfulness-Based Program?

Since Kabat-Zinn (1982) first developed mindfulness-based stress reduction (MBSR), there has been a proliferation of mindfulness-based programs. To support the sustainable development of the field, we contributed to a paper entitled "What Defines a Mindfulness-Based Program?" (Crane et al., 2017). This paper articulates several core, essential ingredients of a mindfulness-based program—these ingredients are summarized in Chapter 6 in Table 6.1.

A mindfulness-based program uses an underpinning model of human experience that draws from Buddhist psychology, science, and the major disciplines of medicine, psychology, and education. They take the best understanding and adapt it for a particular population and context (Hayes, 2016; Hayes, Long, Levin, & Follette, 2013; Kuyken, Padesky, & Dudley, 2009).

Mindfulness-based programs enable people to develop a new relationship with experience characterized by present-moment focus, decentering, and approach motivation. Mindfulness meditation practice is central in mindfulness-based programs as an experiential inquiry-based learning method. Mindfulness-based programs enable us to really see our own minds clearly and the particular ways in which they create our experience. As we practice the mindfulness practices and cognitive-behavioral exercises, we learn to see their potential transformative power as we apply them in our lives (Allen, Bromley, Kuyken, & Sonnenberg, 2009). This is a form of empiricism, practiced by participants in mindfulness programs.[1] Mindfulness-based programs also embrace empiricism at the level of scientific inquiry—that is, what is known or can be investigated through science (Dimidjian & Segal, 2015; Van Dam et al., 2018).

Finally, even though contemporary mindfulness and mindfulness-based programs have an incontrovertible lineage in Buddhist psychology, they are secular in so far as they retain only understandings and practices that are worldly and empirically supported or testable.[2] Contemporary mindfulness-based programs have not retained the religious dimensions of contemplative traditions or the more esoteric ideas or practices. Instead, they retain the deep human understandings, testing them empirically in an ongoing way so new knowledge and understanding is added, and only presents those that pass the test. More than this, mindfulness programs present the understandings and practices in language and formats that are mainstream and accessible.[3] They try to answer questions like:

- "What creates distress and suffering?"
- "How can distress and suffering be ended?"[4]
- "What supports well-being and flourishing?"
- "What mindfulness trainings will support this transformation?"
- "How can this be made as accessible as possible?"

Notes

1. Christina Feldman (2016) gave a keynote about the history of and lineages that informed contemporary mindfulness-based programs. This was transcribed and is available online.

2. This was at the University of Exeter in the United Kingdom, a university where Willem worked for 16 years and close to where Christina cofounded the Gaia House Buddhist Meditation Retreat Centre in 1983.

CHAPTER 1

1. Of course we still have major challenges of world population growth, climate change, various forms of injustice and inequality, and extensive human migration.

2. These cases are composites of people we have worked with, and details have been extensively changed to mask any one person's identity.

3. This is a paraphrasing of the essential teaching in the *Madhupindika Sutta: The Ball of Honey* (MN 18).

4. This term is used in the way neuroscientists use it to connote that our brains show the capacity to change structurally and functionally through learning and practice.

5. We draw on the Pali canon, which is a language developed specifically for these teachings by monks in Sri Lanka circa 200 C.E. We use the Access to Insight website as all the *suttas* are well translated and reproduced here freely. However, the discourses are also produced in full in the series Discourses of the Buddha published as several volumes by Wisdom Press.

6. The Buddha's thinking was both radical and practical. He was radical for suggesting his teachings were available to all, regardless of gender, age, cultural background, or religion. He lived at a time when society was organized by caste and there was political strife, conflict, and profound poverty, as well as relative wealth. A spiritual path was not equally available to men and women. In the midst of all of this, he realized that the insights he had discovered in his own contemplative path that led to inner freedom were universal, concerning the minds of all people. The teachings could be embodied in the midst of life for people of both genders, from all castes, and even across religions. He was radical in proposing that the teachings were universal and available to all to follow and live.

7. Within psychiatry and clinical psychology, the last 50 years have seen the development of psychological therapies that have demonstrated they can help people overcome and recover from a wide range of mental ill health, including depression, anxiety, and substance abuse. These include well-established therapies—such as psychodynamic psychotherapy, behavior therapy, cognitive therapy, and interpersonal therapy—that are now well supported by many hundreds of clinical trials (Gabbard, Beck, & Holmes, 2005). While effective for many people, these therapies are far from a panacea, with some people responding well, some only partially, and some not at all.

8. Richard Burnett, Chris Cullen, and Chris O'Neill adapted the 8-week mindfulness-based cognitive stress reduction and mindfulness-based cognitive therapy curricula for children, and use this analogy in their curriculum.

CHAPTER 2

1. Maps (or theories) can be high level—that is, universally understood representations that apply to all of us and how we attend to and make meaning of our world, as well as how we react and behave in the world. We map our own lives and experiences through our perceptions, using sight, hearing, touch, and so on. These are psychological processes that characterize our species. Maps (or theories) can also be specific to a particular group or set of circumstances. For example, psychologists have developed theories for each of the major mental health problems (e.g., anxiety and depression), and theories that account for particular phenomena (e.g., altruism).

2. Psychology, like any discipline, has subdisciplines, such as cognitive, social, and clinical psychology. Each subdiscipline has tended to develop theoretically and empirically in something of a silo. In reality, to map the mind takes integration across these subdisciplines.

3. These differentiations are in the service of helping people to parse their experience to support greater understanding and responsiveness. In reality, they are often closely interlinked in terms of mental architecture and brain structure/function. Emotion can comprise appraisals (thoughts, images, beliefs) and be closely linked to behavioral impulses, sometimes to the point where the differentiations are

hard to discern. Arguably, these distinctions do not really carve nature at its most exact joints, but they are distinctions that help people to map their minds.

4. LeDoux (2000) hypothesized that this sort of fear-based processing is a chain of quick pattern-matching perception (stick moving = snake moving) that leads to a thalamus–amygdala circuit activation and associated action tendency (to flee) that bypasses the more deliberative, reasoning parts of the brain (the cortex). Only later does the part of the mind that reasons kick in.

CHAPTER 3

1. This quote from Stephen Pinker is preceded by "The two deepest questions about the mind are 'What makes intelligence possible?' and 'What makes consciousness possible?' With the advent of cognitive science, intelligence has become intelligible. It may not be too outrageous to say that at least at the most abstract level of analysis the problem has been solved. But consciousness or sentience, the raw sensation of toothaches and redness and saltiness and middle C, is still a riddle, wrapped in a mystery, inside an enigma."

2. Notably, John Teasdale spent much of his career working on how different ways of knowing the world can drive depression but also provide a way out of depression (Teasdale, 1993, 1999; Teasdale & Barnard, 1993; Teasdale & Chaskalson, 2011a, 2011b). In 2016, John introduced me (WK) to Iain McGilchrist's (2009) seminal book *The Master and His Emissary*, in which the typology of experiential and conceptual ways of being and knowing are articulated in an exceptionally comprehensive and compelling way. These typologies overlap with those mapped out in the Buddhist Four Foundations of Mindfulness that we introduced in Chapter 4 and the work of scientists, such as Daniel Kahneman (2011), Robert Sapolsky (2017), and Frans De Waal (2009). Kahneman's seminal work argues that while humans have at their disposal an immense potential for rational, logical, and systematic thought, our default is a faster, more automatic, intuitive system powerfully shaped by context and emotion. Sapolsky (2017) and De Waal (2009, 2013) argue strongly that both evolution and animal behavior can help us map human experience and behavior. Sapolsky's book *Behave* is a masterful thesis on the influences shaping human behavior, moving from the level of neuron to the wider forces, both in the present and the past of a person's life, including their evolutionary lineage.

3. This model of the dynamic interrelationship of our thoughts, feelings, bodily sensations, and behaviors is supported by much evidence from our own experience and from psychological science. For example, many experiments present information so briefly that we cannot consciously register it—and following, researchers look at the effects on emotional state. Negative words or images create negative moods (sadness, fear), positive words and images create positive moods (happiness), and neutral words and images (e.g., plant) create neutral states. This is dynamic—preexisting

mood states also shape how we perform on these tasks. Someone who is sad tends to bring negative appraisals to even neutral information. The model we present distills a complex field to a level that is readily usable. In reality, much complexity lies behind the model, with dynamic relationships among cognition, emotion, sensations, perception, and the creation of meaning. Any good reference on cognition and emotion outlines this field—for example, Elaine Fox's (2008) excellent text *Emotion Science*.

4. When we use the word *understanding*, we often mean understanding through language. But experiential knowing does not rely on language. Metaphors, images, music, art, nonverbal social cues, and nature can convey meaning powerfully without relying on language. The word *metaphor* stems from the Greek for *meta* meaning across and *phere* meaning carry, so the word *metaphor* literally means *to carry us across to a place of understanding*. Metaphor invokes higher-level meaning making, connections, and looking for the whole beyond the concrete literal meanings. The words *the cat is sitting on the mat* communicate a literal, straightforward meaning. We see and understand a cat sitting on a mat. But the words *she was deflated by his barbed words* connote a richer meaning by invoking imagery and metaphor. Socially, nonverbal cues can have great communicative strength: eye contact, body language, and touch; they all communicate affiliation, safety, power, and hierarchy directly, arguably more emphatically than words. Music is also a powerful form of communication; it may even predate language in our evolution (Dunbar, 2004). What is clear is that there is a great deal of understanding in our nonverbal, even nonconceptual experience. In language, metaphor and poetry are ways of conveying complex, more holistic meaning. Experientially, we can understand states such as safety and connection. Our understanding of the world and the way we react and respond is shaped by these bodily and nonverbal cues (Ackerman, Nocera, & Bargh, 2010).

CHAPTER 4

1. We provide extracts of the *satipatthana* discourse throughout this chapter and in later chapters. The cited translation is used but we substituted references such as he or him and so on, with he or she and them to refer to both men and women. We also refer to people more generally than to "monks" as occurs in places in the discourses.

2. Descartes' error is exposed in our experience; the mind and body are essentially interconnected.

3. The instructions found in the *satipatthana* discourse in establishing mindfulness of the body repeatedly encourage the practitioner to establish a moment-to-moment sensitivity and attention, saying, "the person, breathing in a long breath, knows 'I am breathing in a long breath'; breathing out a long breath, he or she knows 'I am breathing out a long breath'; breathing in a short breath, he or she knows 'I am breathing in a short breath'; breathing out a short breath, he or she knows 'I am

breathing out a short breath.' 'Experiencing the whole body, I shall breathe in,' thus he or she trains him- or herself. 'Experiencing the whole body, I shall breathe out,' thus he or she trains him- or herself. 'Calming the activity of the body, I shall breathe in,' thus he or she trains him- or herself. 'Calming the activity of the body, I shall breathe out,' thus he or she trains him- or herself."

4. In the *satipatthana* discourse it is described this way: "Herein a person when experiencing a pleasant feeling knows 'I experience a pleasant feeling'; when experiencing a painful feeling, he or she knows 'I experience a painful feeling'; when experiencing a neither pleasant nor painful feeling, he or she knows 'I experience a neither pleasant nor painful feeling.'"

5. In the Pali canon, certain words describe complex emergent mental states for which translations are more challenging. For example, the word *Bodhi* describes a state of complete insight into the nature of reality; a liberation from suffering. The word *dukkha* describes the everyday state we have referred to as distress, but also connotes unsatisfactoriness within experience, ranging from a minor itch to excruciating pain. However, it can also connote the distress inherent in change and impermanence, as well as the conditioned distress that can arise when feelings, perceptions, views, and other mental states have become aggregated (e.g., with generalized anxiety).

6. The section of the original discourse on the contemplation of mental states invites knowing states for what they are, to see and understand them as transient states, to step back from elaboration and rumination, and to, as best we can, keep it simple.

7. Buddhist psychology refers to the Four Right Exertions (*cattārimāni sammap- padhānāni*):

- The non-arising (*anuppādāya*) of unwholesome states.
- Abandonment (*pahānāya*) of unwholesome qualities that have arisen.
- Cultivate the arising (*uppādāya*) of wholesome states and skillful qualities that have not yet arisen.
- Maintenance (*ṭhitiyā*) of wholesome states, nonconfusion, increase, pleni- tude, development, and culmination of skillful qualities that have arisen.

CHAPTER 5

1. The source of this quote is unclear. Stephen Covey (1999) used it extensively in his teachings, saying he came across it in a library but was then unable to attribute it. It is sometimes attributed to Viktor Frankl, but there is no verifiable source for this claim either.

2. In cognitive therapy, thoughts and imagery are seen as primary, being the precursor for emotion and behavior. Here the model is less concerned with primacy of one element over another, but rather first being able to disaggregate experience and

then see the dynamic interplay between elements as they are created and re-created in every moment of our experience. Another key difference is that cognitive therapy works to help people identify underlying beliefs that maintain and exacerbate their difficulties. These can be conditional beliefs ("If I teach mindfulness perfectly, people won't see my inadequacies") or unconditional, sometimes called core, beliefs (e.g., "I am inadequate").

3. Sapolsky's (2017) book *Behave* is a masterful thesis of how each of these layers shapes our experience in this moment

4. In actuality, our direct experience can sometimes be more nuanced and unique than the differentiation into sensations, emotions, thoughts, and behavior—the five-factor model is only a shorthand.

CHAPTER 6

1. In one application of protective awareness, Thich Nhat Hanh, a leading mindfulness teacher, encourages us to be discerning about *how much* news we consume and *how* we consume it. A Velcro mind is inclined to consume news on a 24-hour news cycle, and if allowed to do this, it will shape the mind. Moreover, it is possible to read the same news article either with a sense of presence, compassion, and equanimity or with righteous indignation and anger. Thich Nhat Hanh is not suggesting that world news is not important, or that news always evokes unhelpful reactions—simply that we can choose whether, how much, and in what way we consume news.

2. The Buddhist discourses use a range of analogies and terms that are descriptive. For example, a *tangle* or *thicket* gives a sense of their impenetrability and the challenge of untangling.

3. Decentering is sometimes called meta-awareness—being able to use awareness to take a "meta" perspective.

CHAPTER 7

1. We prefer the term *mindfulness practice* because it communicates the broad array of practices that support, train, and cultivate attention imbued with the attitudinal dimensions of curiosity, care, equanimity, and patience.

2. "Near enemy" refers to what can easily be mistaken for befriending but is actually far from befriending. The "far enemy" is the antonym or opposite.

3. Darwin used the word *sympathy*, which seems in English to have been a precursor synonym for *compassion,* as we understand it today.

4. Many people have pointed to this form of gratitude in the interconnectedness of our experience, including Thich Nhat Hanh and Martin Luther King Jr.

CHAPTER 9

1. Frans De Waal (2013) has argued that animal behavior (especially social animals, such as primates) is governed by principles that have evolved to support the well-being of the social unit, and that these behaviors can be framed as moral or ethical.

2. This, of course, is not unique to mindfulness; it is a hallmark of all professions, such as medicine, education, and psychology, as well.

3. This a Sufi saying.

4. We adapted the extract from its original translation to make it as accessible as possible.

APPENDIX 2

1. In many ways, the Buddha and his contemporaries were the first psychologists and scientists, using a systematic approach to studying the mind. Their understanding and prescription for change came through a sustained, in-depth process of examination and testing. Early contemplatives tried different approaches, developing their ideas as new insights emerged and rejecting those that did not work. They worked toward a "theory" and "program" for change.

2. We use the word *secular* to mean worldly and not specifically religious or spiritual. Interestingly, one of its Latin roots (*saeculum*) was used by early Christians to mean "the world," as opposed to the Church (*New Penguin English Dictionary*, 2001).

3. Somewhat ironically, contemporary mindfulness-based approaches have come full circle to the original teachings of the Buddha in rejecting metaphysical questions and positions. The Buddha himself was acutely aware that they tend to galvanize unhelpful views and ideologies.

4. Much of the Buddhist canon uses a medical analogy of symptoms (suffering), diagnosis (what creates and maintains suffering), prognosis (what leads to a good prognosis), and treatment (the path or actions that will end suffering and lead to health).

References

Acharya Buddharakkhita. (1996). The dhammapada: The Buddha's path of wisdom. Retrieved from *www.accesstoinsight.org/tipitaka/kn/dhp/dhp.intro.budd.html*.

Ackerman, J. M., Nocera, C. C., & Bargh, J. A. (2010). Incidental haptic sensations influence social judgments and decisions. *Science, 328*(5986), 1712–1715.

Allen, M., Bromley, A., Kuyken, W., & Sonnenberg, S. J. (2009). Participants' experiences of mindfulness-based cognitive therapy: "It changed me in just about every way possible." *Behavioural and Cognitive Psychotherapy, 37*(4), 413–430.

Alsubaie, M., Abbott, R., Dunn, B., Dickens, C., Keil, T. F., Henley, W., & Kuyken, W. (2017). Mechanisms of action in mindfulness-based cognitive therapy (MBCT) and mindfulness-based stress reduction (MBSR) in people with physical and/or psychological conditions: A systematic review. *Clinical Psychology Review, 55*, 74–91.

Armstrong, K. (2011). *Twelve steps to a compassionate life*. London: Random House.

Baddeley, A. (1996). Exploring the central executive. *Quarterly Journal of Experimental Psychology Section A—Human Experimental Psychology, 49*(1), 5–28.

Baddeley, A. (2012). Working memory: Theories, models, and controversies. *Annual Review of Psychology, 63*, 1–29.

Baer, R. (2015). Ethics, values, virtues, and character strengths in mindfulness-based interventions: A psychological science perspective. *Mindfulness, 6*(4), 956–969.

Baer, R., & Kuyken, W. (2016). Is mindfulness safe? Retrieved from *www.mindful.org/is-mindfulness-safe*.

Bargh, J. A., Chen, M., & Burrows, L. (1996). Automaticity of social behavior: Direct effects of trait construct and stereotype activation on action. *Journal of Personality and Social Psychology, 71*(2), 230–244.

Barks, C., & Moyne, J. (1997). *The essential Rumi*. New York: Penguin.

Barnard, P. J., Duke, D. J., Byrne, R. W., & Davidson, I. (2007). Differentiation in cognitive and emotional meanings: An evolutionary analysis. *Cognition and Emotion, 21*(6), 1155–1183.

Barnard, P. J., & Teasdale, J. D. (1991). Interacting cognitive subsystems: A systemic approach to cognitive–affective interaction and change. *Cognition and Emotion, 5*(1), 1–39.

Barnett, K., Mercer, S. W., Norbury, M., Watt, G., Wyke, S., & Guthrie, B. (2012). Epidemiology of multimorbidity and implications for health care, research, and medical education: A cross-sectional study. *Lancet, 380*(9836), 37–43.

Beck, A. T. (1976). *Cognitive therapy and emotional disorders.* New York: Meridian.

Beck, A. T. (2005). The current state of cognitive therapy: A 40-year retrospective. *Archives of General Psychiatry, 62,* 953–959.

Beck, A. T., & Dozois, D. J. (2011). Cognitive therapy: Current status and future directions. *Annual Review of Medicine, 62,* 397–409.

Beck, A. T., Emery, G., & Greenberg, R. L. (1985). *Anxiety disorders and phobias: A cognitive perspective.* New York: Basic Books.

Beck, A. T., & Haigh, E. A. P. (2014). Advances in cognitive theory and therapy: The generic cognitive model. *Annual Review of Clinical Psychology, 10,* 1–24.

Beck, A. T., Hollon, S. D., Young, J. E., Bedrosian, R. C., & Budenz, D. (1985). Treatment of depression with cognitive therapy and amitriptyline. *Archives of General Psychiatry, 42*(2), 142–148.

Beck, A. T., Rush, A. J., Shaw, B. F., & Emery, G. (1979). *Cognitive therapy of depression.* New York: Guilford Press.

Bhikkhu Analāyo. (2003). *Satipatthana: The direct path to realization.* Birmingham, UK: Windhorse.

Bhikkhu Bodhi. (2005). *In the Buddhas's words: An anthology of discourses from the Pali canon.* Somerville, MA: Wisdom.

Bieling, P. J., Hawley, L. L., Bloch, R. T., Corcoran, K. M., Levitan, R. D., Young, L. T., . . . Segal, Z. V. (2012). Treatment-specific changes in decentering following mindfulness-b;ased cognitive therapy versus antidepressant medication or placebo for prevention of depressive relapse. *Journal of Consulting and Clinical Psychology, 80*(3), 365–372.

Birnie, K., Speca, M., & Carlson, L. E. (2010). Exploring self-compassion and empathy in the context of mindfulness-based stress reduction (MBSR). *Stress and Health, 26*(5), 359–371.

Bishop, S. R., Lau, M., Shapiro, S., Carlson, L., Anderson, N. D., Carmody, J., . . . Devins, G. (2006). Mindfulness: A proposed operational definition. *Clinical Psychology: Science and Practice, 11*(3), 230–241.

Blakemore, S. J. (2018). *Inventing ourselves: The secret life of the teenage brain.* New York: Doubleday.

Blakemore, S. J., & Robbins, T. W. (2012). Decision-making in the adolescent brain. *Nature Neuroscience, 15*(9), 1184–1191.

Bockting, C. L., Hollon, S. D., Jarrett, R. B., Kuyken, W., & Dobson, K. (2015). A lifetime approach to major depressive disorder: The contributions of psychological interventions in preventing relapse and recurrence. *Clinical Psychology Review, 41,* 16–26.

Bohlmeijer, E., Prenger, R., Taal, E., & Cuijpers, P. (2010). Meta-analysis on the effectiveness of mindfulness-based stress reduction therapy on mental health of adults with a chronic disease: What should the reader not make of it? *Journal of Psychosomatic Research, 69*(6), 614–615.

Booth, R. (2017, October 22). Kabat-Zinn, master of mindfulness: "People are losing their minds: That is what we need to wake up." Retrieved from *www.theguardian. com/lifeandstyle/2017/oct/22/mindfulness-jon-kabat-zinn-depression-trump-grenfell.*

Bornemann, B., Herbert, B. M., Mehling, W. E., & Singer, T. (2015). Differential changes in self-reported aspects of interoceptive awareness through 3 months of contemplative training. *Frontiers in Psychology, 5,* 1504.

Bornemann, B., Kok, B. E., Bockler, A., & Singer, T. (2016). Helping from the heart: Voluntary upregulation of heart rate variability predicts altruistic behavior. *Biological Psychology, 119,* 54–63.

Bowen, S., & Vieten, C. (2012). A compassionate approach to the treatment of addictive behaviors: The contributions of Alan Marlatt to the field of mindfulness-based interventions. *Addiction Research and Theory, 20*(3), 243–249.

Breines, J. G., Thoma, M. V., Gianferante, D., Hanlin, L., Chen, X., & Rohleder, N. (2014). Self-compassion as a predictor of interleukin-6 response to acute psychosocial stress. *Brain Behavior and Immunity, 37,* 109–114.

Brewer, J. A., Elwafi, H. M., & Davis, J. H. (2013). Craving to quit: Psychological models and neurobiological mechanisms of mindfulness training as treatment for addictions. *Psychology of Addictive Behaviors, 27*(2), 366–379.

Brewer, J. A., Worhunsky, P. D., Gray, J. R., Tang, Y.-Y., Weber, J., & Kober, H. (2011). Meditation experience is associated with differences in default mode network activity and connectivity. *Proceedings of the National Academy of Sciences of the USA, 108*(50), 20254–20259.

Campbell, J. (1991). *The power of myth.* New York: Anchor.

Cesario, J., Plaks, J. E., Hagiwara, N., Navarrete, C. D., & Higgins, E. T. (2010). The ecology of automaticity: How situational contingencies shape action semantics and social behavior. *Psychological Science, 21*(9), 1311–1317.

Chabris, C., & Simons, D. (2010). *The invisible gorilla: How our intuitions deceive us.* New York: Crown.

Condon, P., Desbordes, G., Miller, W. B., & DeSteno, D. (2013). Meditation increases compassionate responses to suffering. *Psychological Science, 24*(10), 2125–2127.

Cook, J. (2016). Mindful in Westminster: The politics of meditation and the limits of neoliberal critique. *Hau—Journal of Ethnographic Theory, 6*(1), 141–161.

Covey, S. R. (1999). *The 7 habits of highly effective people.* London: Simon & Schuster.

Crane, R. S. (2011). The UK good practice guidelines for mindfulness-based teachers. Retrieved from *http://mindfulnessteachersuk.org.uk.*

Crane, R. S. (2017). Implementing mindfulness in the mainstream: Making the path by walking it. *Mindfulness, 8*(3), 585–594.

Crane, R. S., Brewer, J., Feldman, C., Kabat-Zinn, J., Santorelli, S., Williams, J. M., & Kuyken, W. (2017). What defines mindfulness-based programs? The warp and the weft. *Psychological Medicine, 47*(6), 990–999.

Crane, R. S., Kuyken, W., Hastings, R. P., Rothwell, N., & Williams, J. M. G. (2010).

Training teachers to deliver mindfulness-based interventions: Learning from the UK experience. *Mindfulness, 1*(2), 74–86.

Dalai Lama. (2005). *Science at the crossroads.* Paper presented at the annual meeting of the Society for Neuroscience, Washington, DC. Retrieved from *www. dalailama.com/messages/buddhism/science-at-the-crossroads.*

Dalai Lama. (2011a, February 22). [Facebook post.] Retrieved from *www.facebook. com/DalaiLama/posts/10150096941742616.*

Dalai Lama. (2011b). *Beyond religion: Ethics for a whole world.* London: Random House.

Damasio, A. (1994). *Descartes' error: Emotion, reason, and the human brain.* New York: Putnam.

Darwin, C. (1871). *The descent of man, and selection in relation to sex.* London: John Murray.

Davidson, R. J., & Irwin, W. (1999). The functional neuroanatomy of emotion and affective style. *Trends in Cognitive Sciences, 3*(1), 11–21.

Davidson, R. J., Kabat-Zinn, J., Schumacher, J., Rosenkranz, M., Muller, D., Santorelli, S. F., . . . Sheridan, J. F. (2003). Alterations in brain and immune function produced by mindfulness meditation. *Psychosomatic Medicine, 65*(4), 564–570.

Davidson, R. J., & McEwen, B. S. (2012). Social influences on neuroplasticity: Stress and interventions to promote well-being. *Nature Neuroscience, 15*(5), 689–695.

De Houwer, J., Thomas, S., & Baeyens, F. (2001). Associative learning of likes and dislikes: A review of 25 years of research on human evaluative conditioning. *Psychological Bulletin, 127*(6), 853–869.

De Waal, F. B. M. (2009). *The age of empathy: Nature's lessons for a kinder society.* London: Souvenir Press.

De Waal, F. (2013). *The bonobo and the atheist: In search of humanism among the primates.* New York: Norton.

Desbordes, G., Gard, T., Hoge, E. A., Holzel, B., Kerr, C., Lazar, S. W., . . . Vago, D. R. (2015). Moving beyond mindfulness: Defining equanimity as an outcome measure in meditation and contemplative research. *Mindfulness, 6*(2), 356–372.

Diamond, A. (2013). Executive functions. *Annual Review of Psychology, 64,* 135–168.

Diedrich, A., Grant, M., Hofmann, S. G., Hiller, W., & Berking, M. (2014). Self-compassion as an emotion regulation strategy in major depressive disorder. *Behaviour Research and Therapy, 58,* 43–51.

Dimidjian, S., & Segal, Z. V. (2015). Prospects for a clinical science of mindfulness-based intervention. *American Psychologist, 70*(7), 593–620.

Donovan, W. L., & Leavitt, L. A. (1985). Cardiac responses of mother and infants in Ainsworth's strange situation. In M. Reite & T. Field (Eds.), *The psychobiology of attachment and separation* (pp. 369–387). Orlando, FL: Academic Press.

Dunbar, R. I. M. (2003). The social brain: Mind, language, and society in evolutionary perspective. *Annual Review of Anthropology, 32,* 163–181.

Dunbar, R. I. M. (2004). *The human story: A new history of mankind's evolution.* London: Faber & Faber.

Dunbar, R. I. M., & Shultz, S. (2007). Evolution in the social brain. *Science, 317*(5843), 1344–1347.

Einstein, A. (1956/1999). *The world as I see it.* Secaucus, NJ: Citadel Press.

Eliot, T. S. (1940). *The waste land and other poems.* London: Faber & Faber.

Engen, H. G., & Singer, T. (2015). Compassion-based emotion regulation up-regulates experienced positive affect and associated neural networks. *Social Cognitive and Affective Neuroscience, 10*(9), 1291–1301.

Evans, A., Crane, R., Cooper, L., Mardula, J., Wilks, J., Surawy, C., . . . Kuyken, W. (2015). A framework for supervision for mindfulness-based teachers: A space for embodied mutual inquiry. *Mindfulness, 6*(3), 572–581.

Farb, N. A. S., Anderson, A. K., Mayberg, H., Bean, J., McKeon, D., & Segal, Z. V. (2010). Minding one's emotions: Mindfulness training alters the neural expression of sadness. *Emotion, 10*(1), 25–33.

Farb, N. A. S., Segal, Z. V., Mayberg, H., Bean, J., McKeon, D., Fatima, Z., & Anderson, A. K. (2007). Attending to the present: Mindfulness meditation reveals distinct neural modes of self-reference. *Social Cognitive and Affective Neuroscience, 2*(4), 313–322.

Feldman, C. (2016). The long view: Perils and possibilities of mindfulness. Retrieved from *http://oxfordmindfulness.org/news/long-view-perils-possibilities-3/?insight_type=blog.*

Feldman, C. (2017). *Boundless heart: The Buddha's path of kindness, compassion, joy and equanimity.* Boulder, CO: Shambhala.

Feldman, C., & Kuyken, W. (2011). Compassion in the landscape of suffering. *Contemporary Buddhism, 12*(1), 143–155.

Fergusson, D. M., & Lynskey, M. T. (1996). Adolescent resiliency to family adversity. *Journal of Child Psychology and Psychiatry and Allied Disciplines, 37*(3), 281–292.

Fox, E. (2008). *Emotion science: Cognitive and neuroscientific approaches to understanding human emotions.* New York: Palgrave Macmillan.

Fredrickson, B. L., & Losada, M. F. (2005). Positive affect and the complex dynamics of human flourishing. *American Psychologist, 60*(7), 678–686.

Friedman, R. S., & Forster, J. (2010). Implicit affective cues and attentional tuning: An integrative review. *Psychological Bulletin, 136*(5), 875–893.

Gabbard, G., Beck, J. S., & Holmes, J. (2005). *Concise Oxford textbook of psychotherapy.* Oxford, UK: Oxford University Press.

Garland, E. L., Fredrickson, B., Kring, A. M., Johnson, D. P., Meyer, P. S., & Penn, D. L. (2010). Upward spirals of positive emotions counter downward spirals of negativity: Insights from the broaden-and-build theory and affective neuroscience on the treatment of emotion dysfunctions and deficits in psychopathology. *Clinical Psychology Review, 30*(7), 849–864.

GBD 2015 Disease and Injury Incidence and Prevalence Collaborators. (2016). Global, regional, and national incidence, prevalence, and years lived with disability for 310 diseases and injuries, 1990–2015: A systematic analysis for the Global Burden of Disease Study 2015. *Lancet, 388*(10053), 1545–1602.

Germer, C. K. (2009). *The mindful path to self-compassion: Freeing yourself from destructive thoughts and emotions.* New York: Guilford Press.

Gethin, R. (2011). On some definitions of mindfulness. *Contemporary Buddhism, 12*(1), 16.

Gilbert, P. (2014). The origins and nature of compassion focused therapy. *British Journal of Clinical Psychology, 53*(1), 6–41.

Glasser, M. F., Coalson, T. S., Robinson, E. C., Hacker, C. D., Harwell, J., Yacoub, E., . . . Van Essen, D. C. (2016). A multi-modal parcellation of human cerebral cortex. *Nature, 536*(7615), 171.

Glockner, A., & Witteman, C. (2010). Beyond dual-process models: A categorisation of processes underlying intuitive judgement and decision making. *Thinking and Reasoning, 16*(1), 1–25.

Goetz, J. L., Keltner, D., & Simon-Thomas, E. (2010). Compassion: An evolutionary analysis and empirical review. *Psychological Bulletin, 136*(3), 351–374.

Gold, M. (Director). (2016). The arc of history [television series episode]. In *Inside Obama's White House.* London: BBC.

Goldstein, J., & Kornfield, J. (1987). *Seeking the heart of wisdom.* Boston: Shambhala.

Goldstein, S. (2013). *Mindfulness: A practical guide to awakening.* Boulder, CO: Sounds True.

Goleman, D., & Davidson, R. J. (2017). *Altered traits: Science reveals how meditation changes your mind, brain and body.* New York: Avery.

Good, D. J., Lyddy, C. J., Glomb, T. M., Bono, J. E., Brown, K. W., Duffy, M. K., . . . Lazar, S. W. (2016). Contemplating mindfulness at work: An integrative review. *Journal of Management, 42*(1), 114–142.

Gopher, D., Armony, L., & Greenshpan, Y. (2000). Switching tasks and attention policies. *Journal of Experimental Psychology—General, 129*(3), 308–339.

Gotink, R. A., Chu, P., Busschbach, J. J. V., Benson, H., Fricchione, G. L., & Hunink, M. G. M. (2015). Standardised mindfulness-based interventions in healthcare: An overview of systematic reviews and meta-analyses of RCTs. *PLOS ONE, 10*(4), e0124344.

Greenberg, M. T., & Harris, A. R. (2012). Nurturing mindfulness in children and youth: Current state of research. *Child Development Perspectives, 6*(2), 161–166.

Gregory, R. (1970). *The intelligent eye.* New York: McGraw-Hill.

Grossman, P., Niemann, L., Schmidt, S., & Walach, H. (2004). Mindfulness-based stress reduction and health benefits. *Journal of Psychosomatic Research, 57*(1), 35–43.

Gu, J., Strauss, C., Bond, R., & Cavanagh, K. (2015). How do mindfulness-based cognitive therapy and mindfulness-based stress reduction improve mental health and wellbeing?: A systematic review and meta-analysis of mediation studies. *Clinical Psychology Review, 37,* 1–12.

Gunaratana, B. H. (2002). *Mindfulness in plain English.* Somerville, MA: Wisdom.

Hamilton, J. P., Furman, D. J., Chang, C., Thomason, M. E., Dennis, E., & Gotlib, I. H. (2011). Default-mode and task-positive network activity in major depressive disorder: Implications for adaptive and maladaptive rumination. *Biological Psychiatry, 70*(4), 327–333.

Hanson, R., & Mendius, R. (2009). *Buddha's brain: The practical neuroscience of happiness, love and wisdom.* Oakland, CA: New Harbinger.

Hasenkamp, W., Wilson-Mendenhall, C. D., Duncan, E., & Barsalou, L. W. (2012). Mind wandering and attention during focused meditation: A fine-grained temporal analysis of fluctuating cognitive states. *NeuroImage, 59*(1), 750–760.

Hawton, K., Rodham, K., Evans, E., & Weatherall, R. (2002). Deliberate self harm in adolescents: Self report survey in schools in England. *British Medical Journal, 325*(7374), 1207–1211.

Hayes, S. C. (2004). Acceptance and commitment therapy, relational frame theory, and the third wave of behavior therapy. *Behavior Therapy, 35*(4), 639–665.

Hayes, S. C. (2016). The situation has clearly changed: So what are we going to do about it? *Cognitive and Behavioral Practice, 23*(4), 446–450.

Hayes, S. C., Long, D. M., Levin, M. E., & Follette, W. C. (2013). Treatment development: Can we find a better way? *Clinical Psychology Review, 33*(7), 870–882.

Heffernan, V. (2015, April 14). The muddied meaning of "mindfulness." *New York Times Magazine,* p. 13

Higgins, E. T. (1987). Self-discrepancy: A theory relating self and affect. *Psychological Review, 94*(3), 319–340.

Higgins, E. T. (1996). The "self digest": Self-knowledge serving self-regulatory functions. *Journal of Personality and Social Psychology, 71*(6), 1062–1083.

Higgins, E. T., Bond, R. N., Klein, R., & Strauman, T. J. (1986). Self-discrepancies and emotional vulnerability: How magnitude, accessibility, and type of discrepancy influence affect. *Journal of Personality and Social Psychology, 51*(1), 5–15.

Hofmann, S. G., Grossman, P., & Hinton, D. E. (2011). Loving-kindness and compassion meditation: Psychological interventions. *Clinical Psychology Review, 31*(7), 1126–1132.

Hofmann, W., Schmeichel, B. J., & Baddeley, A. D. (2012). Executive functions and self-regulation. *Trends in Cognitive Sciences, 16*(3), 174–180.

Holmes, E. A., & Mathews, A. (2010). Mental imagery in emotion and emotional disorders. *Clinical Psychology Review, 30*(3), 349–362.

James, W. (1890). *The principles of psychology.* New York: Holt.

Jha, A. P., Krompinger, J., & Baime, M. J. (2007). Mindfulness training modifies subsystems of attention. *Cognitive, Affective, and Behavioral Neuroscience, 7*(2), 109–119.

Johnstone, M. (2007). *I had a black dog.* London: Robinson.

Joyce, J. (1914/1996). *Dubliners.* London: Penguin.

Kabat-Zinn, J. (1982). An outpatient program in behavioral medicine for chronic pain patients based on the practice of mindfulness meditation: Theoretical considerations and preliminary results. *General Hospital Psychiatry, 4*(1), 33–47.

Kabat-Zinn, J. (1990). *Full catastrophe living: How to cope with stress, pain and illness using mindfulness meditation.* New York: Delacorte.

Kabat-Zinn, J. (2005). *Coming to our senses: Healing ourselves and the world through mindfulness.* London: Piatkus Books.

Kabat-Zinn, J. (2006). Mindfulness-based interventions in context: Past, present, and future. *Clinical Psychology: Science and Practice, 10*(2), 144–156.

Kabat-Zinn, J. (2011). Some reflections on the origins of MBSR, skillful means, and the trouble with maps. *Contemporary Buddhism, 12*(1), 281–306.

Kabat-Zinn, J. (2014). Witnessing Hippocratic integrity. *Mindfulness, 5*(4), 460–461.

Kahneman, D. (2011). *Thinking, fast and slow.* London: Penguin Books.

Kallapiran, K., Koo, S., Kirubakaran, R., & Hancock, K. (2015). Review: Effectiveness of mindfulness in improving mental health symptoms of children and adolescents: A meta-analysis. *Child and Adolescent Mental Health, 20*(4), 182–194.

Kanske, P., Bockler, A., Trautwein, F. M., Lesemann, F. H. P., & Singer, T. (2016). Are strong empathizers better mentalizers?: Evidence for independence and interaction between the routes of social cognition. *Social Cognitive and Affective Neuroscience, 11*(9), 1383–1392.

Kanske, P., Bockler, A., Trautwein, F. M., & Singer, T. (2015). Dissecting the social brain: Introducing the EmpaToM to reveal distinct neural networks and brain–behavior relations for empathy and theory of mind. *NeuroImage, 122*, 6–19.

Karl, A., Williams, M. J., Cardy, J., Kuyken, W., & Crane, C. (2018). Dispositional self-compassion and responses to mood challenge in people at risk for depressive relapse/recurrence. *Clinical Psychology and Psychotherapy, 25*(5), 621–633.

Khoury, B., Sharma, M., Rush, S. E., & Fournier, C. (2015). Mindfulness-based stress reduction: A meta-analysis. *Journal of Psychosomatic Research, 78*(6), 519–528.

Killingsworth, M. A., & Gilbert, D. T. (2010). A wandering mind is an unhappy mind. *Science, 330*(6006), 932.

Kings Fund. (2016). Long-term conditions and multi-morbidity. Retrieved from *www.kingsfund.org.uk/time-to-think-differently/trends/disease-and-disability/long-term-conditions-multi-morbidity.*

Klonsky, E. D., Oltmanns, T. F., & Turkheimer, E. (2003). Deliberate self-harm in a nonclinical population: Prevalence and psychological correlates. *American Journal of Psychiatry, 160*(8), 1501–1508.

Kok, B. E., & Singer, T. (2017). Phenomenological fingerprints of four meditations: Differential state changes in affect, mind-wandering, meta-cognition, and interoception before and after daily practice across 9 months of training. *Mindfulness, 8*(1), 218–231.

Krieger, T., Berger, T., & Holtforth, M. G. (2016). The relationship of self-compassion and depression: Cross-lagged panel analyses in depressed patients after outpatient therapy. *Journal of Affective Disorders, 202*, 39–45.

Kuyken, W. (2016). Taking the "long view" on mindfulness and mindfulness-based cognitive therapy. Retrieved from *www.dc.nihr.ac.uk/blog/preventing-depression-with-mindfulness-based-cognitive-therapy-from-evidence-to-practice.*

Kuyken, W., Beshai, S., Dudley, R., Abel, A., Gorg, N., Gower, P., . . . Padesky, C. A. (2016). Assessing competence in collaborative case conceptualization:

Development and preliminary psychometric properties of the Collaborative Case Conceptualization Rating Scale (CCC-RS). *Behavioural and Cognitive Psychotherapy, 44*(2), 179–192.

Kuyken, W., & Evans, A. (2014). Mindfulness-based cognitive therapy for recurrent depression. In R. Baer (Ed.), *Mindfulness-based treatment approaches: Clinicians' guide to evidence and applications* (pp. 27–60). London: Elsevier.

Kuyken, W., Nuthall, E., Byford, S., Crane, C., Dalgleish, T., Ford, T., . . . MYRIAD Team. (2017). The effectiveness and cost-effectiveness of a mindfulness training programme in schools compared with normal school provision (MYRIAD): Study protocol for a randomised controlled trial. *Trials, 18*(1), 194.

Kuyken, W., Padesky, C. A., & Dudley, R. (2009). *Collaborative case conceptualization: Working effectively with clients in cognitive-behavioral therapy.* New York: Guilford Press.

Lakhan, S. E., & Schofield, K. L. (2013). Mindfulness-based therapies in the treatment of somatization disorders: A systematic review and meta-analysis. *PLOS ONE, 8*(8), e71834.

Langer, E. J. (1989). *Mindfulness.* Reading, MA: Addison Wesley Longman.

Lazar, S. W., Kerr, C. E., Wasserman, R. H., Gray, J. R., Greve, D. N., Treadway, M. T., . . . Fischl, B. (2005). Meditation experience is associated with increased cortical thickness. *NeuroReport, 16*(17), 1893–1897.

Lazarus, R. S. (1993). Coping theory and research: Past, present, and future. *Psychosomatic Medicine, 55*(3), 234–247.

LeDoux, J. E. (2000). Emotion circuits in the brain. *Annual Review of Neuroscience, 23,* 155–184.

Leiberg, S., Klimecki, O., & Singer, T. (2011). Short-term compassion training increases prosocial behavior in a newly developed prosocial game. *PLOS ONE, 6*(3), e17798.

Levenson, R. W., Ekman, P., & Ricard, M. (2012). Meditation and the startle response: A case study. *Emotion, 12*(3), 650–658.

Lewin, K. (1951). *Field theory in social science: Selected theoretical papers* (D. Cartwright, Ed.). New York: Harper & Row.

Linehan, M. M. (1993a). *Cognitive-behavioral treatment of borderline personality disorder.* New York: Guilford Press.

Linehan, M. M. (1993b). *Skills training manual for treating borderline personality disorder.* New York: Guilford Press.

Lippold, M. A., Powers, C. J., Syvertsen, A. K., Feinberg, M. E., & Greenberg, M. T. (2013). The timing of school transitions and early adolescent problem behavior. *Journal of Early Adolescence, 33*(6), 821–844.

Loftus, E. F., & Palmer, J. C. (1996). Eyewitness testimony. In P. Banyard & A. Grayson (Eds.), *Introducing psychological research* (pp. 305–309). London: Palgrave.

Lomas, T. (2016). Towards a positive cross-cultural lexicography: Enriching our emotional landscape through 216 "untranslatable" words pertaining to well-being. *Journal of Positive Psychology, 11*(5), 546–558.

Luders, E., Cherbuin, N., & Gaser, C. (2016). Estimating brain age using high-resolution pattern recognition: Younger brains in long-term meditation practitioners. *NeuroImage, 134,* 508–513.

Luders, E., Toga, A. W., Lepore, N., & Gaser, C. (2009). The underlying anatomical correlates of long-term meditation: Larger hippocampal and frontal volumes of gray matter. *NeuroImage, 45*(3), 672–678.

Lumma, A.-L., Kok, B. E., & Singer, T. (2015). Is meditation always relaxing?: Investigating heart rate, heart rate variability, experienced effort and likeability during training of three types of meditation. *International Journal of Psychophysiology, 97*(1), 38–45.

Lutz, A., Brefczynski-Lewis, J., Johnstone, T., & Davidson, R. J. (2008). Regulation of the neural circuitry of emotion by compassion meditation: Effects of meditative expertise. *PLOS ONE, 3*(3), e1897.

Lutz, A., Slagter, H. A., Dunne, J. D., & Davidson, R. J. (2008). Cognitive–emotional interactions: Attention regulation and monitoring in meditation. *Trends in Cognitive Sciences, 12*(4), 163–169.

Lutz, A., Slagter, H. A., Rawlings, N. B., Francis, A. D., Greischar, L. L., & Davidson, R. J. (2009). Mental training enhances attentional stability: Neural and behavioral evidence. *Journal of Neuroscience, 29*(42), 13418–13427.

MacBeth, A., & Gumley, A. (2012). Exploring compassion: A meta-analysis of the association between self-compassion and psychopathology. *Clinical Psychology Review, 32*(6), 545–552.

MacLean, K. A., Ferrer, E., Aichele, S. R., Bridwell, D. A., Zanesco, A. P., Jacobs, T. L., . . . Saron, C. D. (2010). Intensive meditation training improves perceptual discrimination and sustained attention. *Psychological Science, 21*(6), 829–839.

Mann, J., Kuyken, W., O'Mahen, H., Ukoumunne, O. C., Evans, A., & Ford, T. (2016). Manual development and pilot randomised controlled trial of mindfulness-based cognitive therapy versus usual care for parents with a history of depression. *Mindfulness, 7*(5), 1024–1033.

Marlatt, A., & Gordon, J. (1985). *Relapse prevention: Maintenance strategies in the treatment of addictive behaviors.* New York: Guilford Press.

Masicampo, E. J., & Baumeister, R. R. (2007). Relating mindfulness and self-regulatory processes. *Psychological Inquiry, 18,* 255–258.

McCall, C., Steinbeis, N., Ricard, M., & Singer, T. (2014). Compassion meditators show less anger, less punishment and more compensation of victims in response to fairness violations. *Frontiers in Behavioral Neuroscience, 8,* 424.

McGilchrist, I. (2009). *The master and his emissary: The divided brain and the making of the Western world.* New Haven, CT: Yale University Press.

McLaren, I. P. L., & Mackintosh, N. J. (2000). An elemental model of associative learning: I. Latent inhibition and perceptual learning. *Animal Learning and Behavior, 28*(3), 211–246.

Mindfulness All-Party Parliamentary Group. (2015). Mindful Nation UK Report. Retrieved from *https://themindfulnessinitiative.org.uk/publications/mindful-nation-uk-report.*

Mirsky, A. F., & Duncan, C. C. (2001). A nosology of disorders of attention. *Adult Attention Deficit Disorder, 931*, 17–32.

Moffitt, T. E., Arseneault, L., Belsky, D., Dickson, N., Hancox, R. J., Harrington, H., . . . Caspi, A. (2011). A gradient of childhood self-control predicts health, wealth, and public safety. *Proceedings of the National Academy of Sciences of the USA, 108*(7), 2693–2698.

Monteiro, L. M., Musten, R. F., & Compson, J. (2015). Traditional and contemporary mindfulness: Finding the middle path in the tangle of concerns. *Mindfulness, 6*(1), 1–13.

Morrison, A. B., Goolsarran, M., Rogers, S. L., & Jha, A. P. (2014). Taming a wandering attention: Short-form mindfulness training in student cohorts. *Frontiers in Human Neuroscience, 7*, 897.

Mrazek, M. D., Franklin, M. S., Phillips, D. T., Baird, B., & Schooler, J. W. (2013). Mindfulness training improves working memory capacity and GRE performance while reducing mind wandering. *Psychological Science, 24*(5), 776–781.

Nanamoli, B., & Bodhi, B. (Trans.). (1995). Dvehavitakka Sutta: Two kinds of thought. In *The middle length discourses of the Buddha: A translation of the Majjhima Nikaya* (pp. 207–210). Somerville, MA: Wisdom.

Nanamoli, B., & Bodhi, B. (Eds.). (2009). *The middle length discourses of the Buddha: A translation of the Majjhima Nikaya* (4th ed.). Somerville, MA: Wisdom.

National Institute for Health and Care Excellence. (2009). Depression in adults: Recognition and management. Retrieved from *www.nice.org.uk/guidance/cg90*.

Neff, K. D. (2003). Self-compassion: An alternative conceptualization of a healthy attitude toward oneself. *Self and Identity, 2*, 85–101.

Neff, K. D. (2016). The Self-Compassion Scale is a valid and theoretically coherent measure of self-compassion. *Mindfulness, 7*(1), 264–274.

Neff, K. D., & Germer, C. K. (2013). A pilot study and randomized controlled trial of the mindful self-compassion program. *Journal of Clinical Psychology, 69*(1), 28–44.

Neff, K. D., Rude, S. S., & Kirkpatrick, K. L. (2007). An examination of self-compassion in relation to positive psychological functioning and personality traits. *Journal of Research in Personality, 41*(4), 908–916.

Nelson, P. (1993/2012). Autobiography in five short chapters. Retrieved from *https://en.wikipedia.org/wiki/Portia_Nelson*.

The New Penguin English Dictionary. (2001). London: Penguin Books.

Norman, D. A., & Shallice, T. (1986). Attention to action: Willed and automatic control of behavior. In R. J. Davidson, G. E. Schwartz, & D. Shapiro (Eds.), *Consciousness and self-regulation* (pp. 1–18). New York: Plenum Press.

Nyanaponika Thera. (1962). *The heart of Buddhist meditation: A handbook of mental training based on the Buddha's way of mindfulness.* Kandt, Sri Lanka: Buddhist Publication Society.

Ophir, E., Nass, C., & Wagner, A. D. (2009). Cognitive control in media multitaskers. *Proceedings of the National Academy of Sciences of the USA, 106*(37), 15583–15587.

Padesky, C. A., & Mooney, K. A. (1990). Clinical tip: Presenting the cognitive model to clients. *International Cognitive Therapy Newsletter, 6,* 13–14.

Paivio, A. (1969). Mental imagery in associative learning and memory. *Psychological Review, 76*(3), 241–263.

Pamuk, O. (2002). *My name is red* (E. M. Goknar, Trans.). London: Faber & Faber.

Parsons, C. E., Crane, C., Parsons, L. J., Fjorback, L. O., & Kuyken, W. (2017). Home practice in mindfulness-based cognitive therapy and mindfulness-based stress reduction: A systematic review and meta-analysis of participants' mindfulness practice and its association with outcomes. *Behaviour Research and Therapy, 95,* 29–41.

Peacock, J., Baer, R., Segal, Z., Crane, R. S., Kuyken, W., & Surawy, C. (2016). The role of retreats for MBCT teachers. Retrieved from *http://oxfordmindfulness.org/ insight/role-retreats-mbct-teachers.*

Phelps, E. A., Delgado, M. R., Nearing, K. I., & LeDoux, J. E. (2004). Extinction learning in humans: Role of the amygdala and vmPFC. *Neuron, 43*(6), 897–905.

Phelps, E. A., & LeDoux, J. E. (2005). Contributions of the amygdala to emotion processing: From animal models to human behavior. *Neuron, 48*(2), 175–187.

Pinker, S. (1997). *How the mind works.* New York: Norton.

Pinker, S. (2011). *The better angels of our nature: A history of violence and humanity.* New York: Penguin.

Posner, M. I. (1980). Orienting of attention. *Quarterly Journal of Experimental Psychology, 32,* 3–25.

Posner, M. I., Snyder, C. R. R., & Davidson, B. J. (1980). Attention and the detection of signals. *Journal of Experimental Psychology—General, 109*(2), 160–174.

Psychogiou, L., Legge, K., Parry, E., Mann, J., Nath, S., Ford, T., & Kuyken, W. (2016). Self-compassion and parenting in mothers and fathers with depression. *Mindfulness, 7*(4), 896–908.

Raichle, M. E., MacLeod, A. M., Snyder, A. Z., Powers, W. J., Gusnard, D. A., & Shulman, G. L. (2001). A default mode of brain function. *Proceedings of the National Academy of Sciences in the USA, 98*(2), 676–682.

Reinherz, H. Z., Giaconia, R. M., Pakiz, B., Silverman, A. B., Frost, A. K., & Lefkowitz, E. S. (1993). Psychosocial risks for major depression in late adolescence: A longitudinal community study. *Journal of the American Academy of Child and Adolescent Psychiatry, 32*(6), 1155–1163.

Rhys Davids, T. W. (1881). *Buddhist suttas.* Oxford, UK: Clarendon Press.

Rode, S., Salkovskis, P. M., & Jack, T. (2001). An experimental study of attention, labelling and memory in people suffering from chronic pain. *Pain, 94*(2), 193–203.

Rogan, M. T., Staubli, U. V., & LeDoux, J. E. (1997). Fear conditioning induces associative long-term potentiation in the amygdala. *Nature, 390*(6660), 604–607.

Roscoe, G. (1990). *The good life: A Buddhist trilogy.* Bangkok, Thailand: Pacific Rim Press.

Rosling, H., Rosling, O., & Rosling-Ronnlund, A. (2018). *Factfulness: Ten reasons we're wrong about the world—and why things are better than you think*. New York: Flatiron Books.

Salkovskis, P. M., Warwick, H. M. C., & Deale, A. C. (2003). Cognitive-behavioral treatment for severe and persistent health anxiety (hypochondriasis). *Brief Treatment and Crisis Intervention, 3*(3), 353–367.

Sapolsky, R. M. (2004). *Why zebras don't get ulcers* (3rd ed.). New York: St. Martins Griffin.

Sapolsky, R. M. (2017). *Behave: The biology of humans at our best and worst*. London: Penguin Random House.

Schuling, R., Huijbers, M., Jansen, H., Metzemaekers, R., Van den Brink, E., Koster, F., . . . Speckens, A. (2018). The co-creation and feasibility of a compassion training as a follow-up to mindfulness-based cognitive therapy in patients with recurrent depression. *Mindfulness, 9*(2), 412–422.

Schutte, N. S., & Malouff, J. M. (2014). A meta-analytic review of the effects of mindfulness meditation on telomerase activity. *Psychoneuroendocrinology, 42*, 45–48.

Segal, Z. V., Kennedy, S., Gemar, M., Hood, K., Pedersen, R., & Buis, T. (2006). Cognitive reactivity to sad mood provocation and the prediction of depressive relapse. *Archives of General Psychiatry, 63*(7), 749–755.

Segal, Z. V., Williams, J. M. G., & Teasdale, J. D. (2013). *Mindfulness-based cognitive therapy for depression* (2nd ed.). New York: Guilford Press.

Segal, Z. V., Williams, J. M. G., Teasdale, J. D., Crane, R., Dimidjian, S., Ma, H., . . . Kuyken, W. (2018). Mindfulness-based cognitive therapy training pathway. Retrieved from *http://oxfordmindfulness.org*.

Segal, Z. V., Williams, J. M., Teasdale, J. D., & Gemar, M. (1996). A cognitive science perspective on kindling and episode sensitization in recurrent affective disorder. *Psychological Medicine, 26*(2), 371–380.

Seligman, M. E. P., & Csikszentmihalyi, M. (2000). Positive psychology: An introduction. *American Psychologist, 55*(1), 5–14.

Shantideva, A. (1997). *A guide to the Bodhisatva way of life* (V. A. Wallace & A. A. Wallace, Trans.). Ithaca, NY: Snow Lion.

Shapiro, S. L. (2009). The integration of mindfulness and psychology. *Journal of Clinical Psychology, 65*(6), 555–560.

Shapiro, S. L., Astin, J. A., Bishop, S. R., & Cordova, M. (2005). Mindfulness-based stress reduction for health care professionals: Results from a randomized trial. *International Journal of Stress Management, 12*(2), 164–176.

Shonin, E., Van Gordon, W., & Griffiths, M. D. (2013). Mindfulness-based interventions: Towards mindful clinical integration. *Frontiers in Psychology, 4*, 194.

Singer, T. (2006). The neuronal basis and ontogeny of empathy and mind reading: Review of literature and implications for future research. *Neuroscience and Biobehavioral Reviews, 30*(6), 855–863.

Slagter, H. A., Davidson, R. J., & Lutz, A. (2011). Mental training as a tool in the neuroscientific study of brain and cognitive plasticity. *Frontiers in Human Neuroscience, 5*, 17.

Smallwood, J., & Schooler, J. W. (2015). The science of mind wandering: Empirically navigating the stream of consciousness. *Annual Review of Psychology, 66,* 487–518.

Souman, J. L., Frissen, I., Sreenivasa, M. N., & Ernst, M. O. (2009). Walking straight into circles. *Current Biology, 19*(18), 1538–1542.

Strauss, C., Taylor, B. L., Gu, J., Kuyken, W., Baer, R., Jones, F., & Cavanagh, K. (2016). What is compassion and how can we measure it?: A review of definitions and measures. *Clinical Psychology Review, 47,* 15–27.

Teasdale, J. D. (1993). Emotion and 2 kinds of meaning: Cognitive therapy and applied cognitive science. *Behaviour Research and Therapy, 31*(4), 339–354.

Teasdale, J. D. (1999). Metacognition, mindfulness and the modification of mood disorders. *Clinical Psychology and Psychotherapy, 6*(2), 146–155.

Teasdale, J. D. (2016). *Understanding mindfulness and awakening.* Oxford, UK: University of Oxford Mindfulness Centre YouTube Channel.

Teasdale, J. D., & Barnard, P. J. (1993). *Affect, cognition, and change: Re-modeling depressive thought.* Hove, UK: Erlbaum.

Teasdale, J. D., & Chaskalson, M. (2011a). How does mindfulness transform suffering?: I. The nature and origins of dukkha. *Contemporary Buddhism, 12*(1), 89–102.

Teasdale, J. D., & Chaskalson, M. (2011b). How does mindfulness transform suffering?: II. The transformation of dukkha. *Contemporary Buddhism, 12*(1), 103–124.

Teasdale. J. D., Williams, J. M. G., & Segal, Z. (2014). *The mindful way workbook: An 8-week program to free yourself from depression and emotional distress.* New York: Guilford Press.

Thanissaro Bhikkhu. (2013). Madhupindika sutta: The ball of honey (MN 18). Retrieved from *www.accesstoinsight.org/tipitaka/mn/mn.018.than.html.*

Thanissaro Bhikkhu. (2017). Ambalatthika-rahulovada sutta: Instructions to Rahula at Mango Stone. Retrieved from *www.accesstoinsight.org/tipitaka/mn/mn.061. than.html.*

Thich Nhat Hanh. (1975). *The miracle of mindfulness.* Boston: Beacon Press.

Thich Nhat Hanh. (1992). *Touching peace: Practicing the art of mindful living.* Berkeley, CA: Parallax Press.

Van Dam, N. T., van Vugt, M. K., Vago, D. R., Schmalzl, L., Saron, C. D., Olendzki, A., . . . Meyer, D. E. (2018). Mind the hype: A critical evaluation and prescriptive agenda for research on mindfulness and meditation. *Perspectives on Psychological Science, 13*(1), 36–61.

van den Brink, E., & Koster, F. (2015). *Mindfulness-based compassionate living: A new training to deepen mindfulness with heartfulness.* Abingdon, UK: Routledge.

Van Gordon, W., Shonin, E., & Griffiths, M. D. (2016). Are contemporary mindfulness-based interventions unethical? *British Journal of General Practice, 66*(643), 94.

Watkins, E. R. (2008). Constructive and unconstructive repetitive thought. *Psychological Bulletin, 134*(2), 163–206.

Weck, F., Bohn, C., Ginzburg, D. M., & Stangier, U. (2011). Treatment integrity: Implementation, assessment, evaluation, and correlations with outcome. *Verhaltenstherapie, 21*(2), 99–107.

Weng, H. Y., Fox, A. S., Shackman, A. J., Stodola, D. E., Caldwell, J. Z. K., Olson, M. C., . . . Davidson, R. J. (2013). Compassion training alters altruism and neural responses to suffering. *Psychological Science, 24*(7), 1171–1180.

Williams, J. M. G. (2008). Mindfulness, depression and modes of mind. *Cognitive Therapy and Research, 32*(6), 721–733.

Williams, J. M. G., Barnhofer, T., Crane, C., Hermans, D., Raes, F., Watkins, E., & Dalgleish, T. (2007). Autobiographical memory specificity and emotional disorder. *Psychological Bulletin, 133*(1), 122–148.

Williams, J. M. G., Crane, C., Barnhofer, T., Brennan, K., Duggan, D. S., Fennell, M. J. V., . . . Russell, I. T. (2014). Mindfulness-based cognitive therapy for preventing relapse in recurrent depression: A randomized dismantling trial. *Journal of Consulting and Clinical Psychology, 82*(2), 275–286.

Williams, J. M. G., & Penman, D. (2011). *Mindfulness: A practical guide to finding peace in a frantic world.* London: Piatkus.

Williams, M. J., Dalgleish, T., Karl, A., & Kuyken, W. (2014). Examining the factor structures of the Five Facet Mindfulness Questionnaire and the Self-Compassion Scale. *Psychological Assessment, 26*(2), 407–418.

Wittgenstein, L. (2009). *Philosophical investigations* (4th ed.). Chichester, UK: Wiley Blackwell.

Wolever, R. Q., Bobinet, K. J., McCabe, K., Mackenzie, E. R., Fekete, E., Kusnick, C. A., & Baime, M. (2012). Effective and viable mind–body stress reduction in the workplace: A randomized controlled trial. *Journal of Occupational Health Psychology, 17*(2), 246–258.

World Health Organization. (2011). Health statistics and information systems: Disease burden. Retrieved February 23, 2013, from *www.who.int/healthinfo/global_burden_disease/estimates_regional/en/index1.html*.

Yeung, N., & Monsell, S. (2003). Switching between tasks of unequal familiarity: The role of stimulus-attribute and response-set selection. *Journal of Experimental Psychology—Human Perception and Performance, 29*(2), 455–469.

Zenner, C., Herrnleben-Kurz, S., & Walach, H. (2014). Mindfulness-based interventions in schools: A systematic review and meta-analysis. *Frontiers in Psychology, 5*, 603.

Ziegert, D. I., & Kistner, J. A. (2002). Response styles theory: Downward extension to children. *Journal of Clinical Child and Adolescent Psychology, 31*(3), 325–334.

Index

Note. *f*, *t*, *n*, or *b* following a page number indicates figure, a table, a note, or a box.